DISEASES OF THE LUNG

RADIOLOGIC AND PATHOLOGIC CORRELATIONS

DISEASES OF THE LUNG

RADIOLOGIC AND PATHOLOGIC CORRELATIONS

NESTOR L. MÜLLER, M.D., PH.D.

Professor and Chairman
Department of Radiology
University of British Columbia
Head
Department of Radiology
Vancouver Hospital and Health Sciences Centre
Vancouver, British Columbia, Canada

RICHARD S. FRASER, M.D., C.M.

Professor
Department of Pathology
McGill University
Senior Pathologist
McGill University Hospital Center
Montreal, Quebec, Canada

KYUNG SOO LEE, M.D., PH.D.

Professor
Department of Radiology
Sungkyunkwan University School of Medicine
Director of Thoracic Surgery
Department of Radiology
Samsung Medical Center
Seoul, Korea

TAKESHI JOHKOH, M.D., PH.D.

Professor
Department of Medical Physics
Osaka University
School of Allied Health Sciences
Professor
Department of Radiology
Osaka University Medical School
Suita, Osaka, Japan

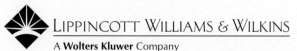

LIPPINCOTT WILLIAMS & WILKINS

A **Wolters Kluwer** Company

Philadelphia · Baltimore · New York · London
Buenos Aires · Hong Kong · Sydney · Tokyo

Acquisitions Editor: Joyce-Rachel John
Developmental Editor: Grace R. Caputo
Production Editor: Deirdre Marino
Manufacturing Manager: Benjamin Rivera
Cover Designer: David Levy
Compositor: Maryland Composition

Library of Congress Cataloging-in-Publication Data

Diseases of the lung: radiologic and pathologic correlations / Nestor L. Müller . . . [et al.].
   p. ; cm.
   Includes bibliographical references and index.
   ISBN 0-7817-3435-5
   1. Lungs—Radiography. 2. Lungs—Pathophysiology. 3. Lungs—Histopathology. I.
Müller, Nestor Luiz, 1948-
   [DNLM: 1. Lung Diseases—pathology. 2. Lung Diseases—radiography. WF 600 D6108 2002]
   RC756 .D575 2002
   616.2′407—dc21

                                                                              2002066095

Care has been taken to confirm the accuracy of the information presented and to describe generally accepted practices. However, the authors and publisher are not responsible for errors or omissions or for any consequences from application of the information in this book and make no warranty, expressed or implied, with respect to the currency, completeness, or accuracy of the contents of the publication. Application of this information in a particular situation remains the professional responsibility of the practitioner.

The authors and publisher have exerted every effort to ensure that drug selection and dosage set forth in this text are in accordance with current recommendations and practice at the time of publication. However, in view of ongoing research, changes in government regulations, and the constant flow of information relating to drug therapy and drug reactions, the reader is urged to check the package insert for each drug for any change in indications and dosage and for added warnings and precautions. This is particularly important when the recommended agent is a new or infrequently employed drug.

Some drugs and medical devices presented in this publication have Food and Drug Administration (FDA) clearance for limited use in restricted research settings. It is the responsibility of the health care provider to ascertain the FDA status of each drug or device planned for use in their clinical practice.

10 9 8 7 6 5 4 3 2 1

To our wives and children—
Ruth, Alison, and Phillip Müller;
Marie-Claire, Nicky, Russell, and Emily Fraser;
Kyung Sook, Joo Hwang, and Joo Young Lee; and
Kayo Johkoh

CONTENTS

PREFACE

The two major aims of *Diseases of the Lung: Radiologic and Pathologic Correlations* are to present a brief overview of the characteristic radiologic and pathologic findings of the most common pulmonary parenchymal and airway diseases and, as much as possible, to relate the radiologic abnormalities to the underlying histologic alterations. Although physicians in the two disciplines often work in isolation from one another, in our opinion this should not be the case. Awareness of the pathologic findings of pulmonary diseases is necessary for the radiologist to fully understand the patterns and distribution of abnormalities on radiologic images. Alternatively, awareness of the radiologic findings, particularly with respect to the overall pattern and distribution of disease, is often helpful, and sometimes essential, to the pathologist in reaching a specific diagnosis.

The radiologic and pathologic diagnosis of many pulmonary abnormalities is based on an assessment of the their pattern and distribution. The pathologist has the advantage of being able to evaluate specimens microscopically and investigate them further with special stains and immunohistochemistry. The radiologist is by necessity limited to an assessment of more gross disease. However, whereas histologic assessment is often confined to small tissue samples, the radiologist is able to evaluate the entire lung and look for additional diagnostic clues in the mediastinum and pleura. Because many diseases have a characteristic distribution that is discernible by examining the entire lung, knowledge of the gross findings is often helpful in arriving at a confident specific diagnosis.

The emphasis of the radiologic images in this book is on high-resolution CT, which provides the best depiction of the anatomic features; the emphasis of the pathologic images is on both gross specimens and histologic manifestations as seen on hematoxylin-eosin stain. Other imaging modalities and stains are included where appropriate to optimally illustrate the characteristic radiologic and pathologic features. *Diseases of the Lung* should prove useful to residents, fellows, and practitioners in radiology, pathology, thoracic surgery, and respiratory medicine.

ACKNOWLEDGMENTS

We would like to express our gratitude to Ms. Jenny Silver for her superb secretarial assistance and to our colleagues who provided many of the illustrations. In particular, we recognize the contributions of Dr. Joungho Han from the Department of Diagnostic Pathology at Samsung Medical Center, Sungkyunkwan University School of Medicine. The other contributors, listed alphabetically, are: Kazuto Ashizawa, Jim Barrie, Maura Brown, Kingo Chida, Jin Mo Goo, Inmaculada Herráez, Osamu Honda, Kazuya Ichikado, Harumi Itoh, Eun-Young Kang, Jin-Hwan Kim, Mi-Young Kim, Sang Jin Kim, Yasuhiro Kondoh, Mitsuhiro Koyama, Takenori Kozuka, Jin Sung Lee, Noboru Maeda, Hiroshi Moriya, Martine Remy-Jardin, Dong Wook Sung, Masashi Takahashi, Hiroyuki Taniguchi, Ukihide Tateishi, and Mitsuko Tsubamoto.

CONGENITAL ABNORMALITIES

PULMONARY SEQUESTRATION
Intralobar Sequestration
Extralobar Sequestration

BRONCHOGENIC CYST

CONGENITAL CYSTIC ADENOMATOID MALFORMATION

CONGENITAL BRONCHIAL ATRESIA

PULMONARY ARTERIOVENOUS MALFORMATION

Congenital anomalies of the lungs can be divided into two major groups: (a) those originating in the primitive foregut or its lung bud (bronchopulmonary or foregut anomalies) and (b) those arising from the sixth aortic arch or venous radicals and their derivatives (pulmonary vascular anomalies). The most common bronchopulmonary anomalies seen in adults are pulmonary sequestration, bronchogenic cyst, congenital cystic adenomatoid malformation, and bronchial atresia. The most common pulmonary vascular anomaly is an arteriovenous malformation.

PULMONARY SEQUESTRATION

The term *pulmonary sequestration* refers to a congenital malformation in which lung tissue lacks communication to the bronchial tree, thus being separated from the remainder of the lung, and is supplied by a systemic artery (1,2). The anomaly may be intralobar or extralobar: the former is surrounded by normal pulmonary tissue, whereas the latter is separate from the normal lung and is enclosed within its own pleural membrane. The arterial supply may arise from the descending thoracic aorta or from the abdominal aorta or one of its branches. The venous return is either by a pulmonary vein (in intralobar sequestration) or by a systemic vein (in extralobar sequestration).

Although widely accepted as a congenital anomaly, it has also been proposed that the abnormality is an acquired lesion (2,3). According to this view the sequestered region represents an area of obstructive pneumonitis that develops following injury to and obliteration of a feeding bronchus. Hypertrophy of small systemic vessels normally present in the pulmonary ligament, then leads to the abnormal vascular supply. In this scenario the cystic spaces observed both pathologically and radiologically represent bronchiectasis.

Intralobar Sequestration

Approximately 75% to 85% of sequestrations are intralobar (1,2). They are diagnosed most commonly in children and young adults (2,4). Most have a history of recurrent pneumonia (4).

Pathologically, intralobar sequestration usually consists of one or more cystic spaces separated by a variable amount of intervening parenchyma that either is fibrotic or shows changes of obstructive pneumonitis (Fig. 1.1). The cysts are filled with mucus or, when infection is present, with pus. The sequestered tissue may be separated from normal lung

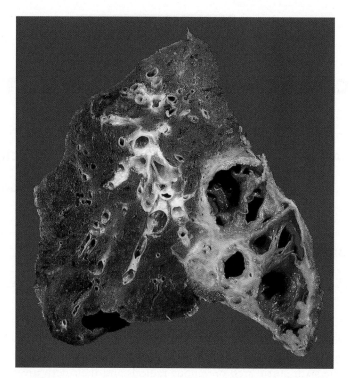

FIGURE 1.1. Intralobar sequestration. A sagittal slice of the left lower lobe shows a well-demarcated focus of parenchymal fibrosis containing several irregularly shaped cysts. Examination of adjacent slices showed the latter to be ectatic bronchi. The abnormal region was supplied by a vessel originating in the descending thoracic aorta. The patient was a 23-year-old woman with a history of repeated pneumonias.

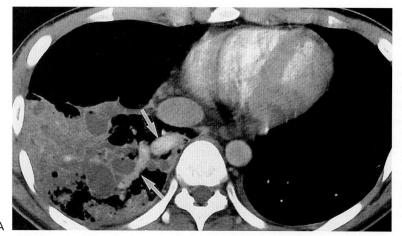
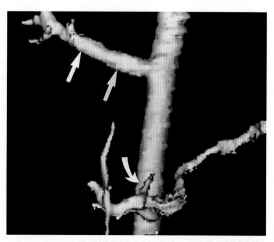

A   B

FIGURE 1.2. Intralobar sequestration. **A:** A contrast-enhanced CT image (7-mm collimation) shows inhomogeneous airspace consolidation and fluid-filled cystic spaces in the right lower lobe. A large vessel (*arrows*) can be seen extending into the consolidated lobe. **B:** A three-dimensional reconstruction image (shaded-surface-display technique) of the lower thoracic and abdominal aorta demonstrates an artery (*straight arrows*) arising from aorta to supply the region of sequestration. The aberrant vessel can be seen to originate several centimeters above level of celiac axis (*curved arrow*).

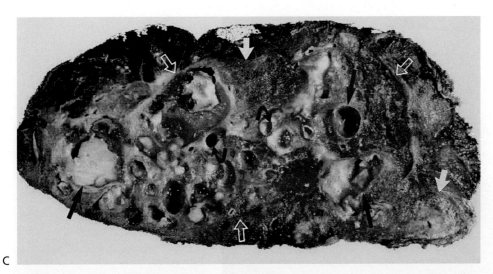

C

FIGURE 1.2. *(continued)* **C:** The excised specimen shows a relatively well-demarcated region of abnormal lung (*open arrows*) characterized by bronchiectasis and obstructive pneumonitis (*solid white arrows*). Many airways are filled with mucus and some are cystic in appearance (*straight black arrows*). The patient was a 22-year-old man.

by a fibrous capsule, or there may be an indistinct transition from one to the other. Microscopically, the cysts resemble dilated bronchi, with respiratory epithelium and occasional mural cartilage plates. The intervening parenchymal tissue often shows abundant intraalveolar macrophages and alveolar septal thickening by fibrous tissue and a mononuclear inflammatory infiltrate (obstructive pneumonitis).

The most common radiographic finding consists of a homogeneous opacity in the posterior basal segment of a lower lobe (usually the left) almost invariably contiguous with the hemidiaphragm. Less commonly, it presents as a cystic mass, area of hyperlucency, recurrent pneumonia, or prominent vessels (2,4,5). The cysts can be single or multiple and are of variable size.

Computed tomography (CT) commonly demonstrates cystic spaces (2,4). In one review of 16 cases (4), the parenchymal abnormalities consisted of cysts with or without fluid (Fig. 1.2) in seven, areas of low-attenuation surrounding cysts or nodules (Fig. 1.3) in six, multiple dilated vessels in two, and a soft-tissue mass (Fig. 1.4) in one. Low-attenuation areas are frequently seen (4,6,7). These can be related to emphysema, thin-walled cysts, or collateral air drift and air trapping resulting from impaired ventilation (4,6,7). Definitive radiologic diagnosis is based on the demonstration of the anomalous systemic arterial supply to the sequestered lobe. In most cases, this can be done by contrast-enhanced spiral CT (2,4,8) (Figs. 1.2 and 1.3). It also may be done by MR imaging or aortography (2,5) (Fig. 1.3).

Extralobar Sequestration

Extralobar pulmonary sequestration is less common than intralobar sequestration, accounting for only 15% to 25% of sequestrations (1). Approximately 70% are located in the left posterior costodiaphragmatic sulcus between the left lower lobe and diaphragm (Fig. 1.5); less commonly, they are located on the right side, within or below the left hemidiaphragm or in the mediastinum or retroperitoneum (1,9). The systemic arterial supply is usually from the abdominal aorta or one of its branches; the vessels may be multiple and small (1,9). In contrast to intralobar sequestration, drainage is usually via the systemic venous system—the inferior vena cava, the azygos or hemiazygos veins, or the portal venous system, resulting in a left-to-right shunt (1,9).

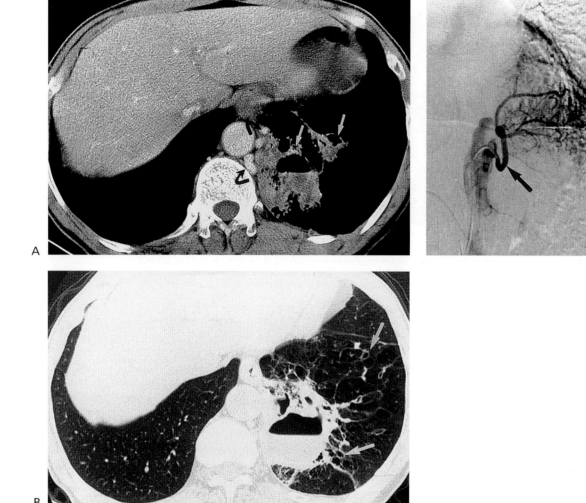

FIGURE 1.3. Intralobar sequestration. **A:** A contrast-enhanced CT image (7-mm collimation) shows focal areas of consolidation and cystic spaces (*white arrows*) in left lower lobe. Enlarged systemic vessels (*black arrows*) can be seen adjacent to the descending thoracic aorta. **B:** Lung windows of HRCT image (1.0-mm collimation) shows consolidation and a large cystic space containing an air–fluid level. Also note evidence of bronchiectasis (*arrows*) and emphysema. **C:** Selective arteriography demonstrates a vessel (*arrow*) arising from the descending aorta (*arrow*) and supplying the sequestered lung. The patient was a 64-year-old man.

Approximately 60% to 70% of patients have other congenital anomalies (1,9). Eventration or paralysis of the ipsilateral hemidiaphragm is present in approximately 60% and left-sided diaphragmatic hernias in approximately 30% (1,9). Because of symptoms related to these congenital anomalies, most cases are diagnosed during infancy or early childhood (1).

Grossly, the sequestered tissue is completely enclosed in its own pleural sac. Airways are usually few in number and the parenchymal tissue often has an immature appearance histologically.

The most common radiographic manifestations consist of a sharply defined, triangular opacity in the posterior costophrenic angle, usually adjacent to the left hemidiaphragm (1) (Fig. 1.5). Less commonly, it appears as a small bump on the left hemidiaphragm, or as a mass in the paravertebral region, mediastinum (Fig. 1.6), upper thorax, or (rarely) subdiaphragmatic region (1,9,10).

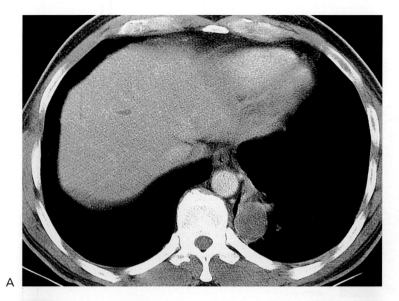

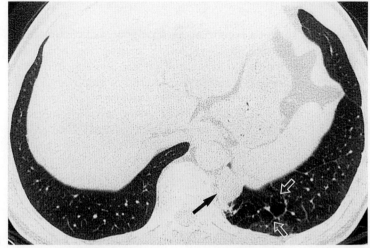

FIGURE 1.4. Intralobar sequestration. **A:** A contrast-enhanced CT image (7-mm collimation) CT scan obtained at the level of the liver dome shows an ovoid, 4-cm-diameter homogeneous mass in left lower lobe. **B:** An HRCT image (1.0-mm collimation) obtained 10 mm inferior to **A** shows a mass (*black arrow*) and surrounding emphysema (*open arrows*). The patient was a 42-year-old man.

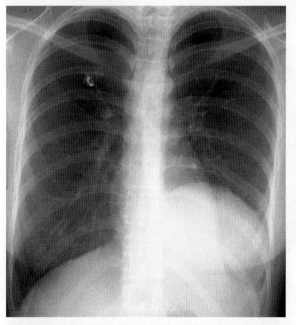

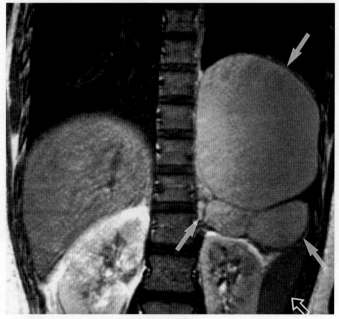

FIGURE 1.5. Extralobar sequestration. **A:** A chest radiograph shows a well-defined mass causing apparent elevation of the left hemidiaphragm. **B:** A gadolinium-enhanced T1-weighted coronal MR image shows a multiloculated cystic lesion (*arrows*) caudad to the left lung and cephalad to the left kidney and spleen (*open arrow*). The patient was a 21-year-old woman with surgically proven extralobar sequestration in left hemidiaphragm.

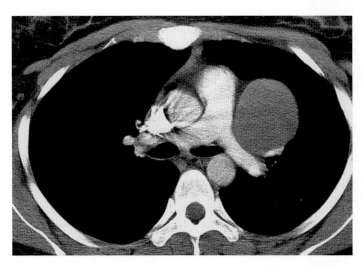

FIGURE 1.6. Extralobar sequestration. A contrast-enhanced (7-mm collimation) CT image at the level of the main bronchi shows a 5-cm-diameter, homogeneous cystic mass adjacent to main and left pulmonary arteries. The excised specimen showed pulmonary parenchyma in the cyst wall, consistent with extralobar sequestration. The patient was a 20-year-old woman.

The CT appearance is usually that of a homogeneous opacity or well-circumscribed mass (1,4). Cystic areas are occasionally seen on CT (4) or MR imaging (Fig. 1.5). In one study of eight patients, areas of low attenuation in the surrounding nonsequestered lung were described in seven (4). These most often correspond to areas of emphysema or dilated airways (4). CT is of limited value in demonstrating the vascular supply; in one review of eight patients, it was identified in only three (37%) (3). Aortography is more useful in this regard; multiple feeding vessels can be demonstrated in about 20% of cases (1,4).

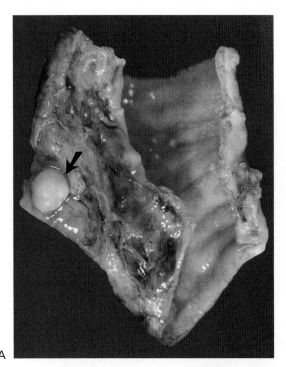

A

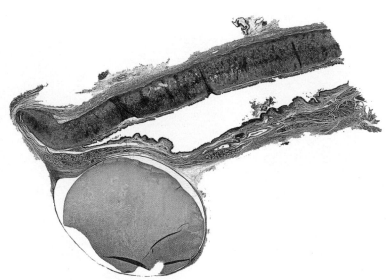

B

FIGURE 1.7. Mediastinal bronchogenic cysts—incidental findings. Gross (**A**) and low-magnification photomicrographic (**B**) images show two bronchogenic cysts discovered incidentally at autopsy. The one in **A** (*arrow*) is somewhat lobulated and located in the connective tissue adjacent to the lower trachea near its bifurcation. The one in **B** was situated in the lower third of the trachea at the junction of its membranous and cartilaginous portions. The cyst is filled with mucus and has a very thin wall. The intimate proximity of these cysts to the tracheal wall supports the hypothesis that they arise by abnormal budding of the tracheobronchial tree during its development.

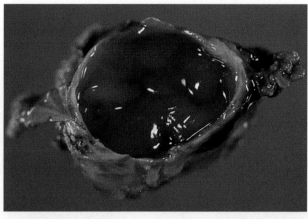
A

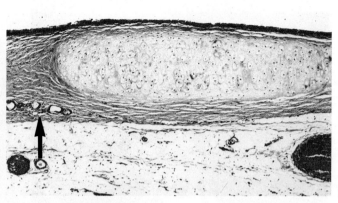
B

FIGURE 1.8. Mediastinal bronchogenic cyst. **A:** A "tumor" excised from the paratracheal region shows a thin-walled cyst filled with thick mucus. **B:** A section of the cyst wall shows it to contain cartilage and seromucinous glands (*arrow*) similar to those found in the normal trachea.

BRONCHOGENIC CYST

Bronchogenic cysts are believed to occur by separation of a bud from the developing tracheobronchial tree *in utero* (Fig. 1.7). The buds are unassociated with pulmonary parenchymal tissue and undergo no additional branching, resulting in a cyst. Approximately 70% to 90% occur in the mediastinum and 10% to 30% in the lungs (11–13).

The cysts are usually solitary, thin-walled, unilocular, and roughly spherical in shape. They may be filled with serous fluid or, more frequently, thick, somewhat inspissated mucoid material (Fig. 1.8A). They do not communicate with the tracheobronchial tree unless they become infected. Histologically, the cyst wall usually is lined by a pseudostratified, ciliated epithelium. The wall contains a variable amount of cartilage, smooth muscle, and seromucinous glands (Fig. 1.8B).

Radiologically, bronchogenic cysts typically present as a sharply circumscribed, round, or oval nodule or mass (12,13). Mediastinal bronchogenic cysts usually are located in the right paratracheal region or just inferior to and slightly to the right of the carina (12,14) (Fig. 1.9).Pulmonary cysts usually are located in the medial third of the lungs (Figs. 1.10 and 1.11); approximately two-thirds are in the lower lobes (14).

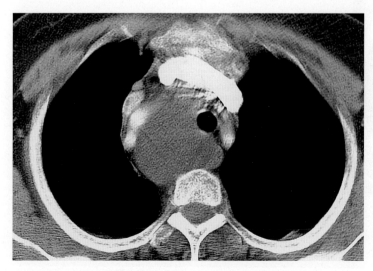

FIGURE 1.9. Mediastinal bronchogenic cyst. A contrast-enhanced CT image (7-mm collimation) at the level of the left innominate vein shows a homogeneous low-attenuation cystic lesion in the right paratracheal region with mass effect. The patient was a 54-year-old woman.

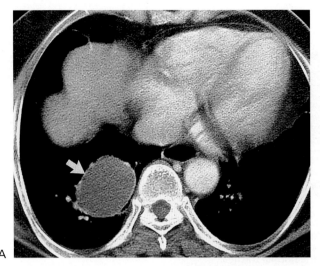
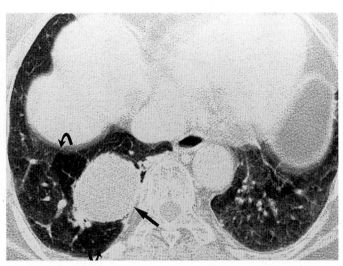

FIGURE 1.10. Intrapulmonary bronchogenic cyst. **A:** A contrast-enhanced CT image (7-mm collimation) at the level of the liver dome shows a 5-cm-sized, ovoid, homogeneous, low-attenuation lesion in the right lower lobe (*arrow*). **B:** An HRCT image (1.0-mm collimation) shows the lesion (*straight arrow*) with surrounding low-attenuation areas due to emphysema (*curved arrows*). The patient was a 50-year-old man.

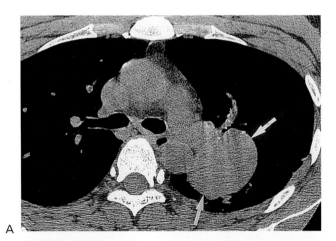

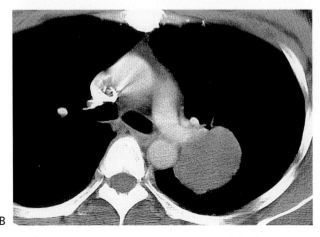

FIGURE 1.11. Intrapulmonary bronchogenic cyst. **A:** An HRCT image (1.0-mm collimation) obtained at the level of the main bronchi shows a homogeneous mass (*arrows*) in the left upper lung zone. **B:** Another image (7-mm collimation) obtained after intravenous administration of contrast shows that the mass does not enhance, consistent with a cyst.

The appearance on CT consists of a cystic mass molded to the adjacent bronchovascular structures. In about half of cases, the cyst shows nonenhancing homogeneous attenuation at or near water density (0 to 20 HU) (13,15) (Figs. 1.9 and 1.10). In the other half, there is a higher-than-water density as a result of the presence of proteinaceous mucoid material or calcium (15,16) (Fig. 1.11). Peripheral calcification is seen in approximately 10% of cases (13). When infected, the cysts may have inhomogeneous enhancement and resemble an abscess (17).

On T2-weighted spin-echo MR images, the cysts characteristically have a homogeneous high signal intensity, which is usually isointense or hyperintense with cerebrospinal fluid (13,18). The high signal intensity reflects the presence of fluid. The signal intensity on T1-weighted images, on the other hand, is variable and can be hypointense, isointense, or hyperintense with skeletal muscle (13). The high signal intensity on T1-weighted images can be related to the proteinaceous mucoid material or, occasionally, blood (17,19). Infected cysts may have intermediate signal intensity on both T1- and T2-weighted images and may be indistinguishable from an abscess (17).

CONGENITAL CYSTIC ADENOMATOID MALFORMATION

The term *congenital cystic adenomatoid malformation* refers to a group of several pathologic abnormalities characterized by architecturally abnormal pulmonary tissue with or without gross cyst formation. When present, the cysts can usually be shown to communicate with normal airways. The vast majority of cases are diagnosed in the neonatal period or early childhood; occasionally, they occur in adults (20,21).

The condition has been classified into three pathologic subtypes (21,22). The *type I* form consists of a large, often multiloculated cyst sometimes associated with several smaller cysts in the adjacent parenchyma (Fig. 1.12). This is the most common type seen in children and adults (21,22). The cyst wall may contain smooth muscle but usually no cartilage and is lined by bronchiolar-type epithelium. The *type II* form is composed of solid areas separated by numerous, fairly evenly spaced cysts measuring 1 to 10 mm, again lined by bronchiolar-type epithelium (Fig. 1.13). The *type III* form is manifested by a more or less solid mass of tissue without gross cyst formation. Microscopically, it is composed primarily of irregularly shaped bronchiolar structures that resemble terminal air spaces of the pseudoglandular period of fetal development.

The radiologic presentation in adults usually consists of a lower lobe mass composed of numerous air-containing cysts scattered irregularly through tissue of unit density. Occasionally, one cyst preferentially expands, creating a single lucent area (22). In one review of the CT findings in seven adults, the abnormalities consisted of multiple thin-walled, complex cystic masses ranging from 4 to 12 cm in diameter (21). Five of the patients had type I lesions with at least one cyst greater than 2 cm in diameter (Fig. 1.12). Two patients had type II malformation with multiple thin-walled cysts ranging from 2 to 20 mm in diameter (Fig. 1.14). In all seven cases, the abnormality involved the lower lobes and was associated with displacement and splaying of vessels in an area of adjacent hyperlucent lung (21).

CONGENITAL BRONCHIAL ATRESIA

Congenital bronchial atresia is an uncommon abnormality characterized by interruption of a bronchus, usually a segmental branch, at or near its origin. The apicoposterior segmental bronchus of the left upper lobe is most commonly affected, followed by segmental bronchi of the right upper lobe, middle lobe, and (occasionally) lower lobe (23). The mean age at diagnosis is 17 years (23).

Pathologically, the airways distal to the point of obliteration are patent and their number normal or near normal. Characteristically, the branches immediately distal to the fo-

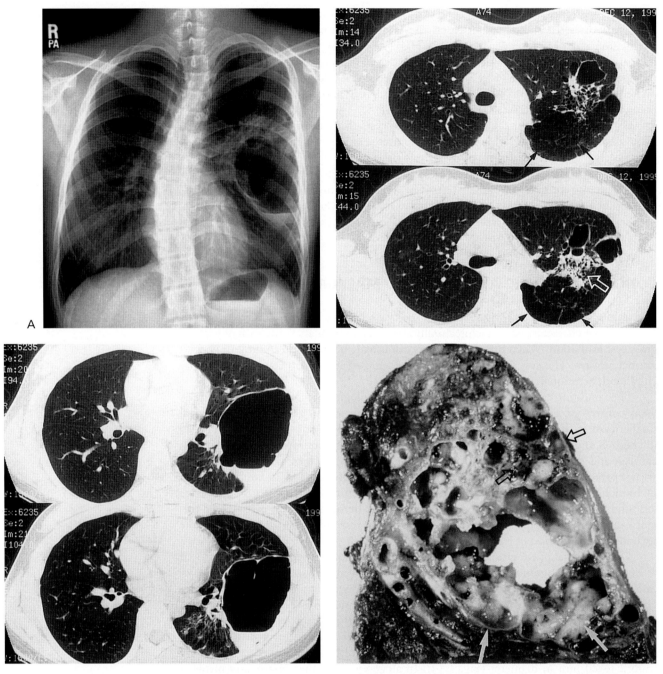

FIGURE 1.12. Congenital cystic adenomatoid malformation type I. **A:** A chest radiograph shows a multiloculated air-filled cystic lesion in the left middle lung zone and consolidation of adjacent lung. **B** and **C:** HRCT images obtained at levels of upper (**B**) and lower (**C**) lung zones, respectively, show extensive multiloculated air-filled cystic lesions in the left lung. Foci of emphysema (*black arrows*) and consolidation (*open white arrow*) are also evident. **D:** A sagittal slice of the excised specimen shows a multiloculated cyst containing mucoid material (*solid arrows*). Foci of parenchymal consolidation are also apparent (*open arrows*). The patient was a 16-year-old woman.

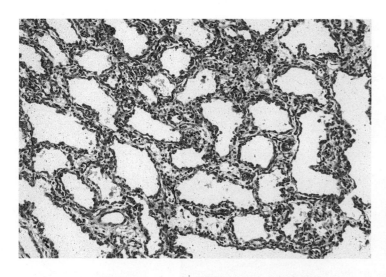

FIGURE 1.13. Congenital cystic adenomatoid malformation, type II. A photomicrograph of a tumor excised from the lower lobe of a 3-month-old infant shows fairly evenly spaced bronchiole-like structures separated by immature-appearing lung parenchyma.

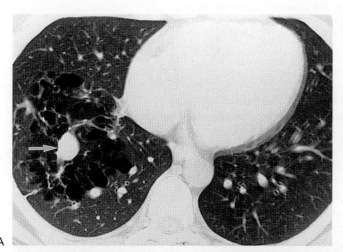

A

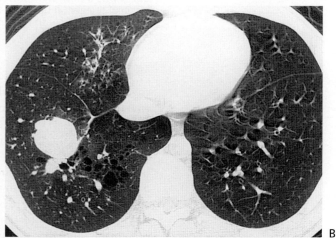

B

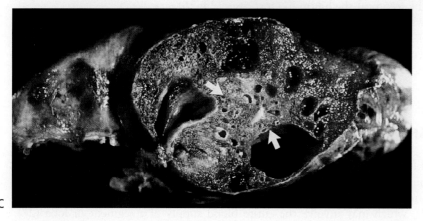

C

FIGURE 1.14. Congenital cystic adenomatoid malformation type II. **A:** An HRCT image (1.0-mm collimation) shows small, air-filled cystic lesions in the right lower lobe. Also note central nodule (*arrow*). **B:** A scan obtained at a more caudad level shows a larger nodule and small, air-filed cystic lesions. **C:** A sagittal slice of the excised lung shows multiple variable-sized intrapulmonary cysts. The nodular lesions in **A** and **B** correspond to foci of obstructive pneumonitis (*arrows* in **C**). The patient was a 39-year-old man.

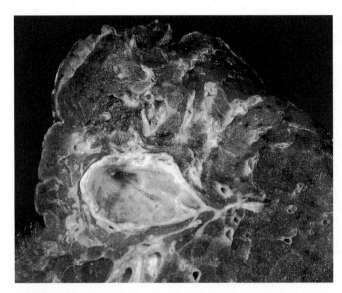

FIGURE 1.15. Bronchial atresia. A sagittal slice of the left upper lobe shows a thick-walled ovoid cyst that was separated from a proximal segmental bronchus by a focus of dense fibrous tissue. The cyst was filled with thick mucus. The patient was a 25-year-old woman.

cus of atresia are dilated and filled with inspissated mucus (Fig. 1.15). Depending on the amount of mucus, these airways may appear linear, ovoid, or spherical and may or may not be branched.

The most common radiographic findings consist of a focal area of hyperlucency (seen in 90% of cases), a perihilar mass (in 80%) (Fig. 1.16), or a combination of both findings (in 70%) (23). The hyperlucency results from a combination of oligemia and an increase in the volume of gas within the affected parenchyma (23). Expiratory radiographs demonstrate air trapping. The presence of gas in lung distal to an atretic bronchus must be related to collateral ventilation; the small size of the airways responsible for this ventilation presumably underlies the hyperexpansion and air trapping. Ovoid or round, branching opacities can be seen near the hilum in most cases (23–25).

CT allows excellent visualization of the segmental overinflation and hypovascularity (24,25). Mucoid impaction is readily recognized by the presence of branching soft-tissue densities in a bronchial distribution, usually associated with bronchial dilation (24,25). The combination of findings is generally considered diagnostic (26) (Fig. 1.16).

PULMONARY ARTERIOVENOUS MALFORMATION

Pulmonary arteriovenous malformations (PAVMs) consist of abnormal, presumably congenital communications between pulmonary arteries and pulmonary veins (27). They can range in size from microscopic to complex aneurysms with multiple feeding arteries and draining veins, which may involve the entire blood supply of a segment or lobe (27). Although it is assumed that the abnormality is present at birth, it seldom becomes manifest clinically until adult life.

Approximately two-thirds of patients have a single pulmonary lesion, and one-third have multiple lesions. Eighty percent to 90% have *hereditary hemorrhagic telangiectasia* (Rendu-Osler-Weber disease), an autosomal dominant vascular dysplasia characterized by the presence of arteriovenous communications in the skin, mucous membranes, and other organs (28).

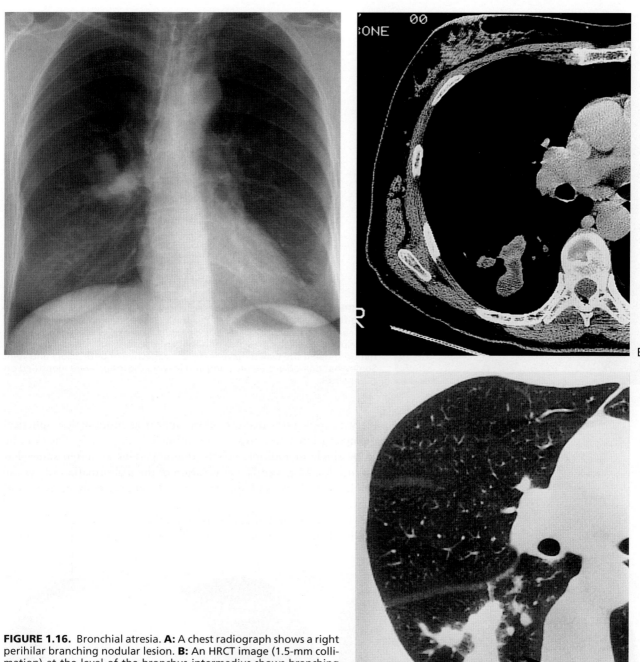

FIGURE 1.16. Bronchial atresia. **A:** A chest radiograph shows a right perihilar branching nodular lesion. **B:** An HRCT image (1.5-mm collimation) at the level of the bronchus intermedius shows branching tubular lesions with low attenuation in right lower lobe. **C:** Lung window shows branching lesion in superior segment of right lower lobe. Decreased attenuation (*arrows*) is evident in the surrounding lung. The patient was a 50-year-old woman.

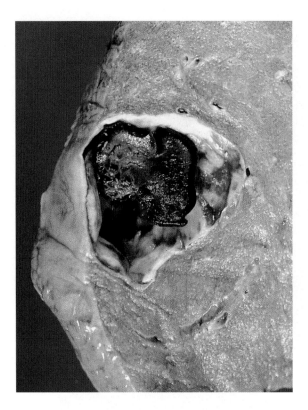

FIGURE 1.17. Pulmonary arteriovenous malformation. A magnified view of a sagittal slice of the left lower lobe shows a well-demarcated cystic structure containing a blood clot. The "cyst" lining is pearly white in appearance, corresponding to the presence of abundant elastic tissue. Histologic examination showed the wall to have features suggestive of both artery and vein. Somewhat dilated vessels entering and leaving the lesion were identified on other slices.

Grossly, pulmonary arteriovenous malformations appear as more or less spherical nodules ranging in diameter from 1 mm to several centimeters (Fig. 1.17). They can be supplied and drained by single or multiple vessels; draining veins are often somewhat larger than the feeding arteries. Microscopic examination of the malformation shows the vessel walls to be variable in thickness and appearance, with some resembling veins and others similar to arteries.

The characteristic radiographic presentation consists of a well-circumscribed homogeneous nodule, somewhat lobulated in contour, usually located in the lower lobe, most

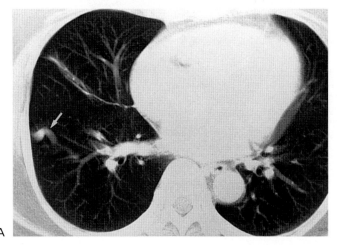
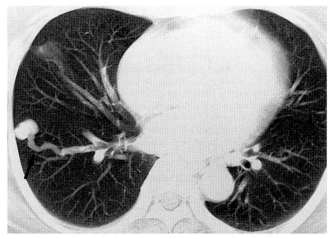

A   B

FIGURE 1.18. Pulmonary arteriovenous malformation. **A:** A CT image (7.0-mm collimation) at the level of the inferior pulmonary veins shows a dilated vessel (*arrow*) in the right lower lobe. Also note linear atelectasis in the middle lobe. **B:** An image immediately adjacent to **A** shows the somewhat dilated malformation itself as well as the draining vein (*arrow*). The patient was a 45-year-old woman.

often in the medial third of the lung. A feeding artery and draining vein can sometimes be seen. However, in many cases the radiographic findings consist of a poorly defined opacity, tortuous tubular opacities, or prominent vessels (28,29).

A confident diagnosis can be made on spiral CT in the vast majority of cases (28,30,31). The characteristic findings consist of a homogeneous, circumscribed nodule or serpiginous mass connected to blood vessels (30,31) (Fig. 1.18). Optimal investigation requires the use of spiral volumetric CT. The procedure allows image reconstruction at various levels within the lesion, thereby facilitating depiction of its center (30,31). Three-dimensional reconstruction can be performed to assess more precisely the architecture of the malformations (31).

REFERENCES

1. Rosado-de-Christenson ML, Frazier AA, Stocker JT, Templeton PA. Extralobar sequestration: radiologic-pathologic correlation. *Radiographics* 1993;13:425–441.
2. Frazier AA, Rosado de Christenson ML, Stocker JT, et al. Intralobar sequestration: radiologic–pathologic correlation. *Radiographics* 1997;17:725–745.
3. Stocker JT, Malczak HT. A study of pulmonary ligament arteries: relationship to intralobar pulmonary sequestration. *Chest* 1986;86:611–615
4. Ikezoe J, Murayama S, Godwin JD, et al. Bronchopulmonary sequestration: CT assessment. *Radiology* 1990;176:375–379.
5. Felker RE, Tonkin ILD. Imaging of pulmonary sequestration. *Am J Roentgenol* 1990;154:241–249.
6. Stern EJ, Webb WR, Warnock ML, et al. Bronchopulmonary sequestration: dynamic, ultrafast, high-resolution CT evidence of air trapping. *Am J Roentgenol* 1991;157:947–949.
7. Ko SF, Ng SH, Lee TY, et al. Noninvasive imaging of bronchopulmonary sequestration. *Am J Roentgenol* 2000;175:1005–1012.
8. Frush DP, Donnelly LF. Pulmonary sequestration spectrum: a new spin with helical CT. *Am J Roentgenol* 1997;169:679–682.
9. Stocker JT. Sequestrations of the lung. *Semin Diagn Pathol* 1986;3:106–121.
10. Sippel JM, Ravichandran PS, Antonovic R, et al. Extralobar pulmonary sequestration presenting as a mediastinal malignancy. *Ann Thorac Surg* 1997;63:1169–1173.
11. St. Georges R, Deslauriers J, Duranceau A. Clinical spectrum of bronchogenic cysts of the mediastinum and lung. *Ann Thorac Surg* 1991;52:6–13.
12. Suen HC, Mathisen DJ, Grillo HC, et al. Surgical management and radiological characteristics of bronchogenic cysts. *Ann Thorac Surg* 1993;55:476–481.
13. Page McAdams H, Kirejczyk WM, Rosado-de-Christenson ML, Matsumoto S. Bronchogenic cyst: Imaging features with clinical and histopathologic correlation. *Radiology* 2000;217:441–446.
14. Rogers LF, Osmer JC. Bronchogenic cyst: a review of 46 cases. *Am J Roentgenol* 1964;91:273–283.
15. Nakata H, Nakayama C, Kimoto T, et al. Computed tomography of mediastinal bronchogenic cysts. *J Comput Assist Tomogr* 1982;6:733–738.
16. Mendelson DS, Rose JS, Efremidis SC, et al. Bronchogenic cysts with high CT numbers. *Am J Radiol* 1983;140:463–465.
17. Naidich DP, Rumancik WM, Ettenger NA, et al. Congenital anomalies of the lungs in adults: MR diagnosis. *Am J Roentgenol* 1988;151:13–19.
18. Nakata H, Egashira K, Watanabe H, et al. MR imaging of bronchogenic cysts. *J Comput Assist Tomogr* 1993;17:267–270.
19. Barakos JA, Brown JJ, Brescia RJ, Higgins CB. High signal intensity lesions of the chest in MR imaging. *J Comput Assist Tomogr* 1989;13:797–802.
20. Hulnick DH, Naidich DP, McCauley DI, et al. Late presentation of congenital cystic adenomatoid malformation of the lung. *Radiology* 1984;151:569–573.
21. Patz EF, Müller NL, Swensen SJ, Dodd LG. Congenital cystic adenomatoid malformation in adults: CT findings. *J Comput Assist Tomogr* 1995;19:361–364.
22. Stocker JT, Madewell E, Drake RM. Congenital cystic adenomatoid malformation of the lung: classification and morphologic spectrum. *Hum Pathol* 1977;8:155–171.
23. Jederlinic PJ, Sicilian LS, Baigelman W, et al. Congenital bronchial atresia: a report of 4 cases and review of the literature. *Medicine* 1986;66:73–83.
24. Pugatch RD, Gale ME. Obscure pulmonary masses: bronchial impaction revealed by CT. *Am J Roentgenol* 1983;141:909–914.
25. Logan PM. Branching parenchymal mass. *Chest* 1998;113:523–524.
26. Rappaport DC, Herman SJ, Weisbrod GL. Congenital bronchopulmonary diseases in adults: CT findings. *Am J Roentgenol* 1994;162:1295–1299.

27. Burke CM, Safai C, Nelson DP, et al. Pulmonary arteriovenous malformations: a critical update. *Am Rev Respir Dis* 1986;134:334–339.
28. Coley SC, Jackson JE. Pulmonary arteriovenous malformations. *Clin Radiol* 1998;53:396–404.
29. Pugash RA. Pulmonary arteriovenous malformations: overview and transcatheter embolotherapy. *Can Assoc Radiol J* 2001;52:92–102.
30. Remy J, Remy-Jardin M, Wattinne L, Defontaines C. Pulmonary arteriovenous malformations: evaluation with CT of the chest before and after treatment. *Radiology* 1992;182:809–816.
31. Remy J, Remy-Jardin M, Giraud F, Wattinne L. Angioarchitecture of pulmonary arteriovenous malformations: clinical utility of three-dimensional helical CT. *Radiology* 1994;191:657–664.

2

PULMONARY INFECTION

PATTERNS OF INFECTION
Lobar Pneumonia
Bronchopneumonia
Interstitial Pneumonia
Septic Embolism
Miliary Infection
Lung Abscess

BACTERIAL PNEUMONIA
Streptococcus pneumoniae
Staphylococcus aureus
Klebsiella pneumoniae
Pseudomonas aeruginosa
Legionella Species
Hemophilus influenzae
Nocardia Species
Actinomyces Species
Mycobacterium tuberculosis
Nontuberculous Mycobacteria

FUNGAL INFECTION
Pulmonary Aspergillosis
Candidiasis
Cryptococcosis
Histoplasmosis
Coccidioidomycosis
Pneumocystis carinii

VIRAL INFECTION
Respiratory Viruses
Varicella-Zoster
Cytomegalovirus

MYCOPLASMA PNEUMONIAE

CHLAMYDIA PNEUMONIAE

**ECHINOCOCCUS GRANULOSUS
(HYDATID DISEASE)**

Pneumonia can be classified in several ways, according to its clinical, microbiologic, or anatomic characteristics. From a clinical point of view, it can be considered to be community acquired or nosocomial (originating or taking place in a hospital) and as occurring in a normal or immunocompromised host. The types of organism responsible for the pneumonia and the course of disease differ in these various settings.

Community-acquired pneumonia is most commonly caused by *Streptococcus pneumoniae, Mycoplasma pneumoniae, Chlamydia pneumoniae, Hemophilus influenzae,* and viruses such as respiratory syncytial virus (1–3). By contrast, the most common pathogens in nosocomial pneumonia are *Staphylococcus aureus* and gram-negative organisms such as *Klebsiella pneumoniae, Pseudomonas aeruginosa,* and *Escherichia coli* (4–6). As might be expected, compared with otherwise normal individuals with pneumonia, immunocompromised patients have an increased incidence and severity of infection caused by all these organisms. In addition, they often have pneumonia caused by organisms not seen in the normal population, including cytomegalovirus, *Pneumocystis carinii,* and *Aspergillus fumigatus.*

PATTERNS OF INFECTION

Pulmonary infection can also be classified into several radiologic and pathologic patterns according to its anatomic features. The three most common such patterns are lobar pneumonia, bronchopneumonia, and interstitial pneumonia. Less common forms of infection include bronchiolitis, septic embolism, miliary infection, and lung abscess. As with the clinical setting, the type of organism responsible for these patterns varies, a feature that is useful in differential diagnosis.

Lobar Pneumonia

Lobar pneumonia is characterized histologically by filling of alveolar airspaces by an exudate of edema fluid and neutrophils, often with relatively little or no tissue damage (Fig. 2.1). This filling is more or less uniform within the affected lung and typically extends across segments (nonsegmental consolidation). It usually begins in the periphery of the lung adjacent to the visceral pleura and spreads via interalveolar pores and small airways centripetally, resulting in a more or less homogeneous area of consolidation (Fig. 2.2). Bronchi that remain filled with gas and become surrounded by the expanding inflammatory exudate are often seen as air bronchograms. The most common causative organisms are *S. pneumoniae, K. pneumoniae,* and *Legionella pneumophila.*

On the radiograph and on CT, homogeneous airspace consolidation involving adjacent segments of a lobe is the predominant finding. On HRCT areas of ground-glass attenuation denoting incomplete filling of alveoli can be seen adjacent to the airspace consolidation (7). The consolidation typically extends across lobular and segmental boundaries (Fig. 2.3).

Bronchopneumonia

Bronchopneumonia is characterized pathologically by patchy, predominantly peribronchiolar inflammation (Fig. 2.4). Why this localization is different from lobar pneumonia is unclear but it may be related to relatively less abundant edema formation (associated with less rapid spread of infection within the lung) and more virulent organisms (resulting in greater tissue destruction) in bronchopneumonia. Although initially patchy, progression of disease often results in lobular and segmental consolidation (confluent bronchopneumonia; Fig. 2.5). The main causative organisms are *S. aureus, H. influenzae, Pseudomonas aeruginosa,* and anaerobic bacteria.

Radiologically, the consolidation is usually multifocal and bilateral. Characteristic findings on HRCT include centrilobular nodules and branching linear structures, airspace

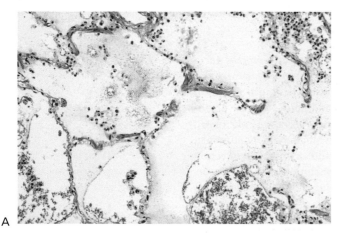 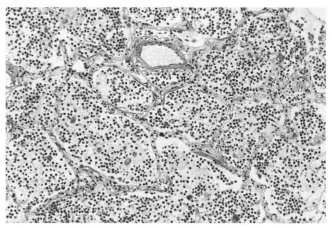

A   B

FIGURE 2.1. Lobar pneumonia. Photomicrographs show early (**A**) and advanced (**B**) stages of lobar pneumonia caused by *S. pneumoniae.* In **A,** the airspaces are filled with edema fluid; only occasional neutrophils are evident. In **B,** neutrophils predominate. The abundant fluid produced in the early stage of disease flows relatively easily from airspace to airspace, resulting in the homogeneous consolidation seen grossly. Note that alveolar septa are intact in both stages of disease (i.e., there is no evidence of irreversible tissue damage).

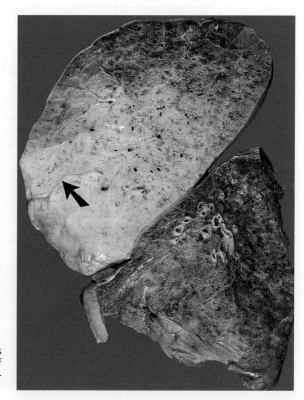

FIGURE 2.2. Lobar pneumonia. Sagittal slice of the right lung shows homogeneous consolidation of the middle lobe and inferior portion of the upper lobe (*arrow* indicates the incomplete minor fissure). *S. pneumoniae* was cultured from the blood premortem.

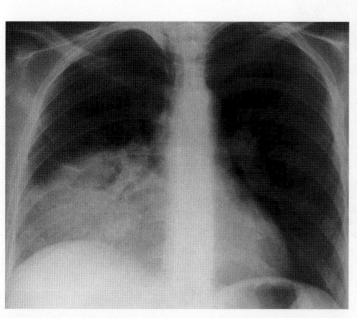

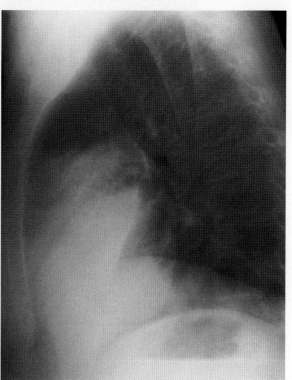

A

B

FIGURE 2.3. Lobar pneumonia. Posteroanterior (**A**) and lateral (**B**) chest radiographs show extensive consolidation of the right middle lobe. The patient was a 34-year-old woman with pneumococcal pneumonia.

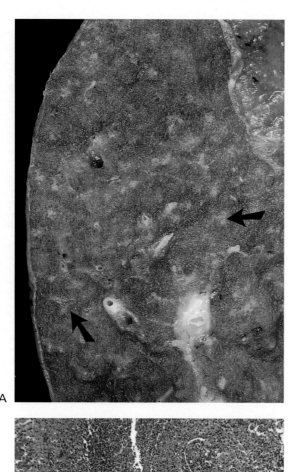

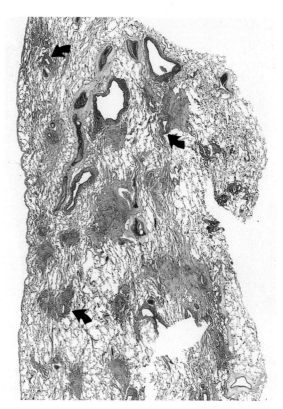

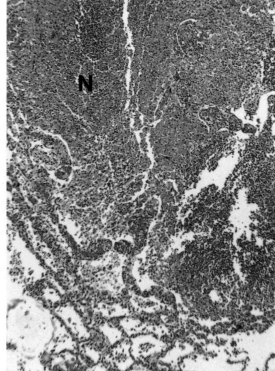

FIGURE 2.4. Acute bronchopneumonia. **A:** Magnified view of a lower lobe shows numerous small foci of whitish consolidation. Many have a nodular appearance; however, some appear to branch (*arrows*), suggesting a relation with small airways. **B:** Low-magnification photomicrograph confirms the patchy nature of the disease, which is clearly located around the lumens of small bronchioles in several foci (*arrows*). **C:** Magnified view of one of the disease foci shows a dense infiltrate of neutrophils associated with necrosis of the underlying pulmonary tissue (*N*).

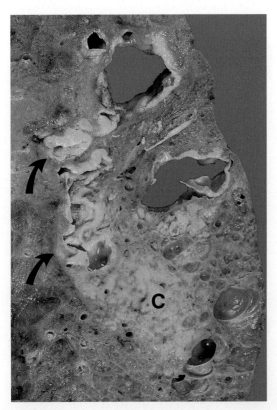

FIGURE 2.5. Confluent bronchopneumonia. Magnified view of a sagittal slice of the right lung shows a focus of consolidation (**C**) associated with several abscesses (*arrows*), some of which are cavitated. Such disease develops by expansion and coalescence of multiple foci of peribronchiolar infection. (The adjacent lung shows interstitial fibrosis with honeycombing.) Postmortem lung culture grew *S. aureus*.

nodules, and multifocal lobular consolidation (7) (Fig. 2.6). The nodules and branching linear opacities result in an appearance resembling a tree in bud and are related to the presence of the inflammatory exudate in the lumen and walls of membranous and respiratory bronchioles and the lung parenchyma immediately adjacent to them. This appearance is similar to bronchiolitis caused by viruses, *Mycoplasma pneumonia,* and chlamydia (7–9). Unlike the latter, however, the tree-in-bud pattern in bacterial bronchopneumonia usually comprises only a small proportion of the radiologic abnormalities.

Interstitial Pneumonia

Interstitial pneumonia is characterized histologically by a mononuclear inflammatory cell infiltrate in the alveolar septa and interstitial tissue surrounding small parenchymal vessels (Fig. 2.7). The most common causes are *Mycoplasma pneumoniae,* viruses, and *Pneumocystis carinii.* Airspace disease is typically absent or minimal (with the exception of *Pneumocystis* infection, in which the organisms reside predominantly in the alveoli). Small airway involvement (bronchiolitis) is often seen with *M. pneumoniae* and viral infection. The common pathogenetic feature of these organisms with respect to disease localization is their association with airway and alveolar epithelium, viruses replicating within epithelial cells, and *Mycoplasma* and *Pneumocystis* attaching to their surface. The ensuing epithelial damage engenders an inflammatory reaction in the adjacent interstitium, causing it to thicken.

The radiologic manifestation of mycoplasmal and viral pneumonia consists most commonly of a patchy or diffuse reticular or reticulonodular pattern (10), reflecting the

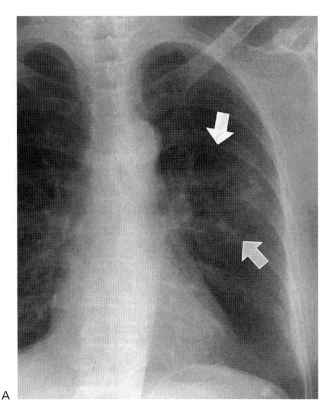

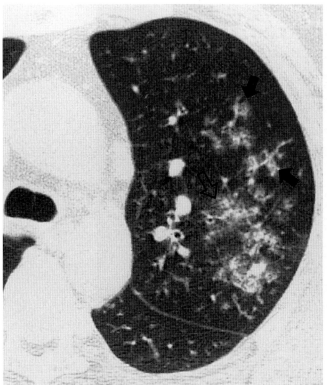

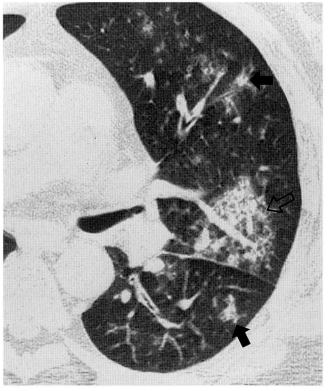

FIGURE 2.6. Acute bronchopneumonia. **A:** Chest radiograph shows focal area of poorly defined consolidation and nodularity in the left upper lobe (*arrows*). **B, C:** HRCT images (1.0-mm collimation) obtained at carinal (**B**) and subcarinal (**C**) levels, respectively, show multiple poorly defined nodular opacities (*solid arrows*) and focal ground glass opacities (*open arrows*) in a predominantly peribronchial distribution in the upper lobe. Also note branching nature of small nodular lesions.

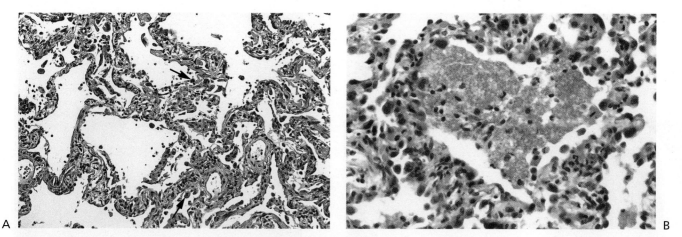

FIGURE 2.7. Interstitial pneumonia. Photomicrographs show a moderate degree of alveolar interstitial thickening that is predominantly the result of an infiltrate of lymphocytes (with the addition of a few neutrophils in **B**). With the exception of a mild increase in macrophages, airspaces are essentially normal in **A**; several enlarged cells (shown on higher magnification to be related to cytomegalovirus) can be seen (*arrows*). The alveolar airspace in **B** is filled with finely vacuolated lightly eosinophilic material related to *Pneumocystis carinii*.

alveolar interstitial thickening (Fig. 2.8). Septal thickening also may be present. Associated bronchiolitis results in centrilobular nodular and branching linear opacities (tree-in-bud pattern) on HRCT (8). *Pneumocystis carinii* pneumonia usually presents with bilateral hazy increased opacity (ground-glass pattern) or a fine reticulonodular pattern on the radiograph. The characteristic HRCT finding consists of extensive bilateral areas of ground-glass attenuation (11,12) (Fig. 2.9).

Septic Embolism

Septic emboli to the lungs originate in a variety of sites, including cardiac valves (endocarditis), peripheral veins (thrombophlebitis), and venous catheters or pacemaker wires. Tricuspid valve endocarditis is the most common cause in intravenous drug abusers. The

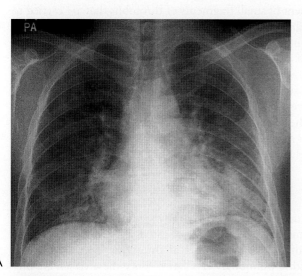
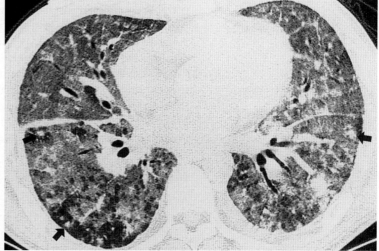

FIGURE 2.8. Interstitial pneumonia. **A:** Chest radiograph shows poorly defined nodular and reticular densities in both lungs and focal areas of consolidation in the lower lobes. **B:** HRCT image (1.5-mm collimation) shows extensive bilateral ground-glass opacities and poorly-defined small nodules (*arrows*). Also note small right pleural effusion (*arrow*). The patient was a 35-year-old man with myelodysplastic syndrome and herpes virus pneumonia.

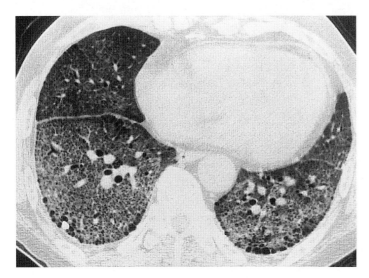

FIGURE 2.9. *Pneumocystis carinii* pneumonia. HRCT image (1.0-mm collimation) shows diffuse bilateral ground-glass opacities and a fine reticular pattern. Focal paraseptal emphysema is evident. The patient was a 64-year-old man undergoing chemotherapy for metastatic adenocarcinoma. (Courtesy of Dr. Jin-Hwan Kim, Department of Radiology, Chungnam National University Hospital, Seoul, Korea.)

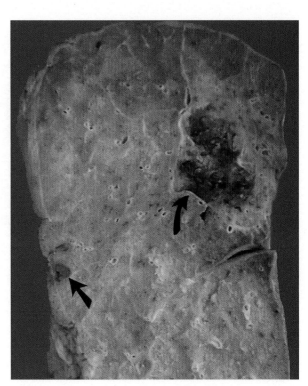

FIGURE 2.10. Septic embolism. Sagittal slice of the right lung shows multiple irregularly shaped foci of yellowish consolidation. Several hemorrhagic lesions are also apparent. One has a wedge shape suggestive of an infarct (*straight arrow*); the other (*curved arrow*) is a cavity lined by granulation tissue. The patient had had staphylococcal septicemia (unknown source) approximately 4 weeks prior to death and had developed radiologic evidence of septic embolism, for which he had been treated.

common feature in all these sites is endothelial damage associated with the formation of friable thrombus containing organisms (usually bacteria, but sometimes fungi). Turbulence of flowing blood results in detachment of small fragments of thrombus that are carried to peripheral pulmonary arteries. Ensuing disease is probably the result of both ischemia and toxins derived from organisms that extend from the thrombus into the adjacent parenchyma. The ischemia may lead to infarction and/or hemorrhage and the toxins from organisms to a neutrophilic exudate and necrosis of lung parenchyma (Fig. 2.10).

The radiologic findings consist of multiple bilateral nodules ranging in size from 0.5 to 3 cm (Fig. 2.11). They often have poorly defined margins and frequently cavitate, reflecting the necrosis. In addition to the nodules and cavitation, CT may show wedge-shaped pleural-based areas of consolidation secondary to infarction or hemorrhage (13,14). The nodules often appear to have a vessel leading into them ("feeding vessel" sign) (13,14).

Miliary Infection

As with septic emboli, miliary infection of the lungs occurs by seeding of microorganisms present in the blood. Unlike the former, however, miliary disease is associated with free organisms rather than organisms contained in fragments of thrombus. Because of their minute size, the organisms lodge within pulmonary capillaries. Since these vessels are present throughout the lung, extension of the organisms into the adjacent alveoli and the ensuing inflammatory reaction are distributed more or less randomly within the parenchyma (although there may be a basal predominance because of gravity-associated blood flow) (Fig. 2.12).

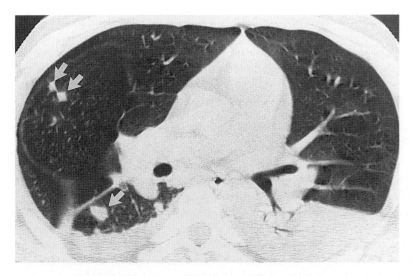

FIGURE 2.11. Septic embolism. CT image (7-mm collimation) shows several nodules (*arrows*) in the right lung and consolidation in the dependent regions of both lower lobes. The patient was a 23-year-old man with staphylococcal endocarditis.

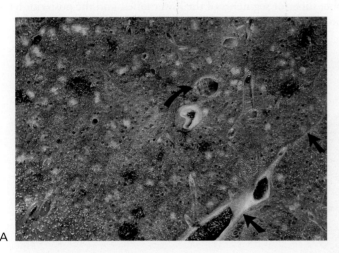

A

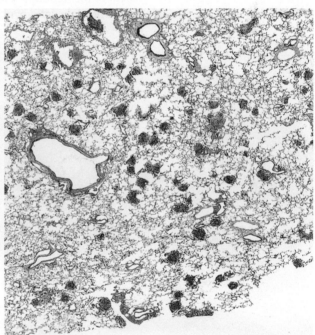

B

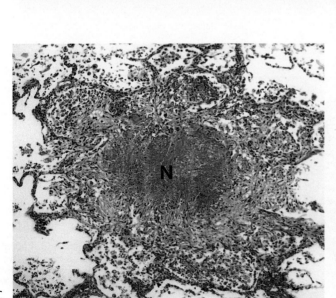

C

FIGURE 2.12. Miliary tuberculosis. **A:** Magnified view of a slice of lung shows numerous white nodules approximately 0.5 to 1 mm in diameter distributed randomly throughout the parenchyma (*straight arrows* = interlobular septum and pulmonary vein; *curved arrow* = centrilobular bronchiole). **B:** Photomicrograph of lung parenchyma from another patient with earlier disease also shows numerous nodules, again with a random distribution. **C:** View of one of the nodules from the previous case shows the presence of granulomatous inflammation filling and obliterating several alveoli; central necrosis (*N*) is evident.

The most common organism responsible for a miliary pattern of infection is *My-cobacterium tuberculosis*. The granulomatous inflammatory reaction that develops in relation to the minute foci of infection tends to be well delimited, resulting in a distinct nodular appearance both pathologically and radiologically (Figs. 2.12 and 2.13). Thus the characteristic radiographic and HRCT findings consist of nodules, 1 to 3 mm in diameter, randomly distributed throughout both lungs (15,16).

Lung Abscess

In most cases, a lung abscess is a complication of a relatively localized focus of bronchopneumonia in which necrotic tissue in the central region is surrounded by granulation and, eventually, fibrous tissue. It may appear grossly as an encapsulated focus of pus (Fig. 2.14) or a cavity (Fig. 2.15). Multiple abscesses associated with more diffuse bronchopneumonia also can be seen (Fig. 2.5). Organizing pneumonia is frequently present in the adjacent lung. Airways and lymph nodes in the drainage area of the abscess may show reactive changes (wall thickening by fibrous tissue/inflammatory cellular infiltrate and hyperplasia, respectively). Common causes include *Staphylococcus aureus, Pseudomonas aeruginosa, Klebsiella pneumoniae,* and anaerobic organisms (17). Infection by the last-named organisms is believed to result from most cases by aspiration of oral secretions contaminated by the bacteria (18). Because such aspiration is gravity dependent, the posterior segment of the right upper lobe, superior segments of the lower lobes, and the posterior basal segment of the left lower lobe are most commonly involved.

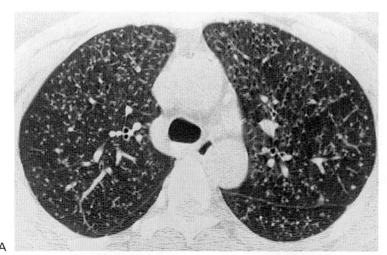

A

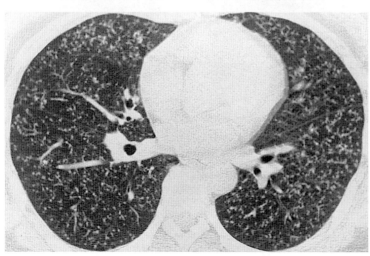

B

FIGURE 2.13. Miliary tuberculosis. HRCT images (1.0-mm collimation) at the levels of azygos arch (**A**) and the right inferior pulmonary vein (**B**) show numerous nodules 1 to 3 mm in diameter distributed randomly throughout both lungs. (Reprinted from Lee JY, et al. *J Comput Assist Tomogr* 2000; 24:691–698, with permission.)

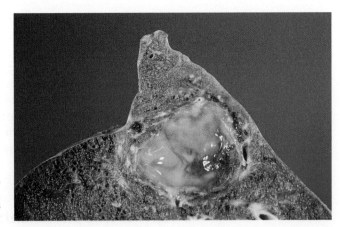

FIGURE 2.14. Lung abscess. Magnified view of the superior segment of a lower lobe shows a well-circumscribed, more or less spherical abscess. Its center is filled with pus and the wall is relatively thin.

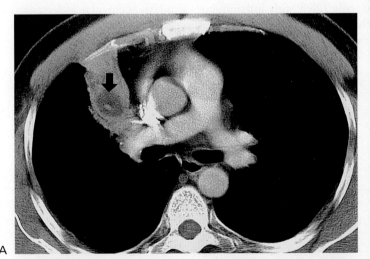

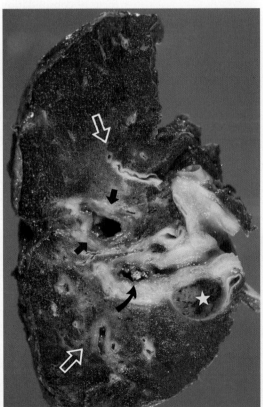

A

B

FIGURE 2.15. Lung abscess. **A:** Contrast-enhanced CT image (7-mm collimation) shows airspace consolidation containing an area of low attenuation (*arrow*) in the anterior segment of the right upper lobe. **B:** View of the excised specimen shows a cavity (*straight black arrows*), the wall of which is composed partly of pinkish granulation tissue and partly of white fibrous tissue. The surrounding lung is consolidated (*open arrows*). The segmental bronchus subtending the area shows thickening of its wall and focal mucosal necrosis (*curved arrow*). A peribronchial lymph node is enlarged (*asterisk*).

As indicated, the characteristic radiologic finding of a lung abscess is a cavity (19). However, the cavity may not be seen when patients are evaluated with supine chest radiography or when the radiographs are obtained before communication is established between the abscess and the bronchial tree allowing the central necrotic material to drain (19). An air–fluid level may be seen when there is incomplete drainage. On CT, an abscess is typically seen as a spherical mass with a wall of irregular thickness. The mass may have central low attenuation or a cavity (Fig. 2.15). The wall shows enhancement following intravenous administration of contrast medium, reflecting the presence of vascularized granulation tissue (supplied predominantly by hypertrophied bronchial arteries) (20).

BACTERIAL PNEUMONIA

Streptococcus pneumoniae

Streptococcus pneumoniae (Pneumococcus) is a gram-positive coccus that grows in pairs or short chains. It is the most common cause of community-acquired pneumonia. Such infection typically results in lobar pneumonia, probably because of the rapid outpouring of edema fluid into the airspaces that is characteristic of the infection (21,22) (Figs. 2.1 to 2.3). However, bronchopneumonia is also common, particularly in patients who have bacteremia (21). Another form of presentation is as a fairly well-circumscribed single, round focus of consolidation "round pneumonia" (23) (Fig. 2.16).

Staphylococcus aureus

Staphylococcus aureus is a gram-positive coccus that grows in clusters. It accounts for only about 3% of all cases of community-acquired pneumonia (24) but is much more common as a cause of nosocomial infection.

The typical pattern at presentation, both pathologically and radiologically, is bronchopneumonia, with patchy areas of airspace consolidation usually involving more than one lobe (Fig. 2.17). Disease is bilateral in approximately 40% of patients (25,26). Because proximal airways are usually filled with inflammatory exudate, segmental atelectasis is common and air bronchograms are infrequent (27). Abscess formation is common histologically and can be identified radiologically in about 15% to 30% of patients. A second,

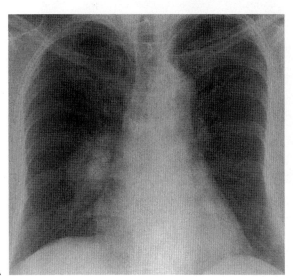
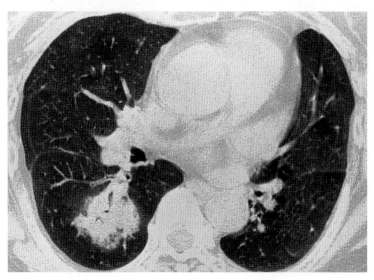

A   B

FIGURE 2.16. Round pneumonia. **A:** Chest radiograph shows an oval mass in right hilar region. **B:** CT image (1.5-mm collimation) shows a round area of consolidation containing an air bronchogram in the superior segment of the right lower lobe. The patient was a 60-year-old woman with *Streptococcus pneumoniae* pneumonia.

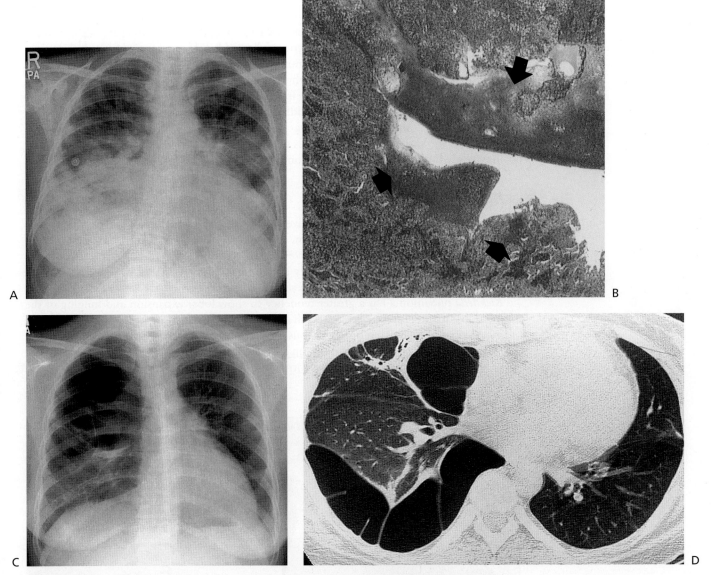

FIGURE 2.17. Staphylococcal pneumonia—pneumatocele formation. **A:** Chest radiograph show numerous nodular opacities, focal areas of airspace consolidation, and bilateral pleural effusions. (The right mediastinal widening is due to mediastinal lipomatosis caused by steroid therapy.) **B:** Photomicrograph of a biopsy obtained from the right lower lobe shows necrotizing pneumonia with focal cavity formation (*arrows*). **C:** Radiograph obtained 22 days later shows multiple pneumatoceles in right upper and middle lung zones. The areas of consolidation and the nodular opacities have almost completely resolved. **D:** HRCT image obtained 1 month later shows multiseptated air-filled cystic lesions in the right middle and lower lobes. Also note parenchymal band in right lower lobe and retracted lung in right middle lobe. The patient was a 26-year-old woman with systemic lupus erythematosus.

less common complication is the formation of a pneumatocele, a thin-walled, gas-filled space that characteristically increases in size over several days to weeks (Fig. 2.17). The abnormality is seen more often in children (40% to 75%) than in adults (15%) (28). It is believed to begin as a focus of consolidation followed by abscess formation and cavitation. Swelling of one or more airways communicating with the cavity or the formation of plugs of partially organized exudate within them results in a check valve mechanism that allows more gas to enter the cavity than leave it, leading to an increase in its size (Fig. 2.18). The reason for the greater incidence in children than adults is unclear.

Hematogenously derived *S. aureus* pneumonia is much less common than that acquired via the airways. The infection is manifested by multiple nodules or masses involving mainly in the lower lobes; cavitation is frequent.

Klebsiella pneumoniae

Klebsiella pneumoniae is a gram-negative bacillus that most frequently infects the elderly, debilitated patients, and alcoholic men. It usually gains entry to the lung by aspiration of oral secretions (29).

The ensuing pneumonia is usually unilateral and involves most commonly the right lung. It is typically lobar in pattern, resembling that caused by *S. pneumoniae*. However, *Klebsiella* pneumonia has a greater tendency to show lobar expansion and bulging of the interlobar fissure, presumably as a result of more abundant inflammatory exudate. On CT, mixed areas of enhancing homogeneous consolidation and predominantly central poorly marginated areas of low attenuation can often be seen (30). The latter reflects the presence of hemorrhagic necrosis and abscess formation (31) (Fig. 2.19).

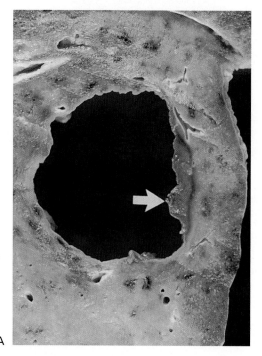
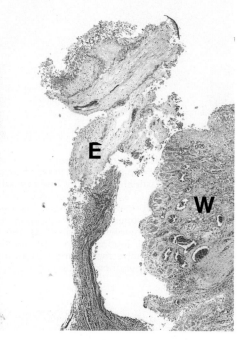

A   B

FIGURE 2.18. Pneumatocele. **A:** Magnified view of an upper lobe shows a well-circumscribed cavity whose wall is mostly smooth; a small amount of necrotic lung is evident on one side (*arrow*). **B:** Photomicrograph of a bronchus that subtended the cavity shows an inflamed wall (*W*) and an elongated plug of mucus and inflammatory cell exudate (*E*). The base of the latter was adherent to the airway wall in the gross specimen. Its distal portion was mobile and was hypothesized to permit air to enter the cavity during inspiration and prevent its egress on exhalation. Radiographs taken before death had shown a focal area of parenchymal consolidation that had undergone cavitation that had subsequently increased in size. Although a pneumatocele is seen most often with *S. aureus* infection, in this case it was felt to be secondary to anaerobes.

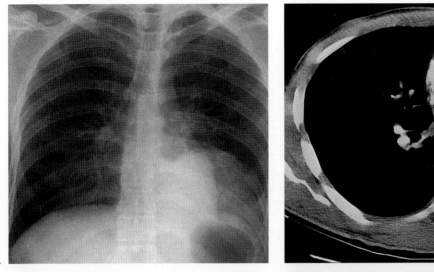

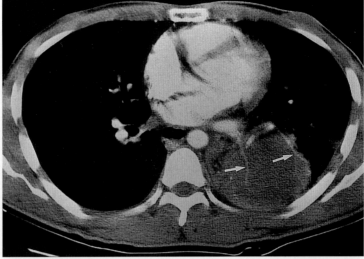

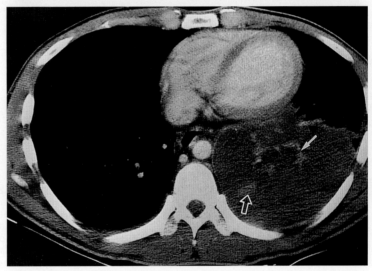

FIGURE 2.19. *Klebsiella pneumoniae* pneumonia. **A:** Chest radiograph shows masslike consolidation of the left lower lobe. **B, C:** Contrast-enhanced CT images (7.0-mm collimation) at the level of the inferior pulmonary veins (**B**) and the ventricles (**C**) show low-attenuation consolidation containing pulmonary vessels (*solid arrows*) (CT-angiogram sign). Focal nodular areas of enhancement (*open arrow*) are evident. A follow-up chest radiograph (not shown) demonstrated cavity formation. The patient was a 29-year-old man.

Pseudomonas aeruginosa

Pseudomonas aeruginosa is a gram-negative bacillus that is the most common cause of nosocomial pulmonary infection (32). It causes confluent bronchopneumonia that is often extensive (Fig. 2.20) and frequently cavitates. The radiologic manifestations are nonspecific and consist most commonly of patchy areas of consolidation and widespread poorly defined nodular opacities. It is often difficult to distinguish *Pseudomonas* pneumonia from underlying disease, particularly adult respiratory distress syndrome (33,34).

Legionella Species

Legionella species, of which there are more than 40, are gram-negative bacilli normally found in aquatic environments. The most common organism responsible for human disease is *L. pneumophila*. The organism causes both community-acquired pneumonia and nosocomial pneumonia.

The most common initial radiographic finding consists of unilateral, nonsegmental, poorly defined airspace consolidation (35–37). Coalescence of the consolidation may lead to segmental or lobar consolidation. Rapid progression is common (36,38), with the full-blown radiographic pattern usually occurring approximately 10 days after the initial presentation. At this time, more than half of the patients have a pattern of lobar pneumonia,

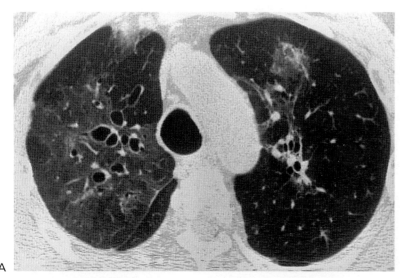

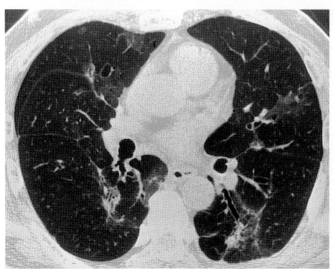

FIGURE 2.20. *Pseudomonas* pneumonia. **A:** An HRCT image (1.0-mm collimation) at the level of the aortic arch shows patchy areas of ground-glass attenuation in both upper lobes. Underlying bronchiectasis is evident. **B:** An image at the level of the lower lobe bronchi shows patchy bilateral areas of ground-glass attenuation and consolidation adjacent to bronchovascular bundles. Bronchiectasis is also present.

and up to 65% have bilateral disease (39) (Fig. 2.21). Pleural effusions are present in 10% to 30% of patients (38,39).

Hemophilus influenzae

Hemophilus influenzae is a gram-negative coccobacillus that is responsible for 5% to 20% of community-acquired pneumonias (40,41). It is also an important cause of nosocomial pneumonia. The radiologic manifestations are those of bronchopneumonia (42). Findings of bronchiolitis alone or in combination with bronchopneumonia are seen in 15% to 30% of patients. The abnormalities consist of poorly defined nodules and patchy unilateral or bilateral areas of consolidation. Cavitation is seen in less than 15% of patients and pleural effusion in about 50% (42).

Nocardia Species

Nocardia species are gram-positive bacilli. The most common human pathogen is *N. asteroides*. Most patients in whom the infection develops have underlying disease or are immunocompromised. The most common pathologic finding is necrotizing bronchopneumonia with multifocal abscess formation (Fig. 2.22).

The radiologic manifestations include lobar consolidation, multifocal consolidation (bronchopneumonia), and multiple nodules or masses often having irregular or poorly de-

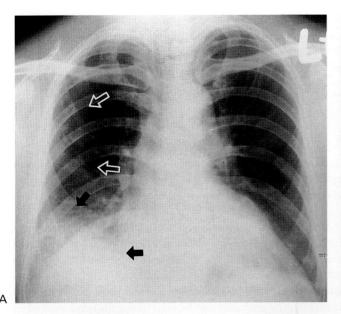

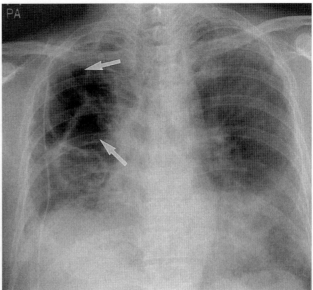

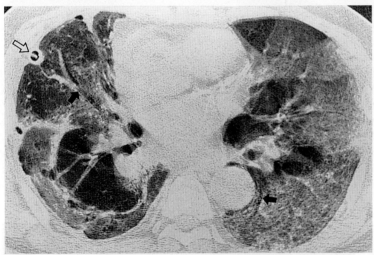

FIGURE 2.21. Legionella pneumonia. **A:** Chest radiograph shows consolidation (*black arrows*) in the right lower lung zone and poorly defined nodules (*open arrows*) in the right upper and middle zones. The parenchymal abnormalities increased rapidly for the next few days. **B:** Radiograph 20 days later shows diffuse bilateral ground-glass opacities and a multiloculated right pneumothorax (*arrows*). A chest tube is in place. **C:** Thin-section (1.0-mm collimation) CT scan obtained at the atrial level shows extensive ground-glass opacities in both lungs. Irregular linear opacity and traction bronchiectasis also can be seen (*arrows*). The findings reflect the presence of acute respiratory distress syndrome (ARDS) and pneumothorax. The patient was a 62-year-old man.

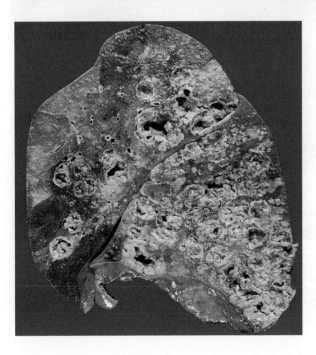

FIGURE 2.22. Nocardiosis. Sagittal slice of the left lung shows extensive necrotizing pneumonia with multifocal abscess formation and cavitation. The patient was a middle-aged man who, unlike most patients with nocardiosis, had no evidence of underlying disease.

fined margins (43,44). Cavitation is common. The infection may spread into the chest wall and result in rib destruction or sinus tract formation. CT findings generally include nodules or masses (45,46). One group of investigators assessed the CT findings in 24 patients (46). One or more nodules or masses was the most common finding, seen in 20 (83%; Fig. 2.23), followed by cavitation in eight (33%), consolidation in eight (33%), and pleural thickening in seven (29%) (46).

Actinomyces Species

Actinomyces species are anaerobic gram-positive bacteria. The most common human pathogen is *A. israelii*. The organisms are normal inhabitants of the oral cavity and are particularly numerous at gingival margins of individuals who have poor oral hygiene and dental caries (47).

Pulmonary infection is characterized pathologically by bronchopneumonia with focal or multifocal abscess formation (Fig. 2.24). The foci of consolidation often are associated with dilated, inflamed bronchi (Fig. 2.25) and may be connected by granulating sinus tracts (48). Disease is often subacute and associated with a variable amount of fibrous tissue. Clumps of basophilic material measuring 100 to 300 μm in diameter and composed of intertwining bacterial filaments (sulfur granules) can be seen in the necrotic areas or in the lumen of dilated bronchi (Fig. 2.25).

The radiographic findings depend on the chronology of the infection. In acute disease, the pattern consists of nonsegmental airspace consolidation. Chronic infection is characterized by abscess formation, fibrosis, and progressive destruction of lung parenchyma (49). Occasionally, the infection extends into the chest wall (49,50).

On CT, disease appears as focal or patchy areas of airspace consolidation or a mass (50,51) (Figs. 2.24 and 2.26). In most cases, both abnormalities have central areas of low attenuation and show rim enhancement following intravenous administration of contrast medium (50,51). The low-attenuation areas represent abscesses or dilated bronchi containing inflammatory exudate; the enhancing rim corresponds to vascular granulation tissue in the abscess wall or hyperplastic bronchial vessels in the mucosa of draining airways (50,51). Pleural thickening (fibrosis) is frequently present.

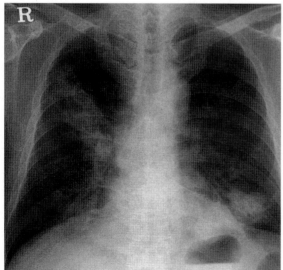
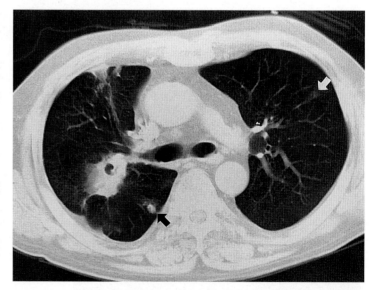

A

B

FIGURE 2.23. Nocardiosis. **A:** Chest radiograph shows multifocal airspace consolidation in the right upper and both lower lung zones. **B:** CT image (7-mm collimation) shows two foci of consolidation, one of which is cavitated in the right upper lobe. Several small nodules (*arrows*) are also present in the right lower and left upper lobes. The patient was a 52-year-old man with non-Hodgkin's lymphoma. (Courtesy of Dr. Jin Mo Goo, Department of Radiology, Seoul National University Hospital, Seoul, Korea.)

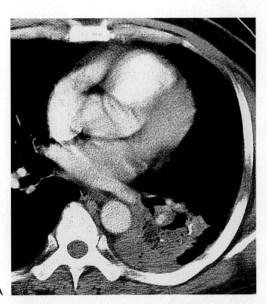

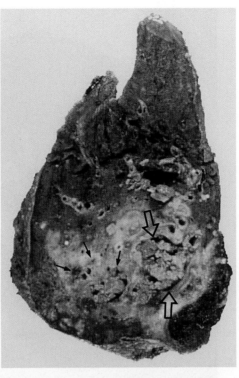

FIGURE 2.24. Actinomycosis. **A:** Contrast-enhanced CT image (7.0-mm collimation) shows consolidation with central low-attenuation area and cavitation in the superior segment of the left lower lobe. The low-attenuation area reflects the presence of necrosis. **B:** Slice of the lobe shows necrotizing pneumonia (*small arrows*) with focal abscess formation (*open arrows*). The patient was a 49-year-old man.

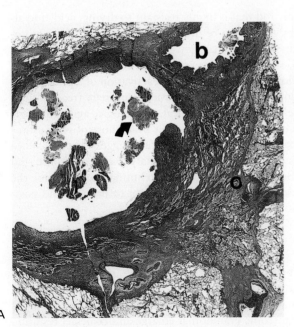

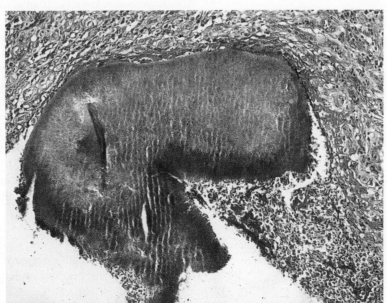

FIGURE 2.25. Actinomycosis. **A:** Photomicrograph shows a chronic abscess that contains several irregularly shaped clumps of basophilic material (*arrow*). The cavity is continuous with a mildly dilated bronchus (b). The adjacent lung shows collapse and obstructive pneumonitis (o). **B:** Magnified view shows the basophilic material to be consistent with a sulfur granule (confirmed by special stains) adjacent to the chronically inflamed cavity wall.

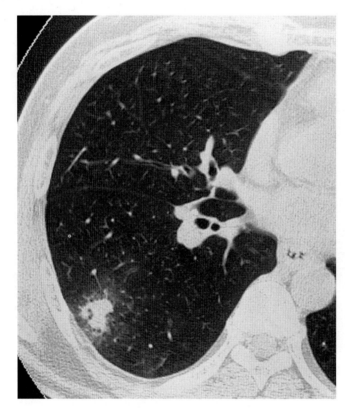

FIGURE 2.26. Actinomycosis. HRCT image (1.0-mm collimation) shows nodular consolidation surrounded by ground-glass attenuation in the right lower lobe. The patient was a 51-year-old man.

Mycobacterium tuberculosis

Mycobacterium tuberculosis is an aerobic rod that is highly resistant to drying, acid, and alcohol. Infection usually is acquired by inhalation of droplet nuclei present in the atmosphere and derived from another individual who has active (usually cavitary) pulmonary tuberculosis. Patients who develop disease after initial exposure are considered to have primary tuberculosis. Patients who develop disease as a result of reactivation of a previous focus of tuberculosis or due to reinfection are considered to have postprimary (reactivation) tuberculosis. Traditionally, it was believed that the clinical, pathologic, and radiologic manifestations of postprimary tuberculosis were quite distinct from those of primary tuberculosis. However, recent studies based on DNA fingerprinting suggest that the radiographic features are similar in patients who apparently have primary disease and those who have postprimary tuberculosis (52). Because these results are preliminary and because the vast majority of published data is based on the traditional concept of primary and postprimary disease, we follow the traditional outline in this book.

Primary Tuberculosis

Inhaled organisms are phagocytosed by alveolar macrophages, which, under the influence of sensitized T-lymphocytes, undergo transformation into epithelioid histiocytes. These aggregate in small clusters (granulomas), which undergo central necrosis (Fig. 2.27). As the disease progresses, individual microscopic granulomas enlarge and coalesce, resulting in a focus of necrotic lung surrounded by a rim of granulomatous inflammatory tissue. This initial parenchymal focus of tuberculosis is known as the Ghon focus. It may enlarge and result in a macroscopically visible area of consolidation and necrosis or, more commonly, undergo healing by envelopment of the granulomatous tissue by mature fibrous tissue (Fig. 2.28). Such healing is often accompanied by dystrophic calcification of the

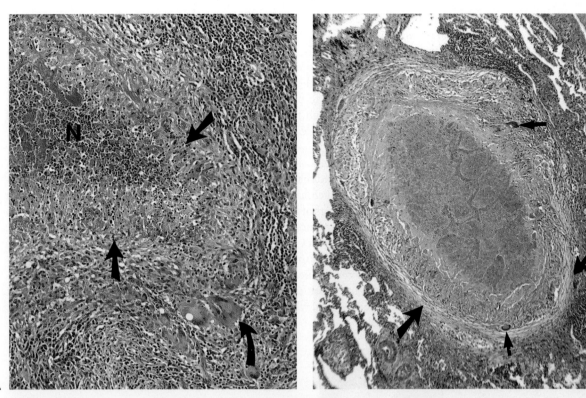

FIGURE 2.27. Tuberculosis—Ghon focus. **A:** Photomicrograph shows a focus of necrotic lung (*N*) surrounded by a layer of epithelioid histiocytes (*straight arrows*) and scattered multinucleated giant cells (*curved arrow*), the two comprising the granulomatous inflammatory component of the lesion. Numerous lymphocytes are evident adjacent to the granulomatous inflammation and there is minimal fibrosis, indicating that this is active disease. **B:** In more advanced (healing) disease, the focus of necrotic tissue is larger and completely surrounded by a layer of granulomatous inflammation (scattered giant cells can be still be identified [*small arrows*]). The lymphocyte infiltrate is less prominent and loose (fibroblastic) connective tissue (*large arrows*) can be seen at the junction of the lesion and uninvolved lung.

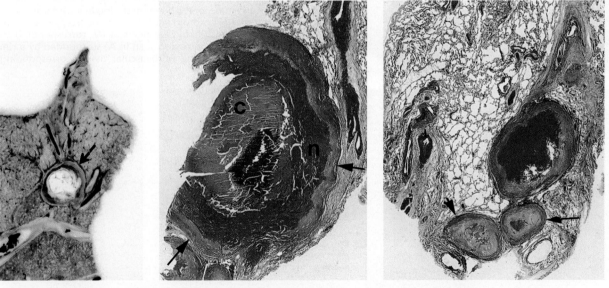

FIGURE 2.28. Tuberculosis—healed granulomas. **A:** Magnified view of a slice of lower lobe shows a well-circumscribed nodule composed of a rim of dense collagen (*arrow*) surrounding chalky white (caseous) necrotic tissue. **B:** Low-magnification view shows the collagenous capsule (*arrows*) and the necrotic material (*n*) (the central purple region [*c*] is calcified). **C:** Low-magnification view of another lesion shows an absence of calcification as well as two satellite granulomas that are almost completely fibrotic (*arrows*).

necrotic tissue. Smaller healed granulomas (satellite nodules) are common adjacent to the principal focus of inflammation.

During the stage of active disease, organisms frequently spread to the regional lymph nodes, where the ensuing granulomatous inflammatory reaction results in lymph node enlargement. The combination of the Ghon focus and affected nodes is known as the Ranke complex. Spread of organisms to other sites in the body via the bloodstream is also common at this time. Although such foci of infection are usually microscopic in extent and rarely cause clinically evident disease, they may be the source of reactivation months or years later.

Although primary tuberculosis occurs most commonly in children, it is being seen with increasing frequency in adults (53,54). There is considerable difference in the prevalence of radiologic findings in children compared with those in adults. The most common abnormality in children consists of lymph node enlargement, which is seen in 90% to 95% of cases (55,56). The lymphadenopathy is most commonly unilateral and located in the hilum or paratracheal region. On CT, the enlarged nodes frequently have inhomogeneous or low attenuation and show peripheral (rim) enhancement (57,58) (Fig. 2.29). The former corresponds to the central necrotic portion of the node, and the latter, to the surrounding vascular inflammatory tissue. The enlarged nodes can compress the adjacent bronchi and result in atelectasis, which is usually lobar and right-sided.

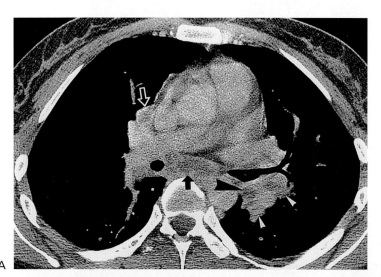

A

FIGURE 2.29. Tuberculous lymphadenitis. **A:** HRCT image (1.0-mm collimation) at the subcarinal level shows enlarged lymph nodes with central areas of low attenuation in subcarinal (*black arrow*), right prevascular (*open arrow*), and left hilar (*arrowheads*) regions. **B:** Photomicrograph of a lymph node obtained at mediastinoscopy shows replacement of the node by confluent granulomas with focal necrosis (*arrows*). **C:** Photomicrograph of a node from another patient shows more extensive necrosis (*N*, corresponding to the low-attenuation region seen in **A**) surrounded by a rim of granulomatous and fibrovascular tissue (corresponding to the enhanced rim).

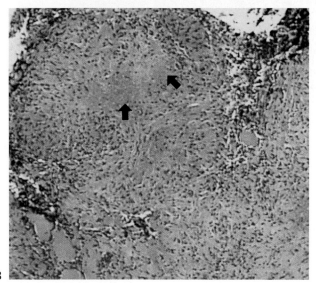

B

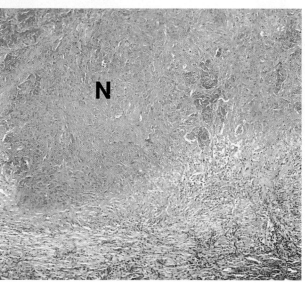

C

Airspace consolidation, related to parenchymal granulomatous inflammation and usually unilateral, is present in approximately 70% of primary disease in children. It shows no predilection for any particular lung zone (56). As compared with children, adults who have primary tuberculosis are less likely to have lymph node enlargement (10% to 30% of patients) and more likely to have parenchymal consolidation (approximately 90% of patients) (59,60) (Fig. 2.30). Pleural effusion is seen in 5% to 10% of children and 30% to 40% of adults (55,56,59).

Postprimary Tuberculosis

Postprimary tuberculosis may result from reinfection or (probably more often) reactivation of organisms in a focus of chronic inflammation/fibrosis acquired during the primary infection. Such reactivation frequently is associated with immunosuppression, malnutrition, and/or debilitation (53,61). It most commonly involves the apical and posterior segments of the upper lobes and the superior segments of the lower lobes (53,61). As with primary disease, the postprimary form is characterized histologically by necrotizing granulomatous inflammation. Coalescence and enlargement of multiple foci of such inflammation lead to consolidation and destruction of the lung parenchyma, often accompanied by fibrosis (fibrocaseous tuberculosis). Erosion into an airway is followed by drainage of necrotic material and the formation of one or more cavities (Figs. 2.31 and 2.32). The expulsed necrotic material frequently spreads via the bronchi to other parts of the lung (endobronchial spread), resulting in the formation of additional foci of tuberculous disease (tuberculous bronchopneumonia); such foci often have a nodular or branched appearance (Fig. 2.33). As might be expected, healing of disease, either following therapy or naturally, is associated with more marked fibrosis; ectatic bronchi are often entrapped within the fibrous tissue (traction bronchiectasis) (Fig. 2.34).

The chest radiograph most commonly shows patchy consolidation and poorly defined nodules involving the upper lobes or the superior segments of the lower lobes (53,62). CT findings include centrilobular nodules and branching linear structures (tree-in-bud appearance) (Fig. 2.35), lobular consolidation, cavitation, and bronchial wall thickening

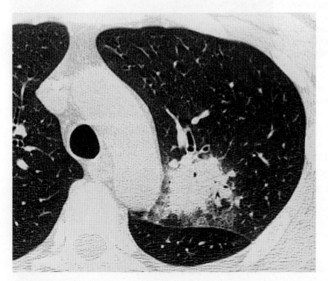

FIGURE 2.30. Primary tuberculous pneumonia. HRCT image (1.0-mm collimation) obtained at level of aortic arch shows consolidation and surrounding ground-glass opacity in left upper lobe. The patient was a 45-year-old man with neutropenia following bone marrow transplantation. (Lee JY, et al. *J Comput Assist Tomogr* 2000;24:691–698, with permission.)

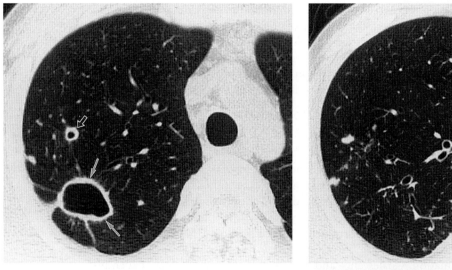

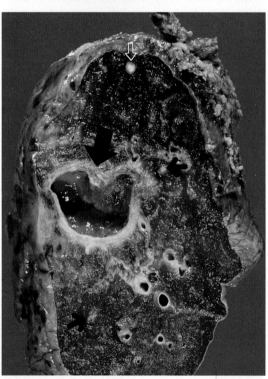

FIGURE 2.31. Cavitary tuberculosis. **A:** HRCT image (1.0-mm collimation) shows a large, thin-walled cavity (*solid arrows*); a smaller cavity (*open arrow*); linear opacities; and a few small nodules in right upper lobe. **B:** Image 30 mm caudad to **A** shows several small nodules and mild bronchial dilatation. **C:** Magnified view of a sagittal slice of the excised specimen shows the cavity (*large arrow*) as well as several calcified (*open arrow*) and uncalcified (*small arrows*) granulomas. The patient was a 30-year-old man with chronic drug resistant tuberculosis. (Lee JY, et al. *J Comput Assist Tomogr* 2000;24:691–698, with permission.)

(53,63). The centrilobular lesions are caused by endobronchial spread of organisms and correspond histologically to necrosis and granulomatous inflammation within and immediately adjacent to bronchioles, as described earlier (63,64). Progression of disease may result in lobular consolidation.

Miliary Tuberculosis

Miliary spread of tuberculosis can occur in both primary and postprimary disease (15,64). In the latter situation, it may be seen in association with typical parenchymal changes, as described earlier, or may be the only pulmonary abnormality. Miliary disease occurs when organisms within the blood are trapped within and exit from small vessels (usually capillaries). The ensuing inflammatory reaction begins in the alveolar interstitium, but rapidly spills over into the adjacent airspaces. Each focus of infection is usually related to a single

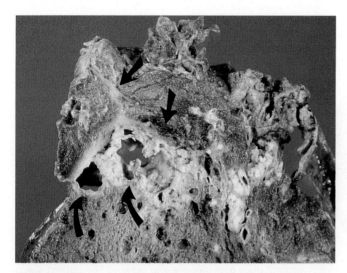

FIGURE 2.32. Cavitary tuberculosis. Magnified view of the apical region of an upper lobe shows poorly delimited foci of caseous necrosis and several irregularly shaped cavities (*curved arrows*). Focal fibrosis (*straight arrows*) is also evident. The appearance is that of chronic active fibrocaseous tuberculosis. The patient was a 76-year-old man who died with undiagnosed disease.

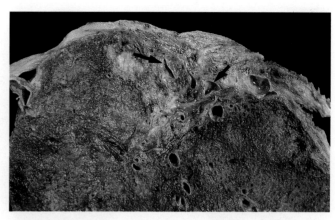

FIGURE 2.34. Healed tuberculosis. Magnified view of the apex of an upper lobe shows an ill-defined area of fibrosis. Several somewhat elongated ectatic bronchi are present within the fibrous tissue (*arrows*).

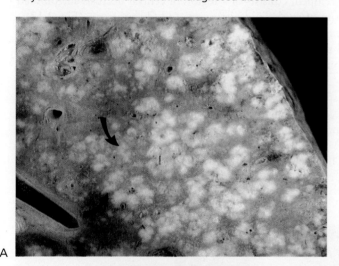

FIGURE 2.33. Tuberculosis—endobronchial spread. **A:** Magnified view of a slice of lower lobe shows multiple foci of consolidation that are distinctly white, consistent with caseous necrosis. Most have a nodular appearance and some appear to be branched (*arrows*), suggesting that they are centered on airways. **B:** Photomicrograph of one of the smaller branched regions shows two well-circumscribed foci of disease, each related to a small membranous bronchiole (*straight arrows* indicate residual airway lumen; *curved arrows* indicate accompanying pulmonary arteries). **C:** Magnified view of one of the foci shows several poorly formed granulomas (*arrows*). Necrosis is absent, presumably because of recent endobronchial spread of tubercle organisms; examination of larger lesions showed typical necrosis. The patient was 38-year-old woman with fulminant pneumonia.

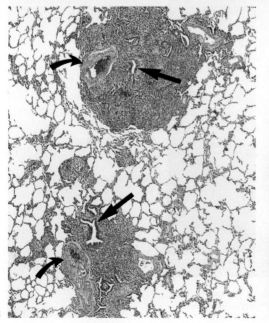

A

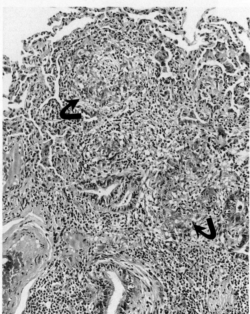

C

B

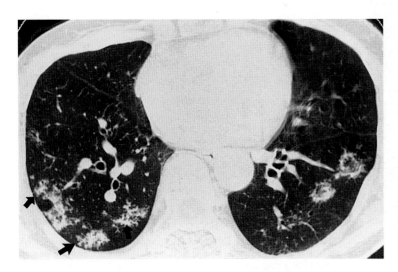

FIGURE 2.35. Pulmonary tuberculosis with endobronchial spread. HRCT image (1.0-mm collimation) shows small nodules and branching linear opacities (tree-in-bud pattern) (*arrows*) in a patchy bilateral distribution. Focal ground glass opacities are also evident. The patient was a 67-year-old woman. (Lee JY, et al. *J Comput Assist Tomogr* 2000;24:691–698, with permission)

granuloma that, when well developed, consists of a region of central necrosis surrounded by a relatively well-delimited rim of epithelioid histiocytes and fibrous tissue (Fig. 2.12).

The characteristic radiographic and HRCT findings consist of 1- to 3-mm-diameter nodules randomly distributed throughout both lungs (15,16) (Fig. 2.13). Thickening of interlobular septa and intralobular fine networks is frequently evident (64).

Tuberculomas

The term *tuberculoma* is often used to refer to a well-delimited, round, or oval focus of parenchymal tuberculosis (65). The central part of lesion consists of caseous material and the periphery of epithelioid histiocytes and multinucleated giant cells and a variable amount of collagen (Fig. 2.36). The collagen becomes more prominent and the cellular re-

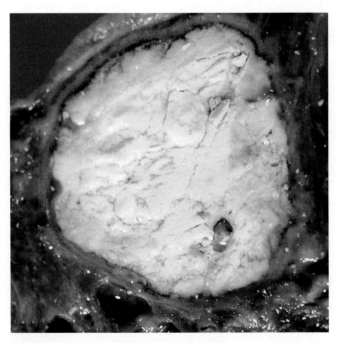

FIGURE 2.36. Tuberculoma. Magnified view of an upper lobe shows a mass of caseous material completely surrounded by a fibrous capsule. The lesion measured approximately 3 cm.

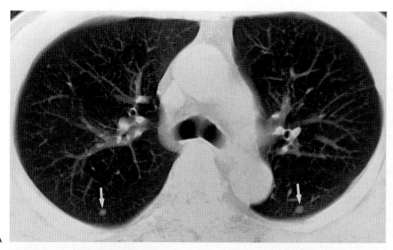

A

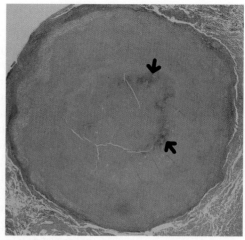

B

FIGURE 2.37. Multiple small tuberculomas simulating metastatic nodules. **A:** CT image (7-mm collimation) shows bilateral, smoothly marginated nodules (*arrows*). **B:** Photomicrograph of a biopsy specimen shows a well-demarcated focus of necrosis with central calcification (*arrows*). The patient was a 66-year-old man. (Lee JY, et al. *J Comput Assist Tomogr* 2000;24:691–698, with permission)

action less evident as healing progresses. Most tuberculomas are less than 3 cm in diameter; however, they may grow up to 5 cm. They are usually seen in the upper lobes and are multiple in about 20% of cases. Satellite nodules histologically identical to the larger focus of disease and measuring less than 1 to 5 mm in diameter are present in most cases (Fig. 2.28).

On CT, tuberculomas are most commonly smoothly marginated (Fig. 2.37); however, fibrosis related to vessels, interlobular septa, or lung parenchyma adjacent to the nodule may result in a spiculated margin (54,65). Calcification within the nodule or satellite nodules around the periphery of the dominant nodule is present in 20% to 30% of cases. Cavitation within the dominant nodule or surrounding satellite nodules also can be seen. Following intravenous administration of contrast, tuberculomas often show ringlike or curvilinear enhancement (Fig. 2.38) (65). The latter corresponds histologically to the granulomatous inflammatory tissue capsule, whereas the nonenhancing area corresponds to the central necrotic material (65).

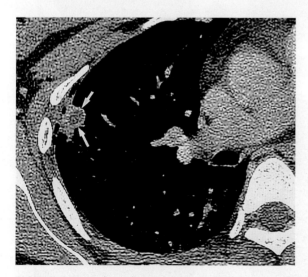

FIGURE 2.38. Tuberculoma. HRCT image (1.0-mm collimation) shows a nodule in right upper lobe with central low attenuation and peripheral enhancing rim (*arrows*).

Tuberculosis in the Acquired Immunodeficiency Syndrome

Patients who have acquired immunodeficiency syndrome (AIDS) are at an increased risk for developing tuberculosis. The radiologic manifestations of the disease in these patients are influenced by the degree of immunosuppression (66,67). The findings in patients who are mildly immunosuppressed (more than 200 CD4 cells/μL) are similar to those of post-primary disease in the normal host (66–68), with focal areas of consolidation and nodular opacities involving mainly the upper lobes. Cavitation occurs in approximately 50% of patients, and lymph node enlargement, in 10%.

Patients who have moderate or severe immunosuppression (less than 200 CD4 cells/μL) have a pattern resembling primary tuberculosis (66–68), the predominant abnormalities consisting of hilar or mediastinal lymph node enlargement and airspace consolidation (Fig. 2.39). In 40% to 60% of patients, the consolidation has a middle or lower lobe predominance. Enlarged hilar or mediastinal nodes are evident on the radiograph in 30% to 60% of patients and on CT in 70% to 90% (67,69,70). As in nonimmunocompromised patients, the enlarged nodes usually have decreased attenuation and often show rim enhancement following intravenous administration of contrast (70). Markedly immunosuppressed individuals have a greater prevalence of miliary tuberculosis (67). It is important to remember that 10% to 20% of severely immunocompromised AIDS patients with tuberculosis have normal radiographs (67).

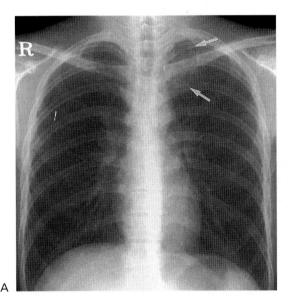

A

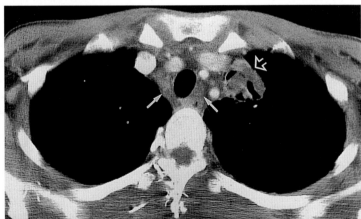

B

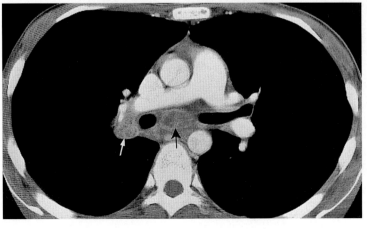

C

FIGURE 2.39. Tuberculosis in association with AIDS. **A:** Chest radiograph shows a poorly defined focal opacity in left upper lobe (*arrows*). **B:** Contrast-enhanced CT image (7-mm collimation) shows an area of consolidation with several cavities (*open arrow*). Mild lymph node enlargement is evident in the paratracheal region (*solid arrows*). **C:** Image at the level of the left main bronchus shows lymph node enlargement in the right hilum and subcarinal area with central low attenuation and peripheral rim enhancement (*arrows*). The patient was a 25-year-old man with AIDS. (Courtesy of Dr. Jin Mo Goo, Department of Radiology, Seoul National University Hospital, Seoul, Korea.)

Nontuberculous Mycobacteria

Nontuberculous (atypical) mycobacteria account for a small but increasing number of pulmonary infections. The most commonly identified pathogen is *M. avium-intracellulare* complex (MAC). In most cases, the pathologic and radiologic features are identical to those of postprimary tuberculosis, with the histologic findings including variable degrees of granulomatous inflammation, necrosis, and fibrosis. The most common radiologic abnormalities consist of heterogeneous nodular and linear opacities involving mainly the apical and posterior segments of the upper lobes (71). Cavitation is seen in approximately 40% of cases (71,72).

A second, more distinctive but less common pattern of presentation consists of small, well-defined bilateral nodular opacities that usually have a patchy distribution but occasionally involve predominantly the upper lobes or middle lobe and lingula (73,74). On HRCT, the nodules have a centrilobular distribution (74,75). Most patients also have bronchiectasis involving several lobes or only the middle lobe and lingular bronchi (76,77) (Fig. 2.40). This form of infection is characteristically indolent clinically and shows a predilection for middle-aged and elderly women.

Disseminated MAC infection occurs in 15% to 25% of patients who have AIDS, usually those who are severely immunocompromised (CD4 counts less than 70/µL) (71).

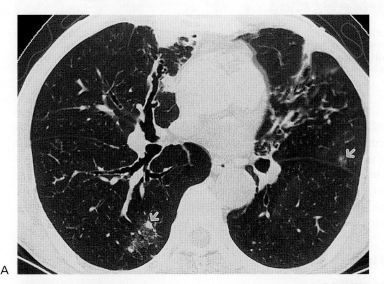

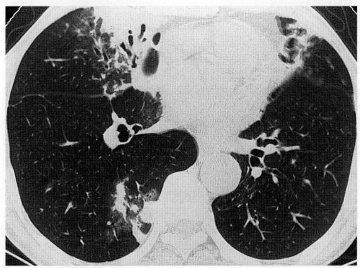

FIGURE 2.40. *Mycobacterium avium-intracellulare* infection. **A:** HRCT image (1.0-mm collimation) at the level of the right middle lobar bronchus shows bronchiectasis in right middle lobe, right lower lobe, and lingula. Small nodules (*arrows*) and focal areas of consolidation can also be seen in the right middle lobe and lingula. **B:** Image at the level of the inferior pulmonary vein shows bronchiectasis in the right middle lobe and lingula. Also note consolidation and ground-glass opacity in right middle lobe and right lower lobe. The patient was a 72-year-old man.

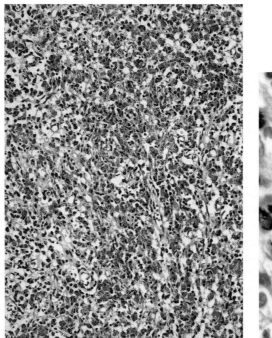
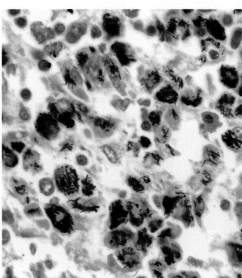

FIGURE 2.41. *Mycobacterium avium intracellulare* infection in AIDS. **A:** Photomicrograph of a biopsy of an enlarged mediastinal lymph node shows replacement of the normal lymphocyte population by numerous histiocytes. **B:** Highly magnified view of the histiocytes stained by the Ziehl-Neelsen method shows numerous intracytoplasmic acid fast rods.

Most of these patients have no pulmonary manifestations; in fact, the radiograph is often normal even in patients who have positive sputum (71). When present, the radiologic findings resemble those of tuberculosis and include focal areas of airspace consolidation, nodules, and mediastinal lymph node enlargement (78). The nodules usually measure less than 10 mm in diameter and have a centrilobular distribution on HRCT (79). Histologic examination of affected lymph nodes shows effacement of the normal architecture by numerous histiocytes containing abundant mycobacteria (Fig. 2.41).

FUNGAL INFECTION

Pulmonary Aspergillosis

Pulmonary aspergillosis may be caused by many species, the most common of which is *Aspergillus fumigatus*. Infection usually is acquired by inhalation of the organisms that are normally present in the environment. It is virtually always seen in individuals who have some underlying abnormality, either structural in the lung (such as a cavity), atopy, or deficiency of the inflammatory or immunologic reactions. The pathologic and radiologic manifestations of disease can be divided into three main forms corresponding to these abnormalities: aspergilloma, allergic bronchopulmonary aspergillosis (ABPA), and invasive aspergillosis. The last named, in turn, can be subdivided into angioinvasive, bronchopneumonic (airway invasive), and chronic necrotizing ("semiinvasive") forms.

Aspergilloma

An aspergilloma (fungus ball) consists of a round to oval conglomeration of fungal hyphae and cellular debris located within a preexisting pulmonary cavity or ectatic bronchus (Figs. 2.42 and 2.43). The most common underlying conditions are tuberculosis and sarcoidosis (80,81). Cavities and ectatic bronchi associated with cystic fibrosis, fungal infection

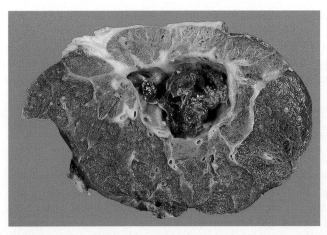
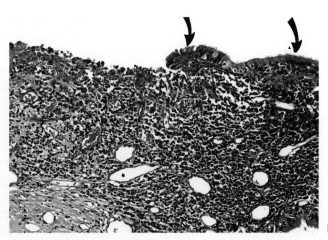

A   B

FIGURE 2.42. Aspergilloma. **A:** Transverse slice of an upper lobe shows a well-circumscribed cavity filled with blood clot and tan-colored aggregates of fungus. **B:** Photomicrograph of the cavity wall shows it to be partially covered by epithelium (*arrows*) and partly ulcerated. The vessels in the stroma under the region of ulceration are particularly prominent; these are derived form the bronchial circulation and are the source of hemoptysis in most cases of aspergilloma. The patient was a 48-year-old man who had a history of repeated hemoptysis.

such as histoplasmosis, abscesses, and carcinoma are seen less commonly. A deficiency of mucociliary- and macrophage-mediated clearance of inhaled organisms within the abnormal space is probably the common factor that permits proliferation of the fungi.

Fungal organisms are almost always identified histologically only in the cavity lumen. However, focal ulceration of the epithelium lining the wall, possibly as a result of secreted toxins, is common (Fig. 2.42). The ulceration results in bleeding from the bronchial vessels located in the cavity wall, which are often markedly hyperplastic, and the principal clinical manifestation, hemoptysis.

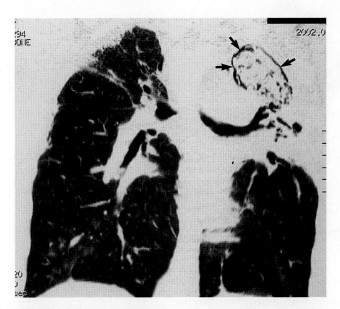

FIGURE 2.43. Aspergilloma. Coronal reconstruction image from volumetric high-resolution CT through the chest shows large oval soft-tissue mass (*arrows*) within a left upper lobe cavity. An air crescent is present between the aspergilloma and the cavity wall. Also noted are left upper lobe bronchiectasis and volume loss. The patient was a 44-year-old man with recurrent hemoptysis.

The characteristic radiologic presentation consists of a discrete, intracavitary mass, usually in the upper lobe (82,83). The mass is easily recognized by the presence of an air crescent between the mass and the wall of the cavity. Because the organisms do not invade the underlying tissue, the fungus ball often can be seen to move following a change in patient position (82,83). Less commonly, the ball is irregular in shape or has a spongelike appearance.

Allergic Bronchopulmonary Aspergillosis

Allergic bronchopulmonary aspergillosis (ABPA) is an uncommon pulmonary disorder seen almost exclusively in asthmatic patients. The pathogenesis is uncertain but is believed to involve both type I and type III allergic reactions (82). Inhaled *Aspergillus* spores may have a propensity to germinate and proliferate in the proximal airways of asthmatics, which often show evidence of asthma-associated mucosal injury (84). The resulting fungal hyphae appear to induce both increased mucus production and additional mucosal injury, eventually resulting in bronchiectasis (82).

Pathologically, segmental and proximal subsegmental bronchi are dilated (Fig. 2.44) and distended with mucus that contains numerous eosinophils and scattered, fragmented fungal hyphae (Fig. 2.45) (82). The adjacent bronchial wall shows fibrosis and chronic inflammation, again with abundant eosinophils. Although there may be focal ulceration of the airway epithelium, tissue invasion by the fungus is not seen. Bronchioles distal to the ectatic bronchi also may be distended with mucus or may show replacement of their epithelium by a granulomatous inflammatory infiltrate and filling of their lumina by necrotic debris (bronchocentric granulomatosis). Patchy filling of alveolar airspaces by eosinophils (eosinophilic pneumonia) may be seen in the adjacent lung parenchyma (83).

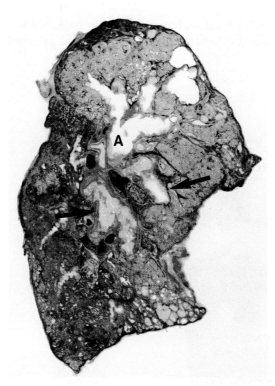

FIGURE 2.44. Allergic bronchopulmonary aspergillosis. Sagittal, paper-mounted slice of the left lung shows moderate ectasia of segmental bronchi in the apico-posterior segment of the upper lobe (**A**) and a milder degree of dilatation in those of the lower lobe and lingula (*arrows*). The airways in the last two sites are filled with mucus. The apicoposterior bronchi have a distinctive "finger-in-glove" appearance.

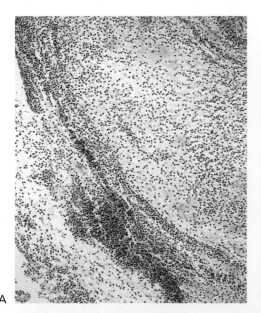
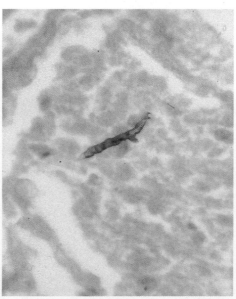

A   B

FIGURE 2.45. Allergic bronchopulmonary aspergillosis—mucus plug. **A:** Photomicrograph of mucus obtained from a segmental bronchus at bronchoscopy shows it to contain numerous cells (confirmed to be eosinophils at higher magnification). **B:** Magnified view stained with silver shows a small hyphal fragment. Branching colonies such as seen in invasive aspergillosis are very unusual in ABPA, presumably reflecting a less severe degree of patient immune abnormality (asthma).

The most common radiographic manifestation consists of fleeting foci of consolidation related to eosinophilic infiltration within the lung parenchyma (83). With progression of disease and the development of bronchiectasis and mucoid impaction, branching Y- and V-shaped ("gloved-finger") opacities can be seen, involving mainly the central regions of the upper lobes (82,83). HRCT shows varicose or cystic bronchiectasis involving mainly segmental and subsegmental upper lobe bronchi (82,85) (Fig. 2.46). Other findings include mucoid impaction and centrilobular nodules, the latter reflecting the presence of dilated bronchioles filled with mucus or necrotic debris. In approximately 25% of cases, the mucous plugs have high attenuation, presumably due to the presence of calcium salts (86).

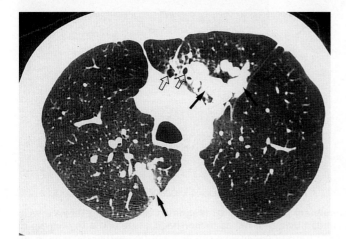

FIGURE 2.46. Allergic bronchopulmonary aspergillosis. HRCT image (1.5-mm collimation) shows mucoid impaction (*arrows*) in dilated bronchi in both upper lobes. Several patent ectatic bronchi (*open arrows*) are also evident, and there is left upper lobe volume loss. The patient was a 46-year-old man with asthma.

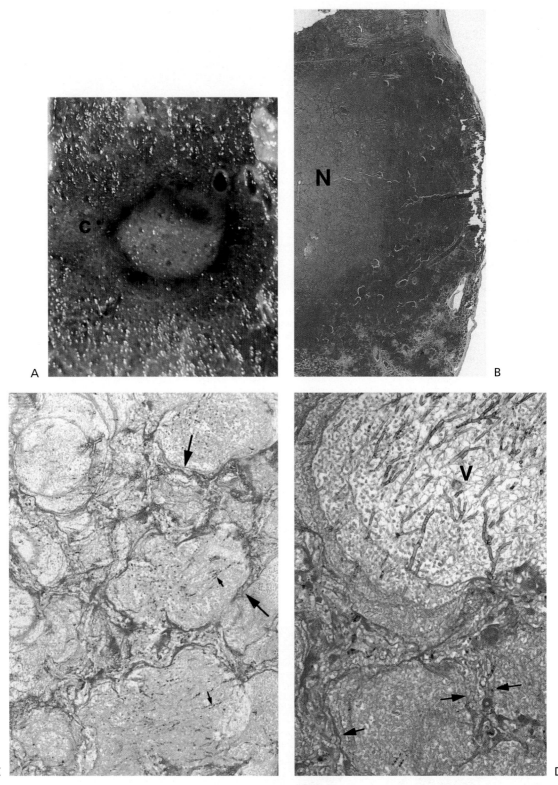

FIGURE 2.47. Angioinvasive pulmonary aspergillosis. **A:** Magnified view of lung shows a well-circumscribed pale nodule surrounded by a thin rim of hemorrhagic tissue and a thicker rim of consolidated lung (c). The lumens of transitional airways can be identified within the nodule, indicating that its underlying structure is intact. **B:** Low-magnification view shows the necrotic central region (N) surrounded by hemorrhage. **C:** View of the central region shows the outline of alveoli and transitional airways (*large arrows* = alveolar septa) with no residual nuclei (coagulative necrosis). Thin fungal hyphae (*small arrows*) can be seen permeating the necrotic tissue. **D:** Magnified view shows the necrotic alveolar septa (*arrows*) and fungal hyphae, the latter within a small pulmonary vessel (V).

Invasive Pulmonary Aspergillosis

Invasive aspergillosis is considered to occur when there is extension of *Aspergillus* into viable tissue. It is seen predominantly in patients who have impaired inflammatory or immune reactions. The most common forms of disease are angioinvasive aspergillosis and acute bronchopneumonia; chronic necrotizing ("semiinvasive") aspergillosis is rare.

Angioinvasive Pulmonary Aspergillosis

Angioinvasive pulmonary aspergillosis is seen most commonly in patients who have severe neutropenia. Predisposing conditions include leukemia, bone marrow and organ transplantation, and the use of corticosteroid and other immunosuppressive agents. The infection is usually multifocal and nodular in appearance. Grossly, the central region of the nodules is typically pale and often shows a relatively intact underlying structure (Fig. 2.47). A rim of hemorrhage and/or consolidated lung is frequently present around the nodule. The characteristic histologic finding consists of coagulative necrosis of the parenchyma and its permeation by numerous fungal hyphae. Infiltration of small to medium-sized pulmonary arteries within the necrotic tissue is common; however, evidence of a reaction, such as vasculitis or thrombosis, is usually absent. Depending on the adequacy of the host inflammatory reaction, the junction between the necrotic and viable parenchyma shows a variably severe neutrophilic infiltrate. Release of enzymes from the latter cells may result in separation of a portion of the necrotic tissue from the adjacent lung, resulting in an intracavitary sequestrum (Fig. 2.48).

Although the presence of vascular infiltration and coagulative necrosis of lung parenchyma have led to the belief that these lesions are infarcts, in fact their spherical shape and the frequent absence of vascular thrombosis argue that they result from injury by toxins secreted by the fungus as it extends from its original focus in all directions into the lung (87). (Despite this, the presence of wedge-shaped, pleural-based foci of parenchymal hemorrhage and/or coagulative necrosis in some cases indicates that there also may be an ischemic component to the lung injury.)

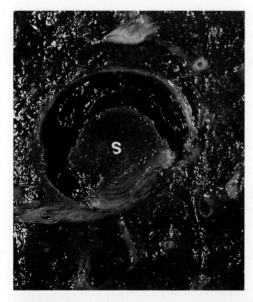

FIGURE 2.48. Angioinvasive pulmonary aspergillosis—sequestrum. Magnified view of lung shows a well-circumscribed nodule composed of a piece of necrotic lung (sequestrum [s]) that has separated from the adjacent viable tissue. In this example, the resulting crescent-shaped space is partially filled with blood.

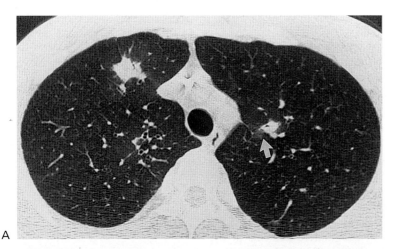

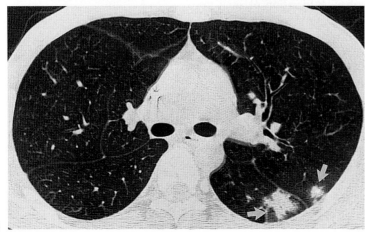

FIGURE 2.49. Angioinvasive pulmonary aspergillosis. HRCT images (1.0-mm collimation) at the level of thoracic inlet (**A**) and the subcarinal region (**B**) show nodules that have irregular margins and adjacent ground-glass opacities (CT halo sign) (*arrows*). The patient was a 27-year-old man with acute myelogenous leukemia.

The radiographic findings consist of poorly defined nodules and focal areas of consolidation that tend to be round; occasionally, there is a segmental or lobar distribution (82,83). The characteristic HRCT findings consist of nodules surrounded by a halo of ground-glass attenuation (Fig. 2.49) and wedge-shaped pleural-based areas of consolidation (88,89) (Fig. 2.50). The former correspond pathologically to the foci of necrotic lung surrounded by viable but hemorrhagic parenchyma (82,90). The latter are related to more extensive intralobular hemorrhage and/or true parenchymal infarction. In approximately 50% of cases the nodules undergo cavitation, manifested as an air crescent surrounding a more or less round, eccentric opacity (sequestrum or "lung ball") (91,92).

Aspergillus Bronchopneumonia

Aspergillus bronchopneumonia, also known as airway invasive aspergillosis, accounts for about 15% to 30% of cases of invasive disease (93). As with bacterial bronchopneumonia, it is characterized histologically by necrosis and a neutrophilic infiltrate that is centered about small bronchi and bronchioles (Fig. 2.51). Infiltration of pulmonary arteries adjacent to the affected airways may be seen and may result in hemorrhage into the adjacent parenchyma; however, coagulative necrosis of lung parenchyma such as that seen in nodular angioinvasive disease is usually absent or minimal in extent.

The most common radiographic presentation consists of patchy unilateral or bilateral areas of consolidation. HRCT demonstrates centrilobular nodules and branching linear opacities (tree-in-bud pattern), and patchy areas of consolidation, often in a peribronchial distribution (82,93) (Fig. 2.52). Histologically, these findings correspond to foci of necrotizing bronchitis and bronchiolitis, typically associated with a neutrophilic inflammatory reaction. *Aspergillus* organisms can be seen to infiltrate the airway walls and immediately adjacent parenchyma (82,93).

Chronic Necrotizing Aspergillosis

Chronic necrotizing (semiinvasive) aspergillosis is a rare variant that resembles a number of other chronic pulmonary diseases, particularly tuberculosis and histoplasmosis (94–96). Patients typically have mildly impaired immunity due to chronic debilitating illness or prolonged corticosteroid therapy or have underlying chronic obstructive pulmonary disease (COPD) (94,95).

Gross examination typically shows ill-defined areas of consolidation and fibrosis containing single or multiple thick-walled cavities (Fig. 2.53) (96,97); some of the latter can be seen to be ectatic bronchi on histologic examination. Aspergillomas may be present within the cavities. Histologically, there is often a mixture of fibrosis and acute or organizing pneumonia. Foci of necrotizing granulomatous inflammation containing fungal hyphae may be seen in the parenchyma or in relation to large or small airways (bronchocentric granulomatosis).

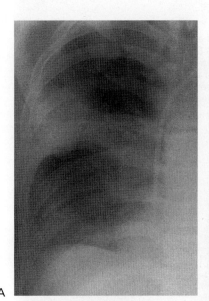

A

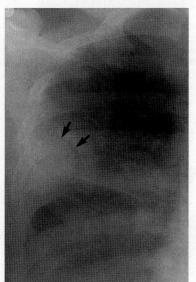

C

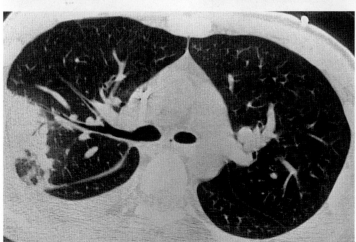

B

FIGURE 2.50. Angioinvasive pulmonary aspergillosis. **A:** Chest radiograph shows a pleura-based focus of airspace consolidation in the right upper lobe. A central venous line is present. **B:** HRCT image (1.0-mm collimation) shows focal consolidation and ground-glass opacity. **C:** Chest radiograph obtained six days after **A** shows an air-crescent (*arrows*) within the area of airspace consolidation. The patient was a 30-year-old man with acute myelogenous leukemia. (Kim MJ, et al. *J Comput Assist Tomogr* 2001;25:305–310, with permission.)

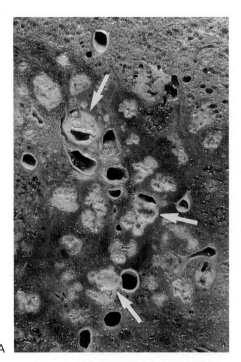
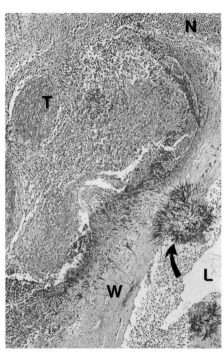

FIGURE 2.51. *Aspergillus* bronchopneumonia. **A:** Magnified view of a slice of lower lobe shows multiple foci of necrosis, some clearly centered on airways (*arrows*) as indicated by their intimate association with pulmonary arteries. The lung parenchyma adjacent to the necrotic regions is hemorrhagic. **B:** Photomicrograph shows small colonies of aspergillus (*arrow*) within a bronchial lumen (*L*) and wall (*W*). Extension of fungus can also be seen into the adjacent pulmonary artery, which is partly occluded by thrombus (*T*). An infiltrate of neutrophils (*N*) is evident in the adjacent lung.

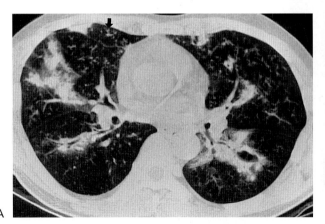
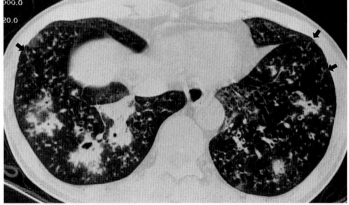

FIGURE 2.52. *Aspergillus* bronchiolitis and bronchopneumonia (airways invasive aspergillosis). HRCT images (1.0-mm collimation) at the level of right middle lobe bronchus (**A**) and liver dome (**B**) show patchy peribronchial consolidation, centrilobular nodules, and branching linear structures (*arrows*). Cavity formation is seen in both lower lobes.

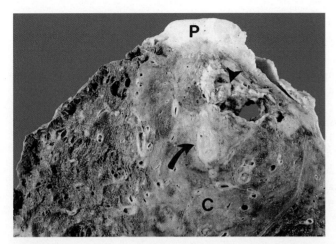

FIGURE 2.53. Chronic necrotizing aspergillosis. Magnified view of a slice of an upper lobe shows a poorly delimited area of consolidation (*C*) and fibrosis. An irregularly shaped cavity containing a fungus ball (*arrowhead*) can be seen anteriorly. A bronchus leading to the cavity (*curved arrow*) shows thickening of its wall and filling of its lumen with necrotic material; histologic examination showed necrotizing bronchitis related to aspergillus. Fungal invasion was also evident in the parenchyma adjacent to the cavity. The apical pleura (*P*) shows dense fibrosis.

The radiologic findings consist of focal areas of consolidation, nodules greater than 1 cm in diameter, or cavities involving predominantly or exclusively the upper lobes (Fig. 2.54) (97,98). The areas of consolidation correspond histologically to foci of inflammation or intraalveolar hemorrhage (97,98). Many of the nodules represent foci of healing granulomatous inflammation, in which a fibrous capsule has developed at the periphery. The cavities tend to have thick walls and to be surrounded by consolidation, the latter related to either organizing pneumonia or granulomatous inflammation (98,99).

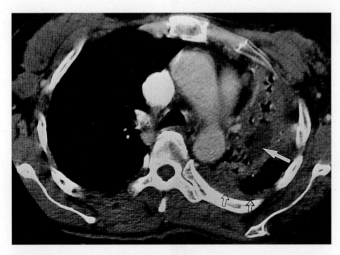

FIGURE 2.54. Chronic necrotizing aspergillosis ("semiinvasive" aspergillosis). Contrast-enhanced CT image (7-mm collimation) demonstrates diffuse consolidation of the left upper lobe. A cavity filled with air and low-attenuation soft tissue (*arrow*) is present. Pleural thickening (*open arrows*) also can be seen. The patient was a 49-year-old woman. (Kim SY, et al. *Am J Roentgenol* 2000;174: 795–798, with permission.)

Candidiasis

Candida albicans is a ubiquitous dimorphic fungus identified in tissue as both oval budding yeast and hyphal forms. Pulmonary infection is uncommon and is invariably seen in debilitated or immunocompromised patients. It usually accompanies widespread infection of the urinary tract, gastrointestinal tract, liver, spleen, or central nervous system (100).

The radiographic manifestations consist of nodules and patchy unilateral or bilateral airspace consolidation (101,102). HRCT shows nodules, ground-glass opacities, and patchy consolidation (103) (Fig. 2.55). The nodules measure from 3 mm to several centimeters in diameter (103). They may be smooth or irregular and may be surrounded by a halo of ground-glass attenuation due to hemorrhage (103). These findings correspond to foci of necrotizing bronchopneumonia, usually with an abundance of neutrophils. Occasionally, miliary infection is seen.

Cryptococcosis

Cryptococcus neoformans is a ubiquitous unimorphic fungus. The majority of infections occur in immunocompromised patients, particularly those with AIDS or lymphoproliferative disorders. The most frequent site is the central nervous system (104).

Pathologic findings are quite variable. Organisms may be abundant or few in number and associated with a granulomatous or lymphocytic inflammatory reaction (Fig. 2.56). In some patients (usually those with AIDS), there is virtually no cellular reaction and the organisms are seen predominantly in the parenchymal interstitium.

The radiologic manifestations include one or more nodules or masses 2 to 10 cm in diameter, poorly defined areas of consolidation, and a diffuse reticulonodular pattern (105,106) (Fig. 2.56). Cavitation occurs in approximately 10% of nodules. Diffuse involvement, including miliary pattern, lymph node enlargement, and cavitation, is seen most commonly in immunocompromised patients (106).

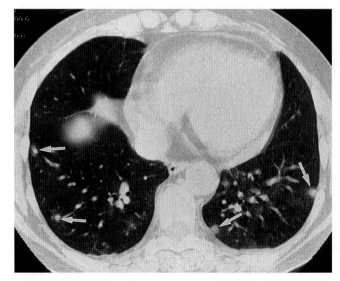

FIGURE 2.55. Candidiasis. HRCT image (1.0-mm collimation) shows multiple small nodules (*arrows*) in both lower lobes. The nodules have poorly defined margins. The patient was a 56-year-old woman with acute myelogenous leukemia.

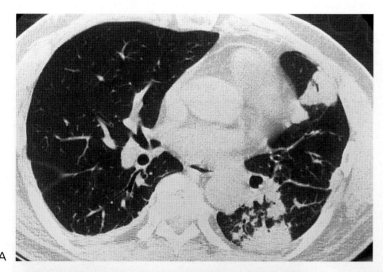

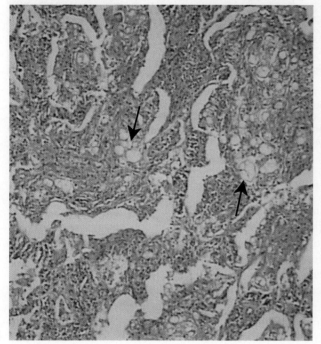

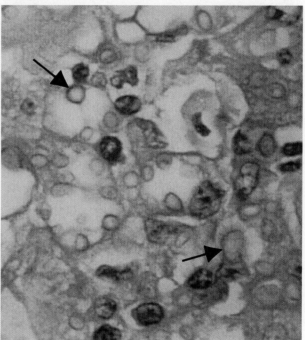

FIGURE 2.56. Cryptococcosis. **A:** HRCT image (1.0-mm collimation) shows peribronchial and subpleural areas of consolidation as well as bilateral pleural thickening. **B:** Photomicrograph of a biopsy specimen shows interstitial pneumonitis. Alveolar airspaces are filled with numerous macrophages containing small, cystlike spaces (*arrows*). **C:** Magnified view shows the spaces to contain clusters of oval to round yeasts that have mucicarmine positive capsules (*arrows*). The patient was a 61-year-old man.

Histoplasmosis

Histoplasmosis is caused by the dimorphic fungus *Histoplasma capsulatum*. It is endemic in the Mississippi and Ohio river valleys in the United States and the St. Lawrence River Valley in Canada. The manifestations of pulmonary disease are quite varied. The most common pathologic abnormality is focal granulomatous inflammation, necrosis, and fibrosis identical to that of tuberculosis (Fig. 2.57). Such disease is usually too limited in extent to be seen on the chest radiograph and is usually unrecognized clinically. Occasionally, enlargement or coalescence of several foci of inflammation results in single or multiple poorly defined areas of airspace consolidation (107) (Fig. 2.58). Most patients with such disease also have ipsilateral hilar lymph node enlargement evident on the radiograph (107).

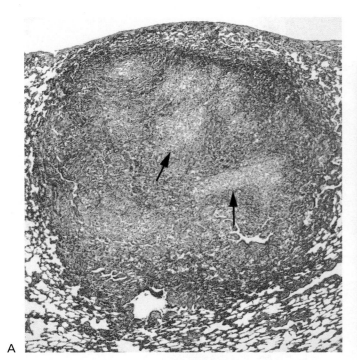
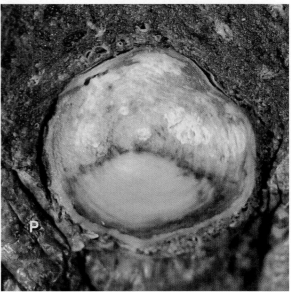

A

B

FIGURE 2.57. Histoplasmosis. **A:** Photomicrograph shows a well-circumscribed focus of inflammation adjacent to the pleura. The paler areas (*arrows*) are foci of granulomatous inflammation, not yet necrotic. This appearance is consistent with disease of a few weeks' duration. **B:** Magnified view of a lower lobe shows an encapsulated 2.5-cm focus of fibrous and necrotic tissue that has a lamellated appearance characteristic of healed histoplasmosis. The abnormality is again adjacent to the pleura (*P*).

A much more common clinical presentation is that of a solitary nodule seen on chest radiography or CT in an asymptomatic patient (107). The nodule corresponds histologically to an encapsulated focus of necrotizing granulomatous inflammation that develops in the same fashion as Ghon focus of tuberculosis. Nodules that have been present for more than a few months frequently show central (target) or diffuse calcification radiologically, as a result of dystrophic calcification of the necrotic material. Enlarged hilar lymph nodes also may be seen (107).

The scenarios described earlier are often unassociated with a clear history of exposure to a source of infection. Exposure to a relatively large number of organisms, such as during excavation of a contaminated worksite, may result in symptoms and multiple areas of consolidation or diffuse nodular opacities on the radiograph. Disseminated disease with a miliary or diffuse reticulonodular pattern occurs mainly in immunocompromised patients (107,108).

Chronic histoplasmosis is a particularly rare manifestation of disease that presents radiologically and pathologically as patchy areas of consolidation, sometimes with cavitation, involving mainly the apical and posterior segments of the upper lobes (107,108). The appearance resembles reactivation tuberculosis. Like the latter condition, healing frequently results in upper lobe scarring, volume loss, and pleural thickening. Calcification of hilar and mediastinal nodes is commonly seen. The nodes may erode into the lumen of adjacent bronchi and result in broncholithiasis (107,108).

Mediastinal lymph node involvement may occur in any form of histoplasmosis. Such nodes may be enlarged or normal in size and are usually well circumscribed. In some patients, however, the inflammatory process extends into the adjacent mediastinum, resulting in fibrosing mediastinitis. Histologic examination in such cases shows dense fibrous tissue containing variable numbers of mononuclear inflammatory cells and granulomas.

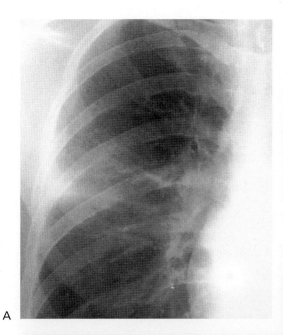
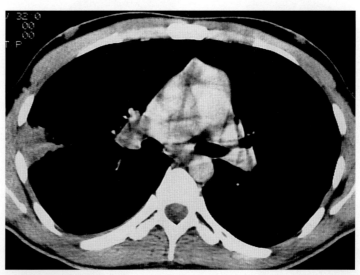
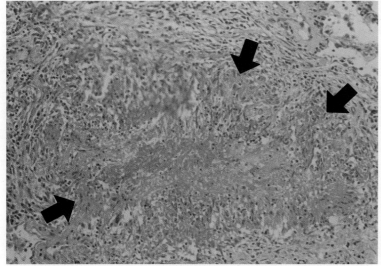

FIGURE 2.58. Histoplasmosis. **A:** Chest radiograph shows focal airspace consolidation in the right upper lobe. **B:** CT image (10-mm collimation) shows a triangular focus of consolidation abutting the lateral chest wall and the right major fissure. **C:** Photomicrograph of a biopsy specimen shows necrotizing granulomatous inflammation (*arrows*); organisms consistent with *H. capsulatum* were identified with special stain. (Courtesy of Dr. Sang Jin Kim, Department of Radiology, Yonsei University Yongdong Severance Hospital, Seoul, Korea.)

Organisms may be difficult to identify. The common radiologic manifestation consists of a focal paratracheal mass of calcified lymph nodes frequently associated with partial or complete obstruction of the superior vena cava (107,108).

Coccidioidomycosis

Coccidioidomycosis is caused by inhalation of spores of the dimorphic fungus *Coccidioides immitis*. It is endemic in the southwestern United States and Mexico. Several patterns of disease can be seen. Acute (primary) infection results in bronchopneumonia, initially associated with a predominantly neutrophilic exudate and subsequently with granulomatous inflammation (109). In most patients, the reaction is mild and the radiograph is normal. Approximately 40% are symptomatic and have patchy areas of consolidation evident on the radiograph (109). Associated hilar lymph node enlargement is seen in 20% of cases. The consolidation usually resolves over several weeks.

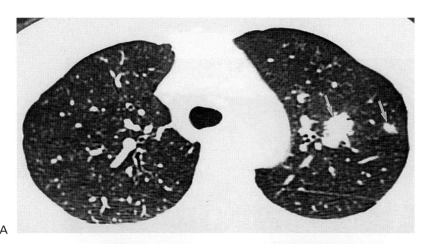

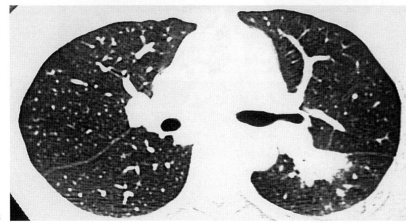

FIGURE 2.59. Coccidioidomycosis. **A:** HRCT image (1.0-mm collimation) at the level of the tracheal carina shows left upper lobe nodules (*arrows*). **B:** Image at the level of the bronchus intermedius shows peribronchial consolidation and small nodules in the superior segment of the left lower lobe. The patient was a 30-year-old woman. (Courtesy of Dr. Jin Sung Lee, Department of Radiology, Asan Medical Center, University of Ulsan, Seoul, Korea.)

Chronic pulmonary coccidioidomycosis is characterized radiologically by nodules or cavities (Fig. 2.59). Most are discovered incidentally in asymptomatic patients; approximately 25% can be seen to result from incomplete resolution of acute bronchopneumonia (109). Most nodules or cavities are solitary and measure 2 to 4 cm in diameter. They may be thin walled ("grape-skin") or thick walled (109), and usually have homogeneous attenuation on CT (110). Histologically, the lesions correspond to foci of necrotizing granulomatous inflammation. Although most often sharply delimited by a well-developed fibrous capsule, inflammation surrounding the necrotic tissue can result in adjacent ill-defined areas of consolidation (110) (Fig. 2.59).

Rarely, disease is progressive and results in unilateral or bilateral upper lobe consolidation, sometimes associated with single or multiple cavities, resembling reactivation tuberculosis. Disseminated disease is seen most commonly in immunocompromised patients and is usually manifested radiologically as a diffuse reticulonodular pattern or miliary nodules.

Pneumocystis carinii

Pneumocystis carinii is a fungus that causes pneumonia only in immunocompromised patients. Individuals who have AIDS, lymphoproliferative disorders, and organ or bone marrow transplants are particularly at increased risk. The organism probably resides normally on the alveolar surface, where it is maintained in low numbers by host defense mechanisms. Infection can be manifested histologically by several patterns. The most common consists of finely vacuolated eosinophilic material within alveolar airspaces accompanied by a variably severe infiltrate of lymphocytes and plasma cells in the adjacent interstitium

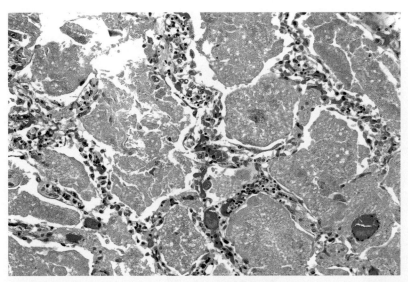 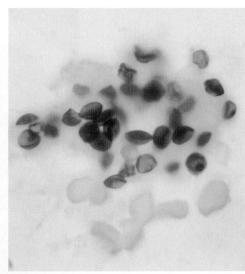

A   B

FIGURE 2.60. *Pneumocystis carinii* pneumonia. **A:** Photomicrograph shows mild alveolar interstitial thickening by a lymphocyte infiltrate and extensive filling of airspaces by finely vacuolated eosinophilic material. **B:** Magnified view of the material in one of the airspaces shows silver positive (black) round or helmet-shaped structures typical of *P. carinii.*

(Fig. 2.60). The foamy material consists of solitary and encysted organisms—which can be detected with special stains as round or helmet-shaped structures—admixed with host-derived material such as surfactant and fibrin. Other histologic reaction patterns include granulomatous inflammation and diffuse alveolar damage (111–113).

The most common radiographic manifestations consist of bilateral hazy increase in density (ground-glass pattern) or a fine reticulonodular pattern (10) (Fig. 2.61). HRCT typically shows bilateral areas of ground-glass attenuation (11,12) (Fig. 2.62). The

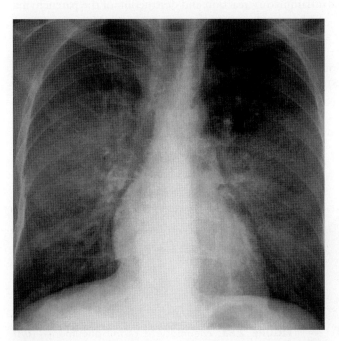

FIGURE 2.61. *Pneumocystis carinii* pneumonia. Chest radiograph shows bilateral hazy ground-glass opacities in a predominantly perihilar distribution. The patient was a 34-year-old man with AIDS.

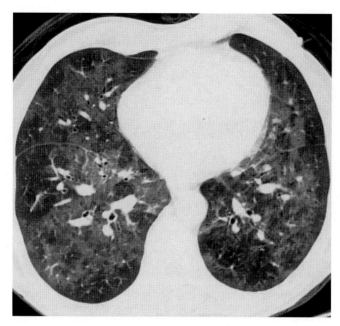

FIGURE 2.62. *Pneumocystis carinii* pneumonia. HRCT image (1.5-mm collimation) shows extensive bilateral ground-glass opacities. The patient was a 46-year-old man with AIDS.

ground-glass attenuation may be patchy, have a geographic or patchwork appearance, be diffuse or involve mainly the perihilar regions or upper lobes. Reticulation or interlobular septal thickening is seen in approximately 20% of patients (Fig. 2.63). The ground-glass opacities reflect the interstitial pneumonitis, whereas the reticulation reflects organization of intraalveolar material or fibrosis. Unusual manifestations include solitary or multiple nodules (Fig. 2.64) and a miliary pattern (114,115). The nodules or masses are often associated with a granulomatous inflammatory reaction and destruction of the parenchyma (114,115).

Cyst formation is seen in about 30% of patients (Fig. 2.63). The cysts are variable in appearance, but most measure 5 mm to 3 cm in diameter, are thin walled, and are located in the upper lobes. Examination of gross specimens shows the inner lining may be smooth or coarsely granular (Fig. 2.65). Some of the former probably correspond to bullae associated with emphysema. However, others, particularly those that have a granular surface, are probably related to infiltration of organisms into the parenchymal interstitium with subsequent necrosis and cavitation (116–118).

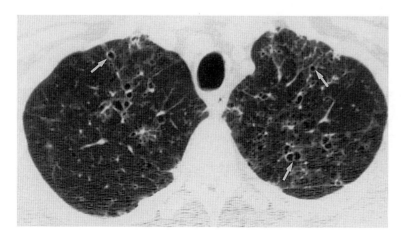

FIGURE 2.63. *Pneumocystis carinii* pneumonia—cyst formation. HRCT image (1.5-mm collimation) shows bilateral cystic changes (*arrows*) and mild emphysema. Small focal reticular and ground-glass opacities are also evident. The patient was a 46-year-old man with AIDS.

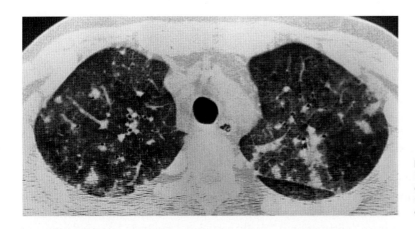

FIGURE 2.64. *Pneumocystis carinii* pneumonia. HRCT image (1.0-mm collimation) shows extensive bilateral ground-glass opacities and several poorly defined nodules. The patient was a 22-year-old man with who had received chemotherapy for non-Hodgkin's lymphoma.

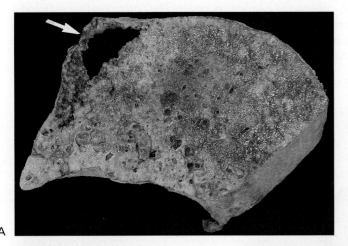

FIGURE 2.65. *Pneumocystis carinii* pneumonia—cyst formation. **A:** Transverse slice of an upper lobe shows extensive consolidation and a cyst (*arrows*) that has a coarsely nodular inner surface. **B:** Photomicrograph of the cavity wall shows filling of alveolar airspaces by typical *P. carinii* exudate (*E*). Alveolar interstitial tissue is absent in the region immediately adjacent to the cyst (*C*). Note that the interstitial tissue around a small vessel has also been infiltrated and replaced by exudate (*arrow*). Although the precise pathogenesis of this effect is unclear, it seems that *P. carinii* is able to infiltrate the parenchymal interstitium and cause its necrosis. Without the pulmonary parenchymal support, the exudate "dissolves" (as illustrated in **C**) and drains via the airways leaving a cyst. The patient was a 27-year-old man with AIDS.

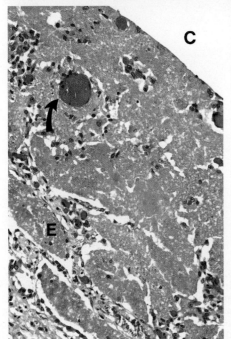

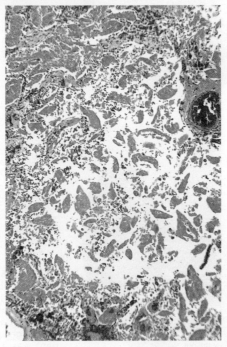

VIRAL INFECTION

Respiratory Viruses

Viruses can result in several clinicopathologic forms of lower respiratory tract infection, the most frequent being tracheobronchitis, bronchiolitis, and pneumonia. The most common pathogens are respiratory syncytial virus, adenovirus, parainfluenza virus, and influenza virus. Infection is usually acquired via the airways, and since the organisms replicate within tissue cells, the most prominent histologic changes are seen in the epithelium and adjacent interstitial tissue.

Tracheobronchitis seldom results in any radiologic abnormalities in the acute stage; however, mucosal injury may manifest many years later as bronchiectasis. Bronchiolitis is particularly important in children and is manifested in the acute stage by epithelial necrosis, a neutrophilic exudate in the airway lumen and a predominantly mononuclear infiltrate in its wall. The airway obstruction is usually partial and results in hyperinflation and poorly defined nodular opacities radiologically (119,120). Parenchymal involvement (pneumonia) initially involves the lung adjacent to the terminal and respiratory bronchioles; however, extension throughout the lobule may occur. The corresponding radiologic manifestations include poorly defined centrilobular nodules and airspace consolidation (119,120). The consolidation can be patchy or confluent. Because of the associated bronchiolitis, hyperinflation is commonly present (119,120).

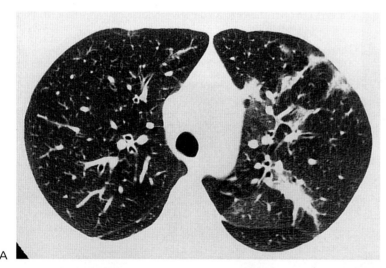

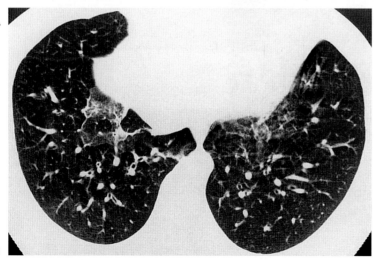

FIGURE 2.66. Influenza virus pneumonia. **A:** HRCT image (1.5-mm collimation) at the level of the aortic arch shows patchy peribronchial and subpleural consolidation and ground-glass opacities involving mainly the left upper lobe. **B:** Image at the level of liver dome shows patchy subpleural ground-glass opacities in both lower lobes. The patient was a 27-year-old woman. (Courtesy of Dr. Jin Mo Goo, Department of Radiology, Seoul National University Hospital, Seoul, Korea.)

Influenza virus may result in rapidly progressive pneumonia, particularly in the elderly and in immunocompromised patients (121,122). Histologically, the lungs show diffuse alveolar damage, characterized by interstitial lymphocyte infiltration, airspace hemorrhage and edema, type 2 cell hyperplasia, and hyaline membrane formation (123,124). The radiologic findings consist of homogeneous or patchy unilateral or bilateral airspace consolidation (125) (Fig. 2.66). Serial radiographs often demonstrate rapid confluence of the areas of consolidation.

Varicella Zoster

Varicella zoster pneumonia has been reported in 5% to 50% of all varicella infections in adults (126,127). More than 90% of cases occur in immunocompromised patients, particularly those with leukemia or lymphoma (127–129). Histologic features are those of diffuse alveolar damage (interstitial mononuclear inflammatory cell infiltrate, intraalveolar proteinaceous exudate, hyaline membranes, and type 2 cell hyperplasia; Fig. 2.67). With recovery, small nodules may be seen scattered randomly throughout the lung parenchyma. Histologically, they are composed of a fibrous capsule that surrounds an area of hyalinized collagen or necrotic tissue.

Cases that show diffuse alveolar damage histologically usually are associated with acute respiratory distress syndrome radiologically—patchy, ill-defined opacities that progress to diffuse airspace consolidation on radiographs and patchy but more or less diffuse ground-glass opacification and consolidation on HRCT. In less severe disease, the radiologic manifestations consist most commonly of bilateral, poorly defined nodular areas of consolidation and 5- to 10-mm-diameter ill-defined nodules (126,127,130). HRCT demonstrates nodules with or without surrounding ground-glass attenuation (Fig. 2.68), and patchy areas of ground-glass attenuation (131). The nodules usually resolve within a week after the disappearance of the skin lesions but may persist for months. They may calcify and result in numerous well-defined, randomly distributed, 2- to 5-mm dense calcifications (126,130).

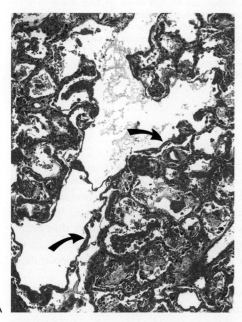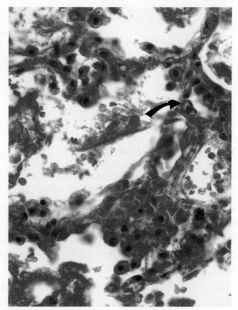

A   B

FIGURE 2.67. Herpes zoster pneumonia. Low- (**A**) and high- (**B**) magnification photomicrographs show filling of most alveolar airspaces by a proteinaceous exudate. There is mild interstitial thickening as a result of capillary congestion and a mild infiltrate of lymphocytes. Hyaline membranes (*arrows*) are evident on the surface of a respiratory bronchiole and its branches in **A.** An intranuclear viral inclusion is present in **B.** The patient was an 8-year-old boy with leukemia who developed chickenpox.

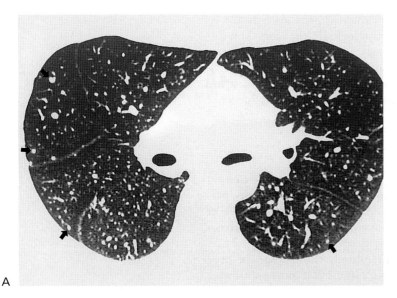

A

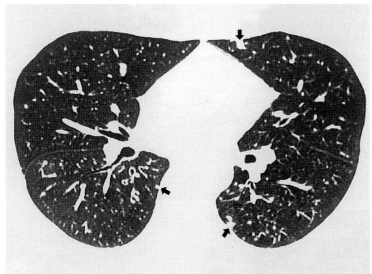

B

FIGURE 2.68. Herpes zoster pneumonia. **A:** HRCT image (1.5-mm collimation) at the level of the main bronchi shows bilateral small nodules (*arrows*) in the subpleural region. **B:** Image at the level of the right middle lobe bronchi shows several small nodules (*arrows*) in both lungs. The patient was a 30-year-old man. (Courtesy of Dr. Dong Wook Sung, Department of Diagnostic Radiology, Kyung Hee University Hospital, Seoul, Korea.)

Cytomegalovirus

Cytomegalovirus (CMV) is an important cause of pneumonia in immunocompromised patients. Histologic findings are variable and can consist of ill-defined nodular foci of airspace hemorrhage, necrosis and inflammation, diffuse alveolar damage, interstitial pneumonitis (Fig. 2.7), or organizing pneumonia (Fig. 2.69). The reaction that occurs may depend on whether the infection develops by seeding of organisms present in the blood (nodules) or by reactivation of latent virus present in the lung (diffuse alveolar damage/pneumonitis).

The radiologic manifestations include poorly defined nodular opacities and patchy bilateral airspace consolidation. CT findings include small nodules, consolidation, and ground-glass opacity (132) (Fig. 2.69). The nodules tend to be bilateral and symmetric, and to have a centrilobular distribution (133). They have been shown to correspond histologically to the hemorrhagic nodules described earlier or to foci of organizing pneumonia (132,134).

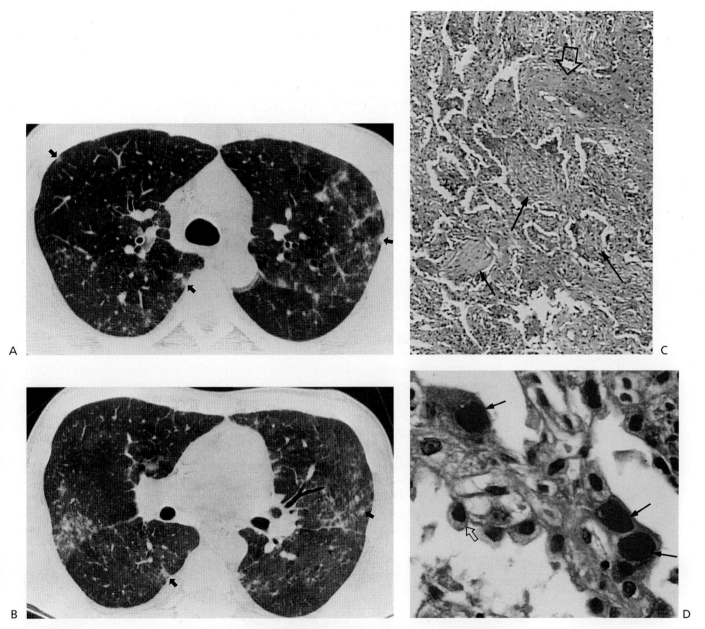

FIGURE 2.69. Cytomegalovirus pneumonia. **A, B:** HRCT images (1.0-mm collimation) at the levels of the azygos arch (**A**) and bronchus intermedius (**B**) show bilateral ground-glass opacities and poorly defined small nodules (*arrows*). A small right pleural effusion is also present. **C:** Photomicrograph of a biopsy specimen shows a moderate degree of interstitial fibrosis and chronic inflammation (*open arrow*) as well as plugs of fibroblastic tissue in the lumens of several airspaces (*solid arrows*). **D:** Highly magnified photomicrograph shows several large cells containing intranuclear inclusions consistent with cytomegalovirus (*solid arrows*). (Compare size with hyperplastic type 2 pneumocytes [*open arrow.*]) The patient was a 28-year-old man with acute myelogenous leukemia.

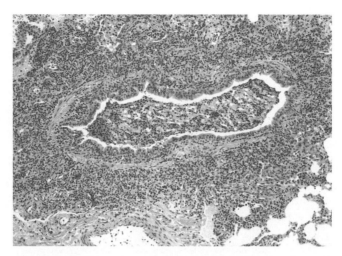

FIGURE 2.70. *Mycoplasma pneumoniae* pneumonia. Photomicrograph of a biopsy specimen shows severe inflammation of the mucosa and submucosal interstitium of a membranous bronchiole. An exudate of inflammatory cells is present in the airway lumen. The adjacent parenchyma shows only mild inflammation.

MYCOPLASMA PNEUMONIAE

Mycoplasma pneumoniae is a common cause of community-acquired pneumonia (135). It is seen most frequently in children and young adults but has been estimated to cause more than 15% of pneumonias in patients older than 40 years (136).

The principal histologic abnormality is bronchiolitis, similar in appearance to that caused by viruses (Fig. 2.70). Extension of infection and the concomitant inflammatory reaction into the parenchyma adjacent to the airways results in pneumonia (137,138). The radiologic manifestations initially consist of interstitial reticular or reticulonodular opacities that progress to a combination of reticulation and patchy airspace consolidation (8). HRCT demonstrates centrilobular nodules and branching lines (tree-in-bud pattern) and unilateral or bilateral lobular areas of consolidation (8), findings that reflect the presence of bronchiolitis and pneumonia, respectively (Fig. 2.71). An-

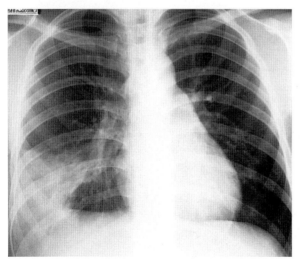

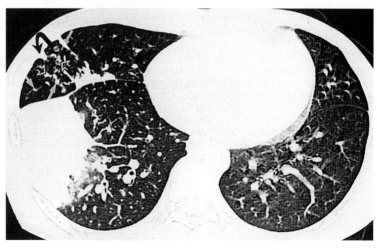

A

B

FIGURE 2.71. *Mycoplasma pneumoniae* pneumonia. **A:** Chest radiograph shows segmental consolidation in the lateral portion of the right lower lung zone. **B:** HRCT image (1-mm collimation) shows segmental consolidation and ground-glass opacities in the anterior and lateral basal segments of right lower lobe. Centrilobular nodules (*white arrows*), branching linear structures (*open arrows*), airspace nodules (*curved arrow*), and subsegmental consolidation are present in the right middle lobe. The patient was a 17-year-old man.

other common abnormality seen on HRCT is thickening of the peribronchial interstitium (8).

CHLAMYDIA PNEUMONIAE

Chlamydia pneumoniae accounts for 5% to 10% of cases of nonbacterial lower respiratory tract infections (139). An increased risk may be present in patients who have AIDS, chronic obstructive pulmonary disease, or cystic fibrosis (140,141). Histologic findings are similar to those of *Mycoplasma pneumoniae* infection.

Radiographic findings consist of airspace consolidation, mixed airspace consolidation, and interstitial opacities or predominantly nodular or reticulonodular opacities (142). Bilateral involvement is seen in half of the patients. Pleural effusion is present in about 15% of patients. HRCT demonstrates centrilobular nodules and branching lines (tree-in-bud pattern) and lobular airspace consolidation (7), representing bronchiolitis and pneumonia, respectively.

ECHINOCOCCUS GRANULOSUS (HYDATID DISEASE)

Echinococcus granulosus is the most common cause of human hydatid disease and occurs in two forms, pastoral and sylvatic. The former is the more common and is seen predominantly in the Middle East, South America, and Russia. The latter is seen in Alaska and northern Canada. The intermediate hosts of the pastoral variety are sheep, cows, horses, and pigs and the definite hosts, dogs. The intermediate hosts of the sylvatic variety are moose, deer, elk, caribou, and bison, and the definite hosts dogs, wolves, arctic foxes, and coyotes (143).

Humans typically acquire the disease by direct contact with definite hosts or by ingestion of eggs present in water, food, or soil (143). The latter hatch in the duodenum into larvae that pass via the portal system to the liver, where most are trapped. Most of those that escape are in turn trapped in alveolar capillaries. In both liver and lung, the larvae develop into cysts that are typically spherical or oval in shape (Fig. 2.72). The cysts are surrounded by a pericyst consisting of fibrous tissue containing a nonspecific chronic inflammatory infiltrate. The surrounding lung usually shows compressive atelectasis. The cyst itself consists of a laminated outer membrane (the exocyst) and a thin inner layer of cells (the endocyst) that produce intracystic fluid and larval protoscoleces. Daughter cysts may develop directly from the exocyst or from free protoscoleces. A multicystic structure may result from serial cyst formation over several generations. Rupture of the cyst with extrusion of its contents into the adjacent parenchyma and/or airways may follow superimposed (usually bacterial) infection.

The radiologic manifestations consist of sharply marginated, spherical, or oval masses 1 to 20 cm in diameter that are surrounded by normal lung (144,145) (Fig. 2.73). Multiple cysts are seen in 20% to 30% of patients. When communication occurs between the cyst and the airways, air may enter the space between the pericyst and exocyst, and produce a thin crescent of air around the periphery of the cyst (meniscus or crescent sign) (145). When there is communication between airways and the inner portion of the cyst through the endocyst, expulsion of cyst contents produces an air–fluid level. Cyst fluid may spill into the surrounding lung, causing an inflammatory reaction that results in consolidation. After the cyst has ruptured into the bronchial tree, the collapsed endocyst–exocyst may be contrasted with surrounding air, resulting in the classic water lily sign (145). On CT, the cysts have homogeneous water density (146,147) (Fig. 2.73).

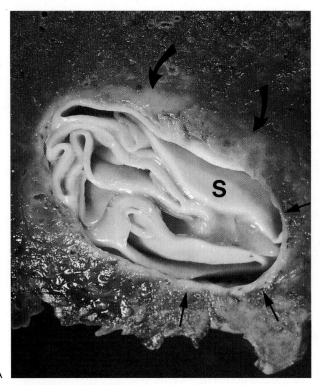

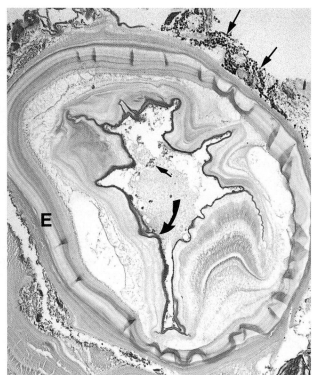

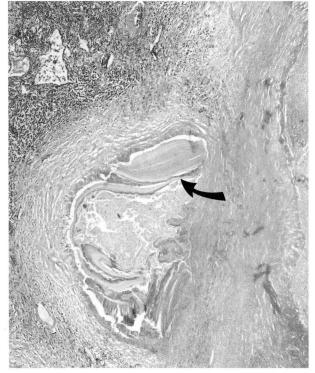

FIGURE 2.72. *Echinococcus granulosus* infection. **A:** Magnified view of a slice of a lower lobe shows a well-demarcated oval cyst near the pleura. The wall of the cyst consists of a thin rim of fibrous tissue (pericyst, *short arrows*) and the adjacent parenchyma appears consolidated focally (*curved arrows*). (The hemorrhagic appearance of the adjacent lung is artifact). The cyst contains complex folds of creamy white membranous material (the exocyst and endocyst of the organism). Focal separation of the exocyst from the pericyst is evident (*S*). **B:** Photomicrograph of a small daughter cyst shows the lamellated exocyst (*E*) and the inner thin germinative layer (endocyst, *curved arrow*). Clusters of minute scolices are evident within the cyst and the pericystic fluid (*short arrows*). **C:** View of the region of consolidation noted grossly shows nonspecific chronic inflammation and fibrous tissue containing small fragments of exocyst (*arrow*), indicating focal rupture of the cyst into the adjacent lung.

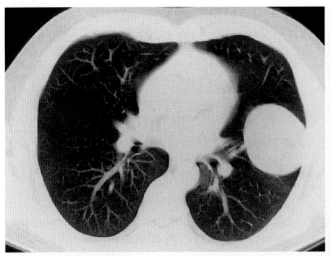 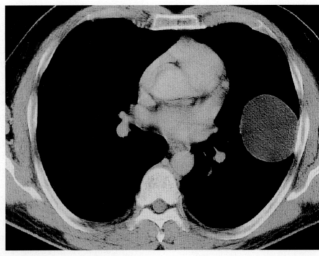

A   B

FIGURE 2.73. *Echinococcus granulosus* infection. **A:** CT image (7-mm collimation) shows smoothly marginated 4-cm-diameter mass in the lingula. **B:** Soft-tissue windows show homogeneous water density, characteristic of hydatid cyst. The patient was a 51-year-old man.

REFERENCES

1. Garibaldi RA. Epidemiology of community-acquired respiratory tract infections in adults: incidence, etiology, and impaction. *Am J Med* 1985;78:32–37.
2. American Thoracic Society. Guidelines for the management of adults with community-acquired pneumonia: diagnosis, assessment of severity, and initial antimicrobial therapy. *Am Rev Respir Dis* 1993;148:1418–1426.
3. Ishida T, Hashimoto T, Arita M, et al. Etiology of community-acquired pneumonia in hospitalized patients. A 3-year prospective study in Japan. *Chest* 1998;114:1588–1593.
4. Lipchik RJ, Kuzo RS. Nosocomial pneumonia. *Radiol Clin North Am* 1996;34:47–58.
5. Bates JH. Campbell GD, Barron AL, et al. Microbial etiology of acute pneumonia in hospitalized patients. *Chest* 1992;101:1005–1012.
6. Rello J, Quintana E, Ausina V, et al. Incidence, etiology, and outcome of nosocomial pneumonia in mechanically ventilated patients. *Chest* 1991;100:439–444.
7. Tanaka N, Matsumoto T, Tatsuya K, et al. High-resolution CT findings in community-acquired pneumonia. *J Comput Assist Tomogr* 1996;20:600–608.
8. Reittner P, Müller NL, Heyneman LH, et al. Mycoplasma pneumoniae pneumonia: radiographic and high-resolution CT features in 28 patients. *Am J Roentgenol* 2000;174:37–41.
9. Colby TV, Swensen SJ. Anatomic distribution and histopathologic patterns in diffuse lung disease: correlation with HRCT. *J Thorac Imaging* 1996;11:1–26.
10. Fraser RS, Müller NL, Colman N, et al. *Diagnosis of diseases of the chest.* Philadelphia: WB Saunders, 1999:979–1032.
11. Bergin CJ, Wirth RL, Berry GJ, et al. *Pneumocystis carinii* pneumonia: CT and HRCT observations. *J Comput Assist Tomogr* 1990;14:756–759.
12. Kuhlman JE, Kavuru M, Fishman EK, et al. *Pneumocystis carinii* pneumonia: spectrum of parenchymal CT findings. *Radiology* 1990;175:711–714.
13. Huang RM, Naidich DP, Lubat E, et al. Septic pulmonary emboli: CT-radiologic correlation. *Am J Roentgenol* 1989;153:41–45.
14. Kuhlman JE, Fishman EK, Teigen C. Pulmonary septic emboli: diagnosis with CT. *Radiology* 1990;174:211–213.
15. Kwong JS, Carignan S, Kang EY, et al. Miliary tuberculosis: diagnostic accuracy of chest radiography. *Chest* 1996;110:339–342.
16. McGuinness G, Naidich DP, Jagirdar J, et al. High resolution CT findings in miliary lung disease. *J Comput Assist Tomogr* 1992;16:384–390.
17. Baker RR. The treatment of lung abscess. Current concepts. *Chest* 1985;87:709–710.
18. Bartlett JG. Anaerobic bacterial pneumonitis. *Am Rev Respir Dis* 1979;119:19–23.
19. Groskin SA, Panicek DM, Ewing DK, et al. Bacterial lung abscess: a review of the radiographic and clinical features of 50 cases. *J Thorac Imaging* 1991;6:62–67.
20. Charan NB, Turk GM, Dhand R. The role of bronchial circulation in lung abscess. *Am Rev Respir Dis* 1985;131:121–124.

21. Kantor HG. The many radiologic faces of pneumococcal pneumonia. *Am J Roentgenol* 1981;137: 1213–1220.
22. Ort S, Ryan JL, Barden G, et al. Pneumococcal pneumonia in hospitalized patients: clinical and radiological presentation. *JAMA* 1983;249:214–218.
23. Rose RW, Ward BH. Spherical pneumonias in children simulating pulmonary and mediastinal masses. *Radiology* 1973;106:179–182.
24. MacFarlane J. An overview of community-acquired pneumonia with lessons learned from the British Thoracic Society Study. *Semin Respir Infect* 1994;9:153–165.
25. Kaye MG, Fox MJ, Bartlett JG, et al. The clinical spectrum of *Staphylococcus aureus* pulmonary infection. *Chest* 1990;97:788–792.
26. Wiita RM, Cartwright RR, Davis JG. Staphylococcal pneumonia in adults: a review of 102 cases. *Am J Roentgenol* 1961;86:1083–1089.
27. MacFarlane J, Rose D. Radiographic features of staphylococcal pneumonia in adults and children. *Thorax* 1996;51:539–540.
28. Dines DE. Diagnostic significance of pneumatocele of the lung. *JAMA* 1968;204:1169–1172.
29. Korvick AJ, Hackett AK, Yu VL, et al. *Klebsiella* pneumonia in the modern era: clinicoradiographic correlations. *South Med J* 1991;84:200–204.
30. Moon WK, Im J-G, Yeon KM, et al. Complications of *Klebsiella* pneumonia: CT evaluation. *J Comput Assist Tomogr* 1995;19:176–181.
31. Genereux GP, Stilwell GA. The acute bacterial pneumonias. *Semin Roentgenol* 1980;15:9–16.
32. Renner RR, Coccaro AP, Heitzman ER, et al. *Pseudomonas* pneumonia: a prototype of hospital-based infection. *Radiology* 1972;105:555–562.
33. Meduri GU, Reddy RC, Stanley T, et al. Pneumonia in acute respiratory distress syndrome: a prospective evaluation of bilateral bronchoscopic sampling. *Am J Respir Crit Care Med* 1998; 158:870–875.
34. Winer-Muram HT, Jennings SG, Wunderink RG, et al. Ventilator-associated *Pseudomonas aeruginosa* pneumonia: radiologic findings. *Radiology* 1995;195:247–252.
35. Evans AF, Oakley RH, Whitehouse GH. Analysis of the chest radiograph in Legionnaire's disease. *Clin Radiol* 1981;32:361–365.
36. Fairbank JT, Mamourian AC, Dietrich PA, et al. The chest radiograph in Legionnaires' disease. Further observations. *Radiology* 1983;147:33–34.
37. Coletta FS, Fein AM. Radiological manifestations of legionella/legionella-like organisms. *Semin Respir Infect* 1998;13:109–115.
38. Hernandez FJ, Kirby BD, Stanley TM, et al. Legionnaires' disease: postmortem pathologic findings of 20 cases. *Am J Clin Pathol* 1980;73:488–495.
39. Fraser DW, Tsai TR, Orenstein W, et al. Legionnaires' disease: description of an epidemic of pneumonia. *N Engl J Med* 1977;297:1189–1197.
40. Bohte R, van Furth R, van den Broek PJ. Aetiology of community-acquired pneumonia: a prospective study among adults requiring admission to hospital. *Thorax* 1995;50:543–547.
41. Neill AM, Martin IR, Weir R, et al. Community-acquired pneumonia: aetiology and usefulness of severity criteria on admission. *Thorax* 1996;51:1010–1016.
42. Pearlberg J, Haggar AM, Saravolatz L, et al. *Hemophilus influenzae* pneumonia in the adult: radiographic appearance with clinical correlation. *Radiology* 1984;151;23–26.
43. Feigin DS. Nocardiosis of the lung: chest radiographic findings in 21 cases. *Radiology* 1986;159:9–14.
44. Conant EF, Wechsler RJ. Actinomycosis and nocardiosis of the lung. *J Thorac Imag* 1992;7:75–84.
45. Yoon HK, Im J-G, Ahn JM, et al. Pulmonary nocardiosis: CT findings. *J Comput Assist Tomogr* 1995;19:52–55.
46. Buckley JA, Padhani AP, Kuhlman JE. CT features of pulmonary nocardiosis. *J Comput Assist Tomogr* 1995;19:726–732.
47. Suzuki JB, Delisle AL. Pulmonary actinomycosis of periodontal origins. *J Periodontol* 1984;55: 581–585.
48. Brown JR. Human actinomycosis: a study of 181 subjects. *Hum Pathol* 1973;4:319–330.
49. Flynn MW, Felson B. The roentgen manifestations of thoracic actinomycosis. *Am J Roentgenol* 1970;110:707–716.
50. Kwong JS, Müller NL, Godwin JD, et al. Thoracic actinomycosis: CT findings in eight patients. *Radiology* 1992;183:189–192.
51. Cheon J-E, Im J-G, Kim MY, et al. Thoracic actinomycosis: CT findings. *Radiology* 1998;209: 229–233.
52. Jones BE, Ryu R, Yang Z, et al. Chest radiographic findings in patients with tuberculosis with recent or remote infection. *Am J Resp Crit Care Med* 1997;156:1270–1275.
53. Lee KS, Song KS, Lim TH, et al. Adult-onset pulmonary tuberculosis: findings on chest radiographs and CT scans. *Am J Roentgenol* 1993;160:753–758.
54. Lee KS, Im JG. CT in adults with tuberculosis of the chest: characteristic findings and role in management. *Am J Roentgenol* 1995;164:1361–1367.

55. Weber AL, Bird KT, Janower ML. Primary tuberculosis in childhood with particular emphasis on changes affecting the tracheobronchial tree. *Am J Roentgenol* 1968;103:123–132.

56. Leung AN, Müller NL, Pineda PR, et al. Primary tuberculosis in childhood: radiographic manifestations. *Radiology* 1992;182:87–91.

57. Im JG, Song KS, Kang HS, et al. Mediastinal tuberculous lymphadenitis: CT manifestations. *Radiology* 1987;164:115–119.

58. Pombo F, Rodriguez E, Mato J, et al. Patterns of contrast enhancement of tuberculous lymph nodes demonstrated by computed tomography. *Clin Radiol* 1992;46:13–17.

59. Choyke PL, Sostman HD, Curtis AM, et al. Adult-onset tuberculosis. *Radiology* 1983;48:357–362.

60. Woodring JH, Vandiviere HM, Fried AM, et al. Update: the radiographic features of pulmonary tuberculosis. *Am J Roentgenol* 1986;146:497–506.

61. Palmer PE. Pulmonary tuberculosis: usual and unusual radiographic presentations. *Semin Roentgenol* 1979;14:204–243.

62. Krysl J, Korzeniewska-Kosela M, Müller NL, et al. Radiologic features of pulmonary tuberculosis: an assessment of 188 cases. *Can Assoc Radiol J* 1994;45:101–107.

63. Im J-G, Itoh H, Lee KS, et al. CT-pathologic correlation of pulmonary tuberculosis. *Crit Rev Diagn Imaging* 1995;36:227–285.

64. Lee JY, Lee KS, Jung K-J, et al. Pulmonary tuberculosis: CT–pathologic correlation. *J Comput Assist Tomogr* 2000;24:691–698.

65. Murayama S, Murakami J, Hashimoto S, et al. Noncalcified pulmonary tuberculomas: CT enhancement patterns with histologic correlation. *J Thorac Imaging* 1995;10:91–95.

66. Perlman DC, El-Sadr WM, Nelson ET, et al. Variation of chest radiographic patterns in pulmonary tuberculosis by degree of human immunodeficiency virus-related immunosuppression. *Clin Infect Dis* 1997;25:242–246.

67. Leung AN. Pulmonary tuberculosis: the essentials. *Radiology* 1999;210:307–322.

68. Keiper MD, Beumont M, Elshami A, et al. CD4 T lymphocyte count and the radiographic presentation of pulmonary tuberculosis: a study of the relationship between these factors in patients with human immunodeficiency virus infection. *Chest* 1995;107:74–80.

69. Laissy JP, Cadi M, Boudiaf ZE, et al. Pulmonary tuberculosis: computed tomography and high-resolution computed tomography patterns in patients who are either HIV-negative or HIV-seropositive. *J Thorac Imaging* 1998;13:58–64.

70. Pastores SM, Naidich DP, Aranda CP, et al. Intrathoracic adenopathy associated with pulmonary tuberculosis in patients with human immunodeficiency virus infection. *Chest* 1993;103:1433–1437.

71. Erasmus JJ, Page McAdams H, Farrell MA, et al. Pulmonary nontuberculous mycobacterial infection: radiologic manifestations. *Radiographics* 1999;19:1487–1503.

72. Albelda SM, Kern JA, Marinelli DL, et al. Expanding spectrum of pulmonary disease caused by nontuberculous mycobacteria. *Radiology* 1985;157:289–296.

73. Woodring JH, Vandiviere H, Melvin IG, et al. Roentgenographic features of pulmonary disease caused by atypical mycobacteria. *South Med J* 1987;80:1488–1497.

74. Miller WT Jr. Spectrum of pulmonary nontuberculous mycobacterial infection. *Radiology* 1994;191:343–350.

75. Moore EH. Atypical mycobacterial infection in the lung: CT appearance. *Radiology* 1993;187:777–782.

76. Lynch DA, Simone PM, Fox MA, et al. CT features of pulmonary *Mycobacterium avium* complex infection. *J Comput Assist Tomogr* 1995;19:353–360.

77. Hartman TE, Swensen SJ, Williams DE. *Mycobacterium avium-intracellulare* complex: Evaluation with CT. *Radiology* 1993;1883:23–26.

78. Marinelli DL, Albelda SM, Williams TM, et al. Non-tuberculous mycobacterial infection in AIDS: clinical, pathologic and radiographic features. *Radiology* 1986;160:77–82.

79. Laissy JP, Cadi M, Cinqualbre A, et al. *Mycobacterium tuberculosis* versus nontuberculous mycobacterial infection of the lung in AIDS patients: CT and HRCT patterns. *J Comp Assist Tomogr* 1997;21:312–317.

80. British Thoracic and Tuberculosis Association. Aspergilloma and residual tuberculosis cavities: the results of a resurvey. *Tubercle* 1970;51:227–245.

81. Wollschlager C, Khan F. Aspergillomas complicating sarcoidosis: a prospective study in 100 patients. *Chest* 1984;86:585–588.

82. Franquet T, Müller NL, Giménez A, et al. Spectrum of pulmonary aspergillosis: histologic, clinical, and radiologic findings. *Radiographics* 2001;21:825–837.

83. Thompson BH, Stanford W, Galvin JR, et al. Varied radiologic appearances of pulmonary aspergillosis. *Radiographics* 1995;15:1273–1284..

84. Bromley IM, Donaldson K. Binding of *Aspergillus fumigatus* spores to lung epithelial cells and basement membrane proteins: relevance to the asthmatic lung. *Thorax* 1996;51:1203–1209.

85. Ward S, Heyneman L, Lee MJ, et al. Accuracy of CT in the diagnosis of allergic bronchopulmonary aspergillosis in asthmatic patients. *Am J Roentgenol* 1999;173:937–942.

86. Logan PM, Müller NL. High-attenuation mucous plugging in allergic bronchopulmonary aspergillosis. *Can Assoc Radiol J* 1996;47:374–377.
87. Fraser RS. Pulmonary aspergillosis: pathologic and pathogenetic features. In: Rosen PP, Fechner RE eds. *Pathology annual,* Part I, Vol. 28. Norwalk, CT: Appleton & Lange, 1993:231.
88. Kuhlman JE, Fishman EK, Siegleman SS. Invasive pulmonary aspergillosis in acute leukemia: characteristic findings on CT, the CT halo sign, and the role of CT in early diagnosis. *Radiology* 1985;157:611–614.
89. Won HJ, Lee KS, Cheon J-E, et al. Invasive pulmonary aspergillosis: prediction at thin-section CT in patients with neutropenia—a prospective study. *Radiology* 1998;208:777–782.
90. Hruban RH, Meziane MA, Zerhouni EA, et al. Radiologic-pathologic correlation of the CT halo sign in invasive pulmonary aspergillosis. *J Comput Assist Tomogr* 1987;11:534–536.
91. Abramson S. The air crescent sign. *Radiology* 2001;218:230–232.
92. Kim MJ, Lee KS, Kim J, et al. Crescent sign in invasive pulmonary aspergillosis: frequency and related CT and clinical factors. *J Comput Assist Tomogr* 2001;25:305–310.
93. Logan PM, Primack SL, Miller RR, et al. Invasive pulmonary aspergillosis of the airways: radiographic, CT, and pathologic findings. *Radiology* 1994;193:383–388.
94. Binder RE, Faling LJ, Pugatch RD, et al. Chronic necrotizing pulmonary aspergillosis: a discrete clinical entity. *Medicine* 1982;61:109–124.
95. George PJ, Boffa PB, Naylor CP, et al. Necrotizing pulmonary aspergillosis complicating the management of patients with obstructive airway disease. *Thorax* 1983;38:478–480.
96. Yousem SA. Histologic spectrum of chronic necrotizing forms of pulmonary aspergillosis. *Hum Pathol* 1997;28:650–656.
97. Franquet T, Müller NL, Giménez A, et al. Semiinvasive pulmonary aspergillosis in chronic obstructive pulmonary disease: radiologic and pathologic findings in nine patients. *Am J Roentgenol* 2000;174:51–56.
98. Gefter WB, Weingrad TR, Epstein DM, et al. "Semiinvasive" pulmonary aspergillosis: a new look at the spectrum of *Aspergillus* infections of the lung. *Radiology* 1981;140:313–321.
99. Kim SY, Lee KS, Han J, et al. Semiinvasive pulmonary aspergillosis: CT and pathologic findings in six patients. *Am J Roentgenol* 2000;174:795–798.
100. Rose HD, Sheth NK. Pulmonary candidiasis: a clinical and pathological correlation. *Arch Intern Med* 1978;138:964–965.
101. Buff SJ, McLelland RM, Gallis HA, et al. *Candida albicans* pneumonia: radiographic appearance. *Am J Roentgenol* 1982;138:645–648.
102. Samuels BI, Bodey GP, Libshitz HI. Imaging in candidiasis. *Semin Roentgenol* 1996;31:76–82.
103. Janzen DL, Padley SPG, Adler BD, et al. Acute pulmonary complications in immunocompromised non-AIDS patients: comparison of diagnostic accuracy of CT and chest radiography. *Clin Radiol* 1993;47:159–165.
104. Kerkering TM, Duma RJ, Shadomy S. Cryptococcosis: clinical implications from a study of 41 patients with and without compromising host factors. *Ann Intern Med* 1981;94:611–616.
105. Feigin DS. Pulmonary cryptococcosis: radiologic-pathologic correlates of its three forms. *Am J Roentgenol* 1983;141:1262–1272.
106. Patz EF, Goodman PC. Pulmonary cryptococcosis. *J Thorac Imaging* 1992;7:51–55.
107. Conces Jr DJ. Histoplasmosis. *Semin Roentgenol* 1996;31:14–27.
108. Gurney JW, Conces Jr DJ. Pulmonary histoplasmosis. *Radiology* 1996;199:297–306.
109. Batra P, Batra RS. Thoracic coccidioidomycosis. *Semin Roentgenol* 1996;31:28–44.
110. Kim KI, Leung AN, Flint JDA, et al. Chronic pulmonary coccidioidomycosis: computed and pathologic findings in 18 patients. *Can Assoc Radiol J* 1998;49:401–407.
111. Weber WR, Askin FB, Dehner LP. Lung biopsy in *Pneumocystis carinii* pneumonia: a histopathologic study of typical and atypical features. *Am J Clin Pathol* 1977;67:11–19.
112. Askin FG, Katzenstein AL. Pneumocystis infection masquerading as diffuse alveolar damage: a potential source of diagnostic error. *Chest* 1981;79:420–422.
113. Bleiweiss IJ, Jagirdar JS, Klein MJ, et al. Granulomatous *Pneumocystis carinii* pneumonia in three patients with the acquired immune deficiency syndrome. *Chest* 1988;94:580–583.
114. Boiselle PM, Crans Jr CA, Kaplan MA. The changing face of *Pneumocystis carinii* pneumonia in AIDS patients. *Am J Roentgenol* 1999;172:1301–1309.
115. Klein JS, Warnock M, Webb WR, et al. Cavitating and noncavitating granulomas in AIDS patients with *Pneumocystis* pneumonitis. *Am J Roentgenol* 1989;152:753–754.
116. Panicek DM. Cystic pulmonary lesions in patients with AIDS. *Radiology* 1989;173:12–14.
117. Kuhlman JE, Knowles MC, Fishman EK, et al. Premature bullous pulmonary damage in AIDS: CT diagnosis. *Radiology* 1989;173:23–26.
118. Gurney JW, Bates FT. Pulmonary cystic disease: comparison of *Pneumocystis carinii* pneumatoceles and bullous emphysema due to intravenous drug abuse. *Radiology* 1989;173:27–31.
119. Han BK, Son JA, Yoon HK, Lee SI. Epidemic adenoviral lower respiratory tract infection in pediatric patients: radiographic and clinical characteristics. *Am J Roentgenol* 1998;170:1077–1080.
120. Palmer Jr SM, Henshaw NG, Howell DN, et al. Community respiratory viral infection in adult lung transplant recipients. *Chest* 1998;113:944–950.

121. Tillett HE, Smith JWG, Clifford RE. Excess morbidity and mortality associated with influenza in England and Wales. *Lancet* 1980;1:793–795.

122. Mullooly JP, Barker WH, Nolan TF. Risk of acute respiratory disease among pregnant women during influenza A epidemics. *Public Health Rep* 1986;101:205–211.

123. Feldman PS, Cohan MA, Hierholzer WJ. Fatal Hong Kong influenza: a clinical microbiological and pathological analysis of nine cases. *Yale J Biol Med* 1972;45:49–63.

124. Yeldandi AV, Colby TV. Pathologic features of lung biopsy specimens from influenza pneumonia cases. *Hum Pathol* 1994;25:47–53.

125. Galloway RW, Miller RS. Lung changes in the recent influenza epidemic. *Br J Radiol* 1959;32:28–31.

126. Feldman S. Varicella-zoster virus pneumonitis. *Chest* 1994;106(Suppl I):22S–27S.

127. Gogos CA, Bassaris HP, Vagenakis AG. Varicella pneumonitis in adults: a review of pulmonary manifestations, risk factors and treatment. *Respiration* 1992;59:339–343.

128. Shirai T, Sano K, Matsuyama S, et al. Varicella pneumonia in a healthy adult presenting with severe respiratory failure. *Intern Med* 1996;35:315–318.

129. Triebwasser JH, Harris RE, Bryant RE, et al. Varicella pneumonia in adults: report of seven cases and a review of literature. *Medicine* 1967;46:409–423.

130. Sargent EN, Carson MJ, Reilly ED. Roentgenographic manifestations of varicella pneumonia with postmortem correlation. *Am J Roentgenol* 1966;98:305–317.

131. Kim JS, Ryu CW, Lee SI, et al. High-resolution CT findings of varicella-zoster pneumonia. *Am J Roentgenol* 1999;172:113–116.

132. Kang EY, Patz EF, Müller NL. Cytomegalovirus pneumonia in transplant patients: CT findings. *J Comput Assist Tomogr* 1996;20:295–299.

133. Moon JH, Kim EA, Lee KS, et al. Cytomegalovirus pneumonia: high resolution CT findings in 10 non-AIDS immunocompromised patients. *Korean J Radiol* 2000;1:73–78.

134. McGuinness G, Scholes JV, Garay SM, et al. Cytomegalovirus pneumonitis: spectrum of parenchymal CT findings with pathologic correlation in 21 AIDS patients. *Radiology* 1994;192:451–459.

135. Mansel JK, Rosenow EC, Smith TF, et al. *Mycoplasma pneumoniae* pneumonia. *Chest* 1989;95:639–646.

136. Talkington DF, Thacker WL, Keller DW, et al. Diagnosis of *Mycoplasma pneumoniae* infection in autopsy and open-lung biopsy tissues by nested PCR. *J Clin Microbiol* 1998;36:1151–1153.

137. Murray HW, Tuazon C. Atypical pneumonias. *Med Clin North Am* 1980;64:507–527.

138. Rollins S, Colby T, Clayton F. Open lung biopsy in *Mycoplasma pneumoniae* pneumonia. *Arch Pathol Lab Med* 1986;110:34–41.

139. Thom DH, Grayston JT, Campbell LA, et al. Respiratory infection with *Chlamydia pneumoniae* in middle-aged and older adult outpatients. *Eur J Clin Microbiol Infect Dis* 1994;13:785–792.

140. Blasi F, Boschini A, Cosentini R, et al. Outbreaks of *Chlamydia pneumoniae* infection in former injection-drug users. *Chest* 1994;105:812–815.

141. Von Hertzen L, Isoaho R, Leinonen M, et al. *Chlamydia pneumoniae* antibodies in chronic obstructive pulmonary disease. *Int J Epidemiol* 1996;25:658–664.

142. McConnell CT, Plouffe JF, File TM, et al. CBPIS Study Group: radiographic appearance of *Chlamydia pneumoniae* (TWRS strain) respiratory infection. *Radiology* 1994;192:819–824.

143. Bhatia G. *Echinococcus. Semin Respir Infect* 1997;12:171–186.

144. Sadrieh M, Dutz W, Navabpoor MS. Review of 150 cases of hydatid cyst of the lung. *Chest* 1967;52:662–666.

145. Beggs I. The radiology of hydatid disease. *Am J Roentgenol* 1985;145:639–648.

146. Saksouk FA, Fahl MH, Rizk GK. Computed tomography of pulmonary hydatid disease. *J Comput Assist Tomogr* 1986;10:226–232.

147. Von Sinner WN, Rifai A, te Strake L, et al. Magnetic resonance imaging of thoracic hydatid disease: correlation with clinical findings, radiography, ultrasonography, CT and pathology. *Acta Radiol* 1990;31:59–62.

3

PULMONARY CARCINOMA

ADENOCARCINOMA
Nonbronchioloalveolar Adenocarcinoma
Bronchioloalveolar Carcinoma

SQUAMOUS CELL CARCINOMA

SMALL CELL CARCINOMA

LARGE CELL CARCINOMA

Pulmonary carcinoma is the most common cause of cancer-related death in both men and women. The most important cause is cigarette smoke (1,2): The relative risk of cancer in smokers compared with nonsmokers is about 10 to 1 and correlates with the duration and amount of smoking.

Several classification schemes of pulmonary neoplasms have been proposed. The most widely accepted is that of the World Health Organization (WHO), published in 1999 (3). According to this classification, there are four main histologic types of pulmonary carcinoma: adenocarcinoma, squamous cell carcinoma, small cell carcinoma, and large cell carcinoma. These four variants constitute about 95% of all pulmonary carcinomas. The remaining types (Table 3.1) are uncommon. Neoplasms other than carcinoma are discussed in Chapter 5.

ADENOCARCINOMA

Adenocarcinoma is the most common type of pulmonary carcinoma, accounting for approximately 40% of cases (4). It is characterized histologically by the formation of glands and papillary structures or by the presence of mucin secretion. In the WHO classification, it is subdivided into acinar, papillary, bronchioloalveolar, solid mucin secreting, and mixed types (Table 3.1) (3). With the exception of the solitary nodule that shows a pure bronchioloalveolar growth pattern and the diffuse form of bronchioloalveolar carcinoma, the usefulness of this subdivision is open to question. As a result, most physicians consider the tumors in two groups: bronchioloalveolar and nonbronchioloalveolar.

Nonbronchioloalveolar Adenocarcinoma

Grossly, nonbronchioloalveolar adenocarcinoma typically presents as a peripheral nodule or mass that is spherical or (more frequently) lobulated in shape (Fig. 3.1). It may be well circumscribed or have spiculated margins; some tumors show both patterns (Fig. 3.2), reflecting the presence of more than one clone of neoplastic cell. Central fibrosis is common, particularly in tumors adjacent to the pleura. Frequently, this results in retraction of the pleura into the tumor and a distinctive puckered appearance (Figs. 3.1 and 3.3). Similar retraction can also be seen in tumors not in direct contact with the pleura, in which case a band of collapsed lung or fibrous tissue may be seen to extend from the pleural indentation to the periphery of the tumor (pleural tag) (Fig. 3.4). Grossly evident necrosis is often minimal or absent in tumors less than 3 cm in diameter; it is more frequent in larger ones. Presumably, because of the peripheral location of most tumors, drainage of such necrotic tissue via the airways is limited, and cavitation is uncommon. Peripheral tumors may directly invade the pleura and chest wall; rarely, subsequent pleural spread results in circumferential growth around the lung, resembling mesothelioma (5).

TABLE 3.1. 1999 WHO CLASSIFICATION OF LUNG CARCINOMA

Squamous cell carcinoma
  Variants
    Papillary
    Clear Cell
    Small cell
    Basaloid

Small cell carcinoma
  Variant
    Combined small cell carcinoma

Adenocarcinoma
  Acinar
  Papillary
  Bronchioloalveolar carcinoma
    Nonmucinous
    Mucinous
    Mixed mucinous and nonmucinous or indeterminate
  Solid adenocarcinoma with mucin
  Adenocarcinoma with mixed subtypes
  Variants
    Well-differentiated fetal adenocarcinoma
    Mucinous ("colloid") adenocarcinoma
    Mucinous cystadenocarcinoma
    Signet ring adenocarcinoma
    Clear cell adenocarcinoma

Large cell carcinoma
  Variants
    Large cell neuroendocrine carcinoma
      Combined large cell neuroendocrine carcinoma
    Basaloid carcinoma
    Lymphoepithelioma-like carcinoma
    Clear cell carcinoma
    Large cell carcinoma with rhabdoid phenotype

Adenosquamous carcinoma
Carcinomas with pleomorphic, sarcomatoid, or sarcomatous elements
  Carcinomas with spindle and/or giant cells
    Pleomorphic carcinoma
    Spindle cell carcinoma
    Giant cell carcinoma
  Carcinosarcoma
  Pulmonary blastoma
  Other

Carcinoid tumor
  Typical carcinoid
  Atypical carcinoid

Carcinomas of salivary gland type
    Mucoepidermoid carcinoma
    Adenoid cystic carcinoma
    Others

Unclassified carcinoma

From Travis WD, Colby TV, Corrin B, et al. *Histological typing of lung and pleural tumours: international histological classification of tumours*, 3rd ed. Berlin: Springer-Verlag, 1999.

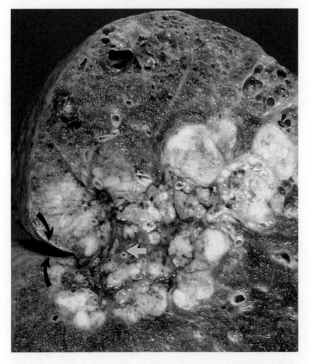

FIGURE 3.1. Adenocarcinoma. A magnified view of an upper lobe shows a coarsely lobulated tumor that has a focus of dense fibrous tissue in its central portion (*white arrow*), resulting in retraction of the adjacent pleura (*black arrows*). Focal emphysema is evident in the lung apex.

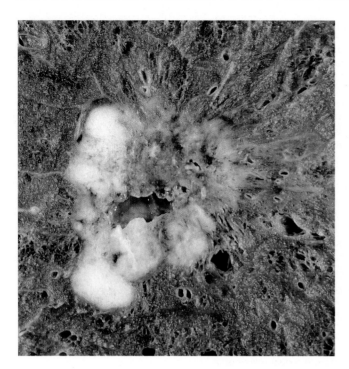

FIGURE 3.2. Adenocarcinoma—variable appearance. A magnified view of a peripheral adenocarcinoma shows two patterns. Tumor on the left side is white and has a lobulated contour; that on the right has a gray appearance and a spiculated margin. Histologically, the former was a moderately differentiated acinar adenocarcinoma with minimal tissue reaction. The right-sided tumor was poorly differentiated and was associated with a prominent lymphocytic and fibroblastic reaction. The admixture of the inflammatory tissue with the tumor is responsible for the gray appearance; retraction of the fibrous tissue and its extension into the adjacent parenchyma led to the spiculation. This variable pattern is common in pulmonary adenocarcinoma and is probably related to the emergence of more than one clone of tumor cell.

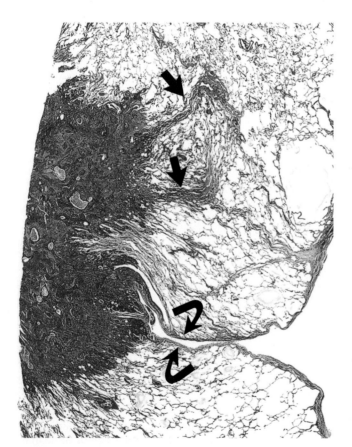

FIGURE 3.3. Adenocarcinoma–pleural puckering. A low-magnification photomicrograph of a peripheral adenocarcinoma shows deep indentation of the pleura into the mid-portion of the tumor (*curved arrows*). Two small foci of subsegmental atelectasis (*straight arrows*) are also evident, corresponding to radiologic foci of spiculation.

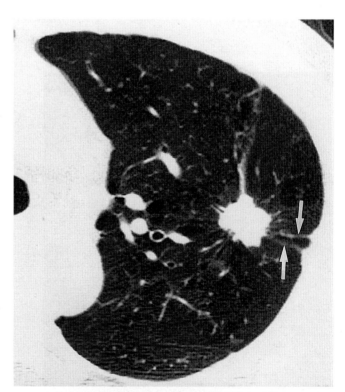

FIGURE 3.4. Adenocarcinoma. A CT image (1.0-mm collimation) shows a 2-cm-diameter nodule in left upper lobe. The tumor has both lobulated and spiculated margins. Two pleural tags are evident (*arrows*).

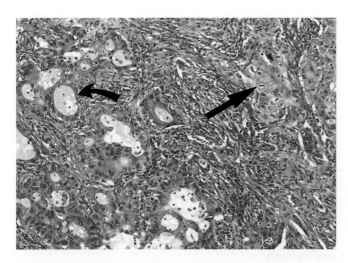

FIGURE 3.5. Adenocarcinoma. The photomicrograph shows a typical nonbronchioloalveolar adenocarcinoma, composed of irregularly shaped glandular structures (some containing mucus; *curved arrow*) and sheets of cells that have no clearcut differentiation (*straight arrow*). No underlying lung structure is evident, and there is a moderately severe inflammatory reaction.

Histologically, most nonbronchioloalveolar adenocarcinomas show a mixture of patterns, including acini, tubules, and sheets of cells without structural evidence of glandular differentiation (Fig. 3.5); intracellular or extracellular mucin may or may not be evident. All these patterns are associated with destruction of the underlying parenchyma and a variable inflammatory/fibroblastic reaction. Foci of neoplastic cells that have a bronchioloalveolar pattern are common at the expanding edge of nonbronchioloalveolar tumors. Although usually limited in extent, they are sometimes sufficient in amount to be clearly visible in both gross specimens and CT images (Fig. 3.6). Nonbronchioloalveolar adeno-

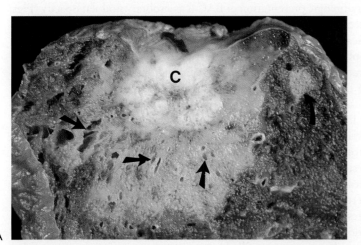

A

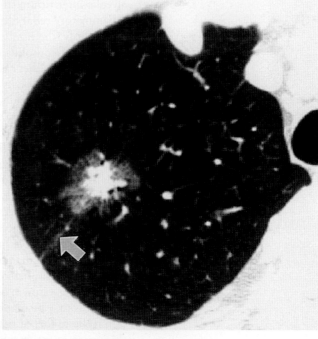

B

FIGURE 3.6. Adenocarcinoma—mixed bronchioloalveolar and nonbronchioloalveolar patterns. **A:** A sagittal slice of an upper lobe shows a subpleural white nodule approximately 2 cm in diameter (*C*). Normal lung structures are not evident within it, indicating that it is both invasive and destructive. The tumor is surrounded by a rim of tan-colored tissue in which such structures are identifiable. (*Straight arrows* indicate bronchioles.) Histologic examination confirmed the white tumor to be an acinar adenocarcinoma and the tan-colored one to have a bronchioloalveolar pattern. A satellite nodule of bronchioloalveolar carcinoma is present on the right (*curved arrow*). **B:** HRCT image (1.0-mm collimation) of another tumor shows a nodular area of ground-glass opacity with central soft-tissue attenuation in right upper lobe. The margin is lobulated and spiculated. A pleural tag (*arrow*) is evident. (**B** from Lee KS, et al. *Radiographics* 1997;17: 1345–1357, with permission.)

carcinomas commonly have spread to regional lymph nodes at presentation; the prevalence of such spread appears to be greater than that associated with bronchioloalveolar and squamous cell carcinoma (6).

The characteristic radiologic presentation of adenocarcinoma consists of a solitary nodule or mass with a lobulated or spiculated margin (5,7) (Figs. 3.4 and 3.7). The histologic correlate of the spiculation is variable and may correspond to strands of fibrous tissue that extend from the tumor margin into the lung, to direct infiltration of tumor into the adjacent parenchyma, to small foci of parenchymal collapse as a result of bronchiolar obstruction by the expanding tumor, or to spread of tumor in lymphatic channels and interstitial tissue of adjacent vessels, airways, or interlobular septa (lymphangitic spread) (7) (Fig. 3.8). The nodules enhance following intravenous administration of contrast. The enhancement is greater than 15 HU on CT and presumably reflects the vascular stroma of the tumor (8) (Fig. 3.9).

Bronchioloalveolar Carcinoma

Bronchioloalveolar carcinoma (BAC) is characterized histologically by spread of tumor cells on the surface of the lung parenchyma without its destruction (Fig. 3.10) (9). (As indicated previously, foci of such growth are common in many nonbronchioloalveolar carcinomas; to be classified as BAC, such growth must be the predominant pattern [more than 90%].) Tumor cells may be arranged in a single layer or may form small papillary projections into the alveolar air spaces. They also may grow along the surface of transitional airways; however, extension into membranous bronchioles is unusual. Intraalveolar mucus or proteinaceous fluid (surfactant-like material) may be secreted by the tumor cells (Fig. 3.11); in some cases, it accounts for the major proportion of a tumor's volume. The alveolar interstitium adjacent to the tumor cells is often thickened by fibrous tissue and an inflammatory cell infiltrate (Fig. 3.10); occasionally, this is marked ("sclerosing" subtype).

Grossly, the tumors may appear as a peripheral nodule (Fig. 3.12) or as a poorly defined area of consolidation, with the latter sometimes affecting an entire segment or lobe (Fig. 3.13). In either case, normal structures such as interlobular septa, membranous bronchioles, and pulmonary vessels are identifiable within the tumor.

The most common radiologic presentation of BAC is as a solitary nodular opacity (Figs. 3.14 to 3.16), a pattern seen in 60% of cases (10). CT demonstrates either a peripheral soft-tissue nodule or a focal area of ground-glass attenuation (Fig. 3.14) or consolidation (10,11) (Figs. 3.15 and 3.16). Bubblelike areas of low attenuation within the nodule ("bubble lucencies"), air bronchograms, heterogeneous attenuation, and spiculated margins are frequently present (12,13). Bubblelike lucencies are observed more frequently with BAC (50%) than with other carcinomas (Figs. 3.15 and 3.16) (7). They are usually related to small patent bronchioles incorporated within the nodule; occasionally, they represent small cystic structures of uncertain origin lined by papillary tumor projections (7). Incorporation of larger membranous bronchioles or small bronchi within areas of lung consolidated by tumor cells may be manifested as an air bronchogram (Figs. 3.17 and 3.18) (14). The presence of ectatic bronchioles in a focus of fibrosis in the center of the tumor may result in the same finding. Growth of tumor cells around preexisting areas of emphysema or cysts related to fibrosis may be manifested as pseudocavitation (15,16). Areas of ground-glass attenuation relate to foci of tumor associated with minimal interstitial thickening. More marked thickening or foci in which the airspaces are filled by tumor cells or their secretions tend to be manifested as consolidation (10,13). Spiculation is frequently seen in focal BAC (Fig. 3.16). As with nonbronchioloalveolar tumors, it may be related to fibrotic strands radiating from the tumor (7, 13) or lymphangitic spread of the tumor itself. Pleural tags are also common, and usually correspond to an interlobular septum thickened by fibrous tissue or tumor, or to a focus of parenchymal invasion that extends to the pleural surface (7,13).

The second most common radiographic presentation of BAC is an area of ground-glass opacification or airspace consolidation (Figs. 3.19 and 3.20). Air bronchograms are commonly present. Production of copious amounts of mucin may result in lobar expansion and bulging of the interlobar fissure (17,18). Mucin has a lower CT density than tu-

(*text continues on page 87*)

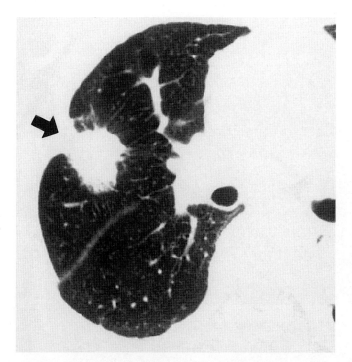

FIGURE 3.7. Adenocarcinoma. HRCT image (1.0-mm collimation) at the level of the bronchus intermedius shows a 3-cm diameter nodule in the right upper lobe. It has lobulated and spiculated margins and is associated with a moderate degree of pleural puckering (*arrow*).

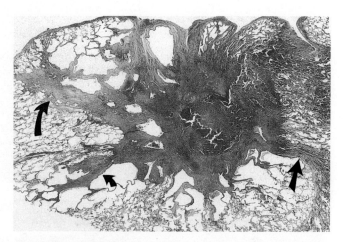

FIGURE 3.8. Adenocarcinoma showing spiculation. A low-magnification photomicrograph shows a spiculated adenocarcinoma adjacent to the pleura. The spicules are the result of subsegmental atelectasis (*straight arrow*), interlobular septal thickening by fibrous tissue (*long curved arrow*) and peribronchiolar thickening by tumor infiltration (*short curved arrow*).

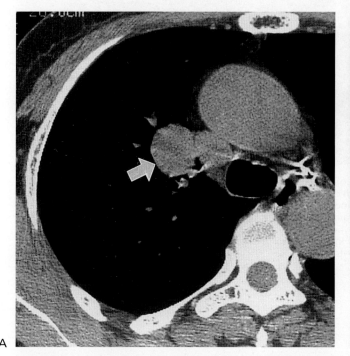

A

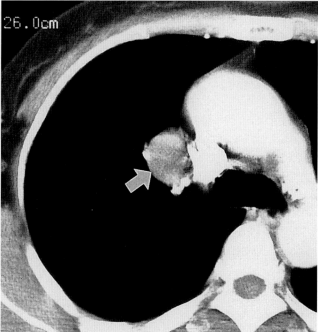

B

FIGURE 3.9. Adenocarcinoma showing enhancement after administration of intravenous contrast medium. **A:** A CT image (1.0-mm collimation) at the level of the carina shows a 3-cm-diameter nodule (*arrow*) in the right upper lobe. The attenuation value of nodule was 26 HU. **B:** An image taken after intravenous administration of contrast shows nodule enhancement (*arrow*). The attenuation value was 51 HU.

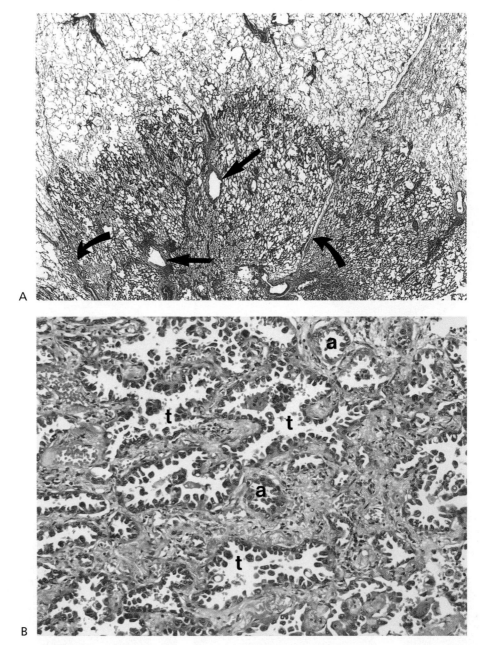

FIGURE 3.10. Bronchioloalveolar carcinoma. Low- (**A**) and high- (**B**) magnification photomicrographs show two tumors, each characterized by spread of neoplastic cells on the airspace surface with preservation of underlying lung architecture. In **A,** interlobular septa (*curved arrows*) and membranous bronchioles (*straight arrows*) are clearly seen; the lumen of transitional airways is less obvious but still evident when compared with the adjacent normal lung. In **B** there is a moderate degree of parenchymal interstitial fibrosis; however, the lumen of transitional airways (t) and alveoli (a) can still be identified.

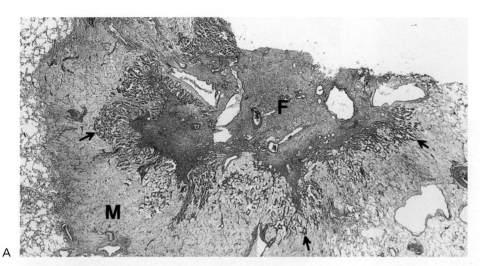

A

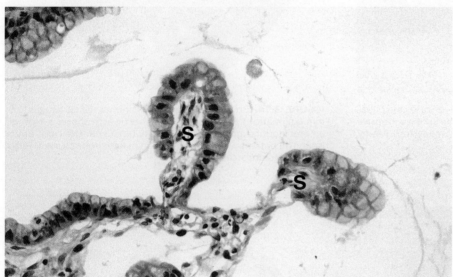

B

FIGURE 3.11. Bronchioloalveolar carcinoma—mucinous type. **A:** A low-magnification view of an ill-defined 2.5-cm nodule shows it to consist of a central region of mature fibrous tissue (*F*) surrounded by a rim of tumor cells located on the airspace surface in the fashion of bronchioloalveolar carcinoma (*arrows*). The most peripheral (lightly stained) part of the tumor consists of airspaces filled with mucus (*M*). **B:** A magnified view shows the tumor cells with apical mucus-containing cytoplasm lining alveolar septa (*S*). Lightly stained mucus is evident in the adjacent airspaces. The mucus is so abundant that it has spread beyond the confines of the neoplastic cells themselves to form approximately half of the tumor bulk.

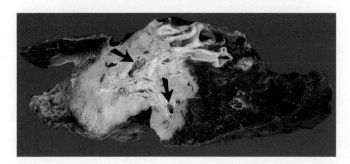

FIGURE 3.12. Bronchioloalveolar carcinoma—solitary nodule. A transverse slice of an upper lobe shows a well-demarcated, slightly lobulated tumor extending from the anterior to the posterior pleura (the latter being retracted). Several membranous bronchioles and vessels (*arrows*) can be identified within the tumor.

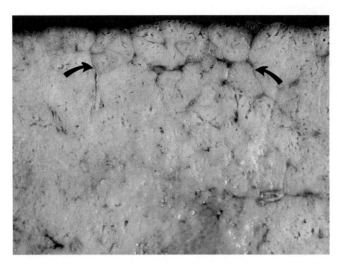

FIGURE 3.13. Bronchioloalveolar carcinoma—diffuse consolidation. A magnified view of a slice of lower lobe shows extensive consolidation. Interlobular septa (*arrows*) and many transitional airways can be recognized within the tumor.

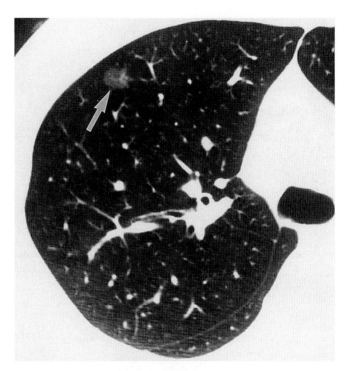

FIGURE 3.14. Bronchioloalveolar carcinoma. HRCT image (1.0-mm collimation) at the level of the aortic arch shows a 1-cm diameter nodular ground-glass opacity (*arrow*) in the right upper lobe. The patient was a 55-year-old man with nonmucinous bronchioloalveolar carcinoma.

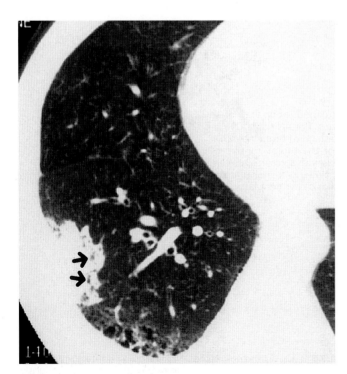

FIGURE 3.15. Bronchioloalveolar carcinoma. HRCT image (1.0-mm collimation) shows peripheral consolidation associated with bubblelike lucencies (*arrows*) in the right lower lobe. The patient was a 68-year-old man with a mucinous bronchioloalveolar carcinoma. (From Lee KS, et al. *Radiographics* 1997;17:1345–1357, with permission.)

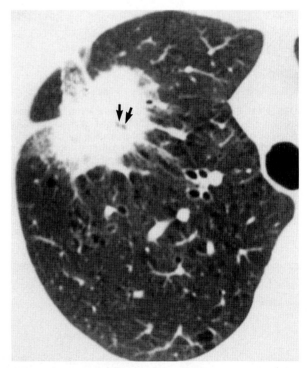

FIGURE 3.16. Bronchioloalveolar carcinoma. HRCT image (1.5-mm collimation) shows a spiculated right upper lobe nodule with bubble lucencies (*arrows*). The patient was a 58-year-old-woman.

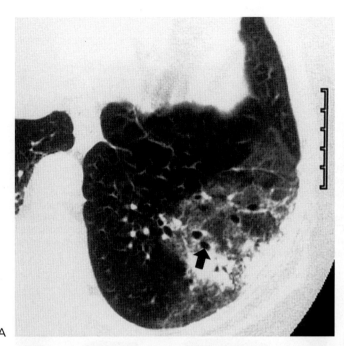
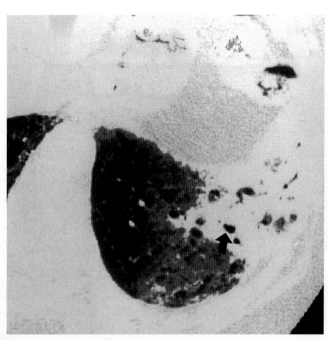

A   B

FIGURE 3.17. A, B: Mucinous bronchioloalveolar carcinoma–air bronchogram. CT images (1.0-mm collimation) obtained at level of basal segments of left lower lobe show areas of ground-glass opacity and airspace consolidation. Patent, somewhat dilated airways are evident within the tumor (*arrows*). (From Jang HJ, et al. *Radiology* 1996;199:485–488, with permission.)

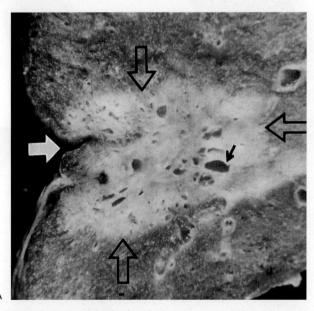
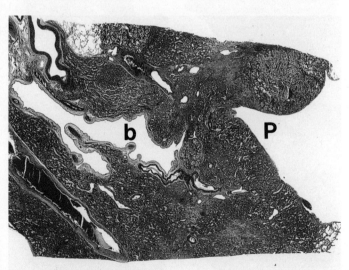

A   B

FIGURE 3.18. Bronchioloalveolar carcinoma—air bronchogram. **A:** A magnified view of a lower lobe shows a well-demarcated tumor (*open arrows*) adjacent to the pleura. The latter is retracted (*white arrow*). A patent airway is evident within the tumor (*small arrow*). **B:** A view of another tumor shows a patent membranous bronchiole (*b*) surrounded by lung parenchyma that is consolidated by neoplastic cells. Spread of such cells around but not into these airways is characteristic of bronchioloalveolar carcinoma and is responsible for the presence of an air bronchogram on CT. *P* indicates the retracted pleural space.

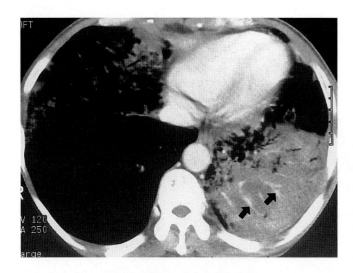

FIGURE 3.19. Bronchioloalveolar carcinoma–airspace consolidation and CT angiogram sign. A contrast-enhanced CT image (7-mm collimation) shows extensive consolidation in the left lower lobe and patchy consolidation in the right middle lobe. Contrast-enhanced vessels can be seen within the area of consolidation in the lower lobe (CT angiogram sign) (*arrows*). The patient was a 63-year-old man with mucinous bronchioloalveolar carcinoma. (From Lee KS, et al. *Radiographics* 1997;17:1345–1357, with permission.)

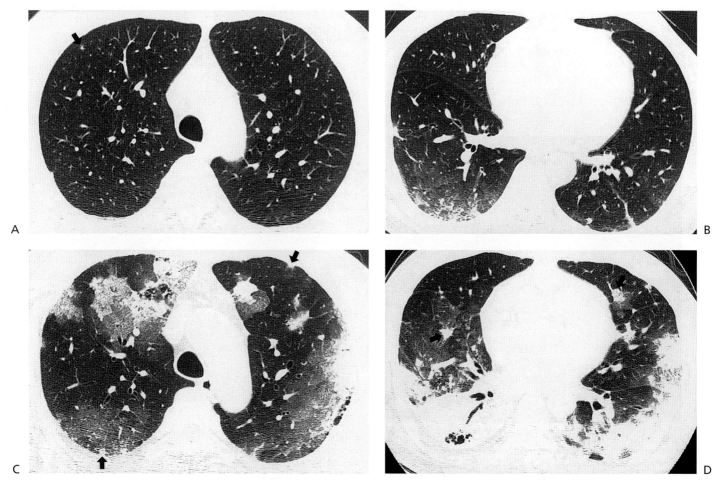

FIGURE 3.20. Progression of bronchioloalveolar carcinoma over time. **A,B:** CT images at the levels of the azygos arch and the inferior pulmonary veins, respectively, show a small nodule in the right upper lobe (*arrow* in **A**) and patchy ground-glass opacities in both lower lobes. **C, D:** Follow-up CT scans obtained at similar levels to **A** and **B** 1 year later show multiple nodules (*arrows*), progression of the ground-glass opacities, and extensive airspace consolidation. The patient was a 54-year-old man with mucinous bronchioloalveolar carcinoma.

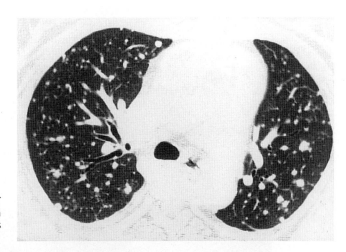

FIGURE 3.21. Multinodular bronchioloalveolar carcinoma. HRCT (1.0-mm collimation) image shows small nodules throughout both lungs. A small right pleural effusion is also present. The patient was a 55-year-old woman.

mor. Therefore BACs containing large amounts of mucin have relatively low attenuation. Following intravenous administration of contrast the pulmonary vessels can be clearly seen within the low-attenuation areas (CT-angiogram sign) (18) (Fig. 3.19). It should be noted, however, that this sign can be observed in various other conditions, including lobar pneumonia, lymphoma, lipoid pneumonia, infarction, and edema (19–21).

A third and relatively uncommon radiologic pattern of BAC is multiple nodules (13,17) (Fig. 3.21). On CT, these may be well or poorly defined and are sometimes cavitated. They may consist of poorly defined areas of ground-glass attenuation, consolidation, or both (13,17).

SQUAMOUS CELL CARCINOMA

Squamous cell carcinomas account for about 25% to 30% of pulmonary carcinomas. They are characterized histologically by keratinization and/or prominent intercellular bridges (Fig. 3.22). Most originate in lobar, segmental, or proximal subsegmental bronchi (Fig. 3.23) (5). They tend to grow into the airway lumen as polypoid or papillary tumors and

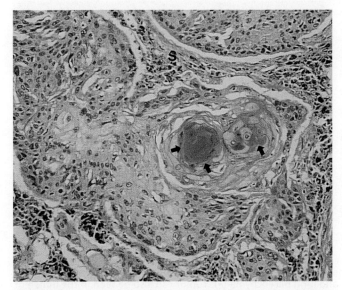

FIGURE 3.22. Squamous cell carcinoma. A photomicrograph of a moderately differentiated squamous cell carcinoma shows a transition between relatively small cells adjacent to fibrovascular stroma (*S*) and larger, more pale staining cells in the central region. Two densely eosinophilic foci (*arrows*), corresponding to intracellular keratinization, are apparent.

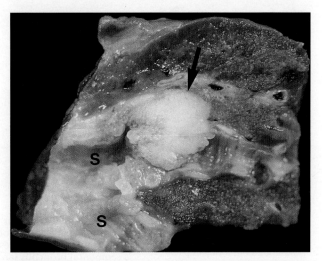

FIGURE 3.23. Squamous cell carcinoma. A highly magnified view of a portion of a lower lobe shows two basal segmental bronchi (*S*). The origin of one is occluded by a polypoid squamous cell carcinoma. Early extension into the adjacent parenchyma is evident (*arrow*).

therefore are usually associated with features of airway obstruction in the distal lung. These consist of a combination of atelectasis, bronchiectasis and mucus plugging, and obstructive pneumonitis. The relative proportion of each of these varies with individual tumors. The most prominent in surgically excised specimens is usually obstructive pneumonitis, which consists of alveolar airspace filling by proteinaceous fluid (in the early stage) and foamy macrophages (later on), and alveolar interstitial thickening by fibrous tissue and a predominantly lymphocytic inflammatory infiltrate (Fig. 3.24). Histologic evidence of infection (necrosis and a neutrophil infiltrate) is usually absent. The foamy macrophages contain lipid secreted by alveolar and bronchiolar epithelial cells that is normally extruded

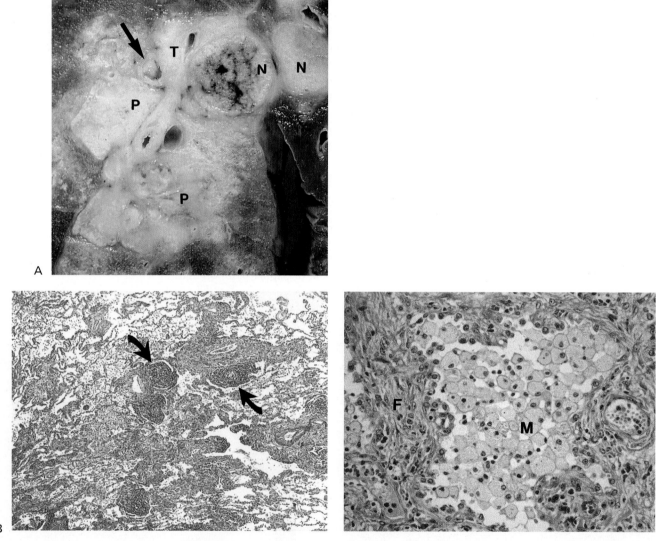

FIGURE 3.24. Squamous cell carcinoma—obstructive pneumonitis. **A:** A magnified view of a sagittal slice of a lower lobe shows a poorly delimited white carcinoma in peribronchial interstitial tissue (*T*), lymph nodes (*N*), and lung parenchyma (*P*). Tumor can also be seen in the lumen of a segmental bronchus (*arrow*). The parenchyma adjacent to the carcinoma has a finely granular yellow appearance. Low- (**B**) and high- (**C**) magnification views of the latter region show patchy chronic inflammation (*arrows*), alveolar interstitial fibrosis (*F*), and airspace filling by finely vacuolated macrophages (*M*). The vacuoles contain lipid (which is responsible for the yellow gross appearance) that cannot be extruded from the alveoli via the mucociliary escalator because of the proximal airway obstruction.

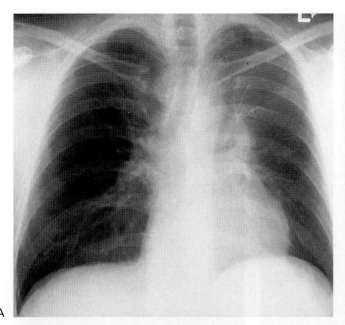

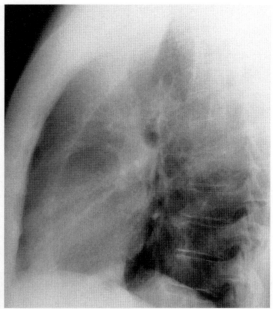

A

B

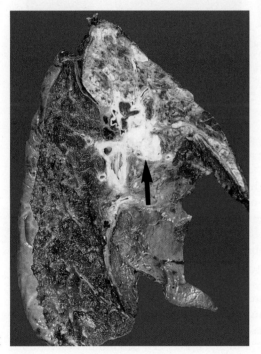

C

FIGURE 3.25. Squamous cell carcinoma—chronic obstructive pneumonitis. Posteroanterior (**A**) and lateral (**B**) chest radiographs show left upper lobe atelectasis. **C:** A sagittal slice of the left lung shows marked collapse of the upper lobe and obstruction of its bronchus by a 2-cm carcinoma (*arrow*). The upper lobe parenchyma has a gray and black appearance as a result of fibrosis and concentration of anthracotic (carbon) pigment, respectively.

via the airway mucocilliary escalator. In long-standing obstructive pneumonitis, airspace macrophages decrease in number and interstitial fibrous tissue increases in amount, resulting in more marked atelectasis (Fig. 3.25). Occasionally, bronchiectasis with mucus plugging is more prominent than either atelectasis or obstructive pneumonitis (Fig. 3.26).

Most squamous cell carcinomas also extend through the bronchial wall into the adjacent lung parenchyma. Necrosis of the central portion of the tumor is common, particularly in larger ones. Possibly because of their intimate association with proximal airways, the

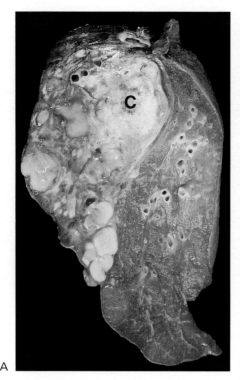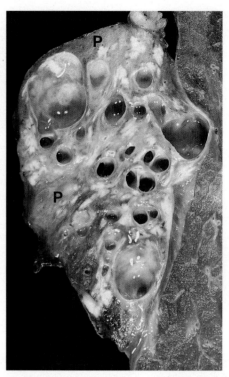

FIGURE 3.26. Squamous cell carcinoma—bronchiectasis and mucus plugging. **A:** Sagittal slice of left lung shows a proximal white carcinoma (*C*) without clear airway origin in the upper lobe. Airways throughout the lobe are distended with yellowish mucus. **B:** A magnified view of the reverse side of the lobe following removal of the mucus more clearly shows the bronchial dilatation. Only a few small foci of obstructive pneumonitis (*P*) are evident.

necrotic material can drain relatively easily and cavity formation is common (Fig. 3.27). Occasionally, a cavity results from infection and abscess formation in an area of obstructive pneumonitis.

The most common radiologic abnormality consists of atelectasis and obstructive pneumonitis involving a segment, a lobe, or the entire lung (Figs. 3.25 and 3.28). The combination of a hilar bulge due to a large central mass and atelectasis secondary to the airway obstruction results in an inverse S configuration, a finding known as the S-sign of Golden (5). Distinction of tumor from obstructive pneumonitis can usually be readily made on contrast-enhanced CT, the atelectatic portion typically showing greater enhancement than the tumor (22,23).

A small percentage of squamous cell carcinomas presents as intraparenchymal nodules that lack apparent connection to a bronchus (Fig. 3.29). Grossly and radiologically, these are similar to peripheral adenocarcinomas (4). The borders of the nodule are often irregular or lobulated. Approximately 10% of squamous cell carcinomas cavitate (5) (Fig. 3.27). The cavities are usually thick walled and have a nodular inner surface. The latter is probably related to local differences in necrosis and growth rate within the tumor.

SMALL CELL CARCINOMA

Small cell lung cancer (SCLC) accounts for about 20% of pulmonary carcinomas (4,5). Approximately 90% to 95% occur centrally, apparently arising in a lobar or main bronchus (5) (Fig. 3.30). Early in its course, SCLC grows predominantly in the airway wall and adjacent peribronchial interstitium (Fig. 3.31). The overlying airway epithelium is often intact, although focal areas of squamous metaplasia or ulceration may be seen.

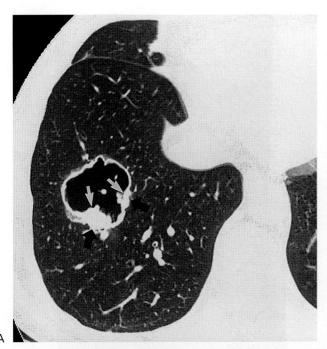
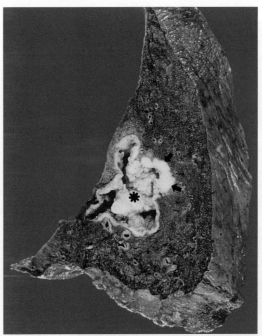

A

B

FIGURE 3.27. Squamous cell carcinoma—cavitation. **A:** HRCT image (1.0-mm collimation) shows a 4-cm-diameter thin-walled cavitary lesion in the right lower lobe. Note focal nodular thickening (*arrows*) of cavity wall. **B:** A sagittal slice of the excised specimen confirms the presence of a cavitated carcinoma with focal intracavitary (*asterisk*) and intraparenchymal (*arrows*) extension. The patient was a 53-year-old man.

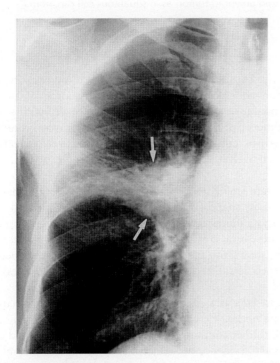

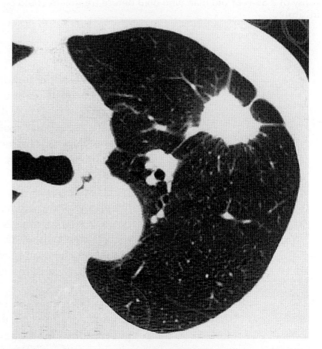

FIGURE 3.28. Squamous cell carcinoma—obstructive pneumonitis. A chest radiograph shows a poorly defined mass (*arrows*) and mild distal consolidation due to obstructive pneumonitis. The patient was a 61-year-old man.

FIGURE 3.29. Squamous cell carcinoma presenting as peripheral nodule. HRCT (1.0-mm collimation) image shows a 3-cm left upper lobe nodule with lobulated and spiculated margins and several pleural tags. Histologic examination showed moderately differentiated squamous cell carcinoma. The patient was a 67-year-old man.

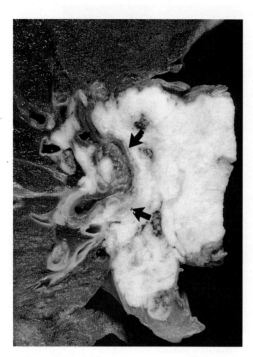

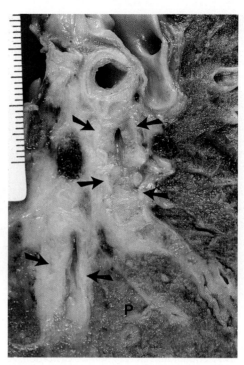

FIGURE 3.30. Small cell carcinoma. A magnified view of a sagittal slice of the right lung at the hilum shows a poorly delimited neoplasm located in the bronchial mucosa and peribronchial interstitial tissue (*arrows* indicate cartilage plates). Direct extension into peribronchial and hilar lymph nodes as well as mediastinal adipose tissue is evident. (The residua of the nodes can be seen as foci of black pigmentation.) The specimen was obtained at autopsy of a 55-year-old man who died before treatment could be instituted.

FIGURE 3.31. Small cell carcinoma. A magnified view of a lower lobe shows marked stenosis of two segmental bronchi by a fleshy tumor. (*Arrows* indicate cartilage plates enveloped by tumor.) The tumor extends into the adjacent peribronchial interstitial tissue, several lymph nodes, and the adjacent basal segmental parenchyma (P). The airway narrowing is the result of more or less diffuse mucosal infiltration by the tumor cells, rather than a localized polypoid tumor, as in squamous cell carcinoma.

Infiltration of the tumor into the adjacent lung parenchyma occurs as it increases in size. Involvement of peribronchial lymph nodes by direct extension or metastasis is almost invariable (Fig. 3.30). The combination of sites involved by tumor usually results in a lobulated, perihilar mass at the time of presentation. As the tumor grows, bronchial lumens may be obstructed by extrinsic compression (Fig. 3.31); however, atelectasis and obstructive pneumonitis are relatively uncommon and usually indicate advanced disease.

Histologically, the tumor cells are small (two to three times the size of a mature lymphocyte) and round or fusiform in shape (Fig. 3.32). Cytoplasm is minimal and necrosis is common. Neurosecretory granules resembling those found in normal neuroendocrine cells of the airway epithelium are found in most tumors. Similarly, immunohistochemical study typically shows the presence of nonspecific neuroendocrine markers such as chromogranin or specific substances such as ACTH or gastrin-releasing peptide.

Radiologically, SCLC usually presents as a central mass formed by the combination of primary tumor and affected lymph nodes. Mediastinal lymph node enlargement is also present in the most cases (Fig. 3.33). Other common findings include narrowing and displacement of major vessels and bronchi, evidence of mediastinal invasion, and pleural effusion. In 5% to 10% of cases, SCLC presents as a peripheral nodule without associated lymphadenopathy (24,25) (Fig. 3.34). Most of these lesions have smooth but lobulated margins. Spiculation may occur due to local lymphatic invasion (25). Marginal ground-glass attenuation is seen in some cases, reflecting the presence of edema and hemorrhage (25).

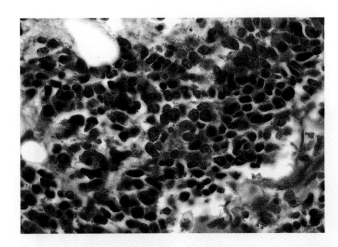

FIGURE 3.32. Small cell carcinoma. The photomicrograph shows cells that have hyperchromatic, moderately pleomorphic nuclei, and minimal cytoplasm (the latter indicated by the close approximation of adjacent nuclei).

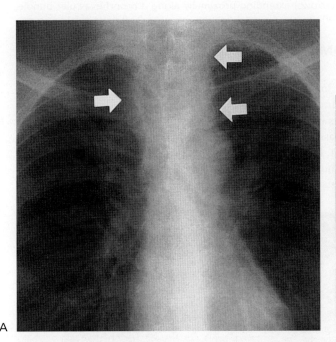

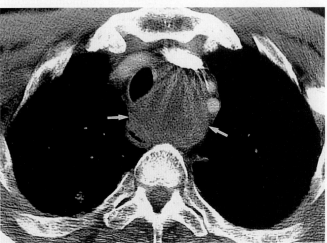

A

B

FIGURE 3.33. Small cell carcinoma—lymph node enlargement. **A:** A chest radiograph shows bilateral superior mediastinal widening (*arrows*) associated with a shift of the trachea to the right. **B:** A contrast-enhanced CT image (7-mm collimation) at the level of the thoracic inlet shows marked lymph node enlargement (*arrows*) in left paratracheal area, again with displacement of trachea and esophagus to the right.

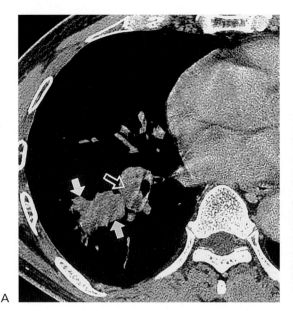
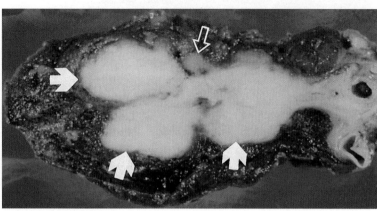

FIGURE 3.34. Small cell carcinoma presenting as peripheral branching mass. **A:** A CT image (1.0-mm collimation) at the level of the right inferior pulmonary vein shows a tubular mass (*solid arrows*) in right lower lobe. Hilar nodal enlargement (*open arrow*) is evident. **B:** The resected specimen shows a lobulated tumor (*arrows*) extending proximally along a bronchovascular bundle. The patient was a 61-year-old man.

LARGE CELL CARCINOMA

Large cell carcinomas account for approximately 5% of all lung carcinomas (4,5). Grossly, they are often large, well-circumscribed masses with extensive necrosis (Fig. 3.35). Histologically, they consist of sheets of cells that have large, often vesicular, nuclei; prominent nucleoli; and abundant cytoplasm (Fig. 3.35). By definition, features of squamous or glandular differentiation are absent. However, evidence of neuroendocrine differentiation may be seen, in which case the tumor is classified as large cell neuroendocrine carcinoma. Although multiple foci of necrosis are characteristic, cavitation is uncommon.

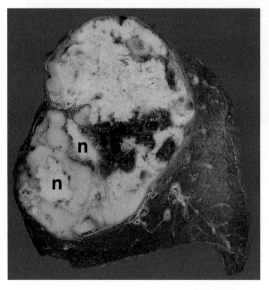
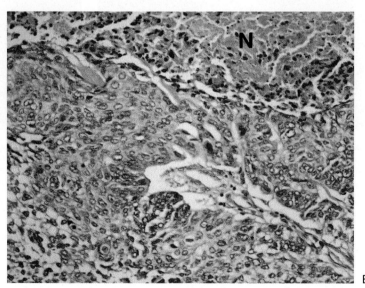

FIGURE 3.35. Large cell carcinoma. **A:** A sagittal slice of the right lower lobe shows a well-circumscribed tumor measuring approximately 10 cm in greatest dimension. Multiple foci of necrosis (*n*) and hemorrhage are evident. **B:** A photomicrograph of the tumor shows it to consist of sheets of cells with abundant cytoplasm and vesicular nuclei. Foci of necrosis (*N*) are present.

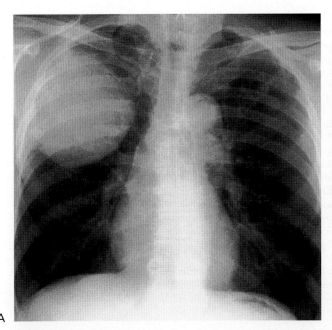
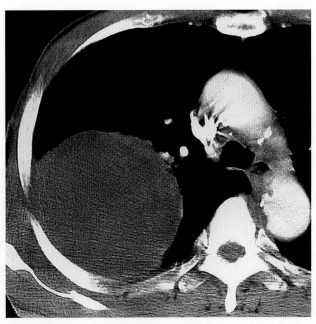

A

B

FIGURE 3.36. Large cell carcinoma. **A:** A chest radiograph shows a 10-cm-diameter mass in the right upper lobe. **B:** A contrast-enhanced CT image (7-mm collimation) demonstrates a large low-attenuation mass. The patient was a 66-year-old man.

About 70% present radiologically as a parenchymal mass usually measuring greater than 3 cm in diameter (4,5) (Fig. 3.36). The margins of the mass are usually poorly defined and lobulated (26).

REFERENCES

1. Beckett WS. Epidemiology and etiology of lung cancer. *Clin Chest Med* 1993; 14:1–15.
2. Bartecchi CE, MacKenzie TD, Schrier RW. The human costs of tobacco use. *N Engl J Med* 1994; 330: 907–912
3. Travis WD, Colby TV, Corrin B, et al. *Histological typing of lung and pleural tumors: international histological classification of tumors,* 3rd ed. New York: Springer Verlag, 1999.
4. Quinn D, Gianlupi A, Broste S. The changing radiographic presentation of bronchogenic carcinoma with reference to cell types. *Chest* 1996;110:1474–1479.
5. Rosado-de-Christenson ML, Templeton PA, Moran CA. Bronchogenic carcinoma: radiologic-pathologic correlation. *Radiographics* 1994;14:429–446.
6. Tateishi M, Fukuhama Y, Hamatake M, et al. Characteristics of non-small cell lung cancer 3 cm or less in diameter. *J Surg Oncol* 1995;59:251–254.
7. Zwirewich CV, Vedal S, Miller RR, et al. Solitary pulmonary nodule: high-resolution CT and radiologic-pathologic correlation. *Radiology* 1991;179:469–476.
8. Swensen SJ, Viggiano RW, Midthun DE, et al. Lung nodule enhancement at CT: multicenter study. *Radiology* 2000;214:73–80.
9. Haque AK. Pathology of carcinoma of lung: an update on current concepts. *J Thorac Imaging* 1991; 7:9–20.
10. Shah RM, Balsara G, Webster M, et al. Bronchioloalveolar cell carcinoma: impact of histology on dominant CT pattern. *J Thorac Imaging* 2000;15:180–186.
11. Jang HJ, Lee KS, Kwon OJ, et al. Bronchioloalveolar carcinoma: focal area of ground-glass attenuation at thin-section CT as an early sign. *Radiology* 1996;199:485–488.
12. Kuriyama K, Tateishi R, Doi O, et al. Prevalence of air bronchograms in small peripheral carcinomas of the lung on thin-section CT: comparison with benign tumors. *Am J Roentgenol* 1991;156: 921–924.
13. Lee KS, Kim Y, Han J, et al. Bronchioloalveolar carcinoma: clinical, histopathologic, and radiologic findings. *Radiographics* 1997;17:1345–1357.
14. Wong JSL, Weisbrod GL, Chamberlain D, et al. Bronchioloalveolar carcinoma and the air bronchogram sign: a new pathologic explanation. *J Thorac Imag* 1994;9:141–144.

15. Weisbrod GL, Chamberlain D, Herman SJ. Cystic change (pseudocavitation) associated with bronchioloalveolar carcinoma: a report of four patients. *J Thorac Imag* 1995;10:106–111.
16. Weisbrod GL, Towers MJ, Chamberlain DW, et al. Thin-walled cystic lesions in bronchioloalveolar carcinoma. *Radiology* 1992;185:401–405.
17. Adler B, Padley S, Miller RR, et al. High-resolution CT of bronchioloalveolar carcinoma. *Am J Roentgenol* 1992;159:275–277.
18. Im J-G, Han MC, Yu EJ, et al. Lobar bronchioloalveolar carcinoma: "angiogram sign" on CT scans. *Radiology* 1990;176:749–753.
19. Walykey MM. And what is your sign? *Radiology* 1991;178:894.
20. Senac JP, Bousquet C, Giron JM, Cousine OS. "Angiogram sign": semiotic value in 60 cases. *Radiology* 1992;185:243.
21. Vincent JM, Ng YY, Norton AJ, et al. CT "angiogram sign" in primary pulmonary lymphoma. *J Comput Assist Tomogr* 1992;16:829–931.
22. Naidich DP, McCauley DI, Khouri NF, et al. Computed tomography of lobar collapse: endobronchial obstruction. *J Comput Assist Tomogr* 1983;7:745–757.
23. Onitsuka H, Tsukuda M, Araki A, et al. Differentiation of central lung tumor from postobstructive lobar collapse by rapid sequence computed tomography. *J Thorac Imaging* 1991;6:28–31.
24. Quoix E, Fraser R. Wolkove N, et al. Small cell lung cancer presenting as a solitary pulmonary nodule. *Cancer* 1990;66:577–582.
25. Yabuuchi H, Murayama S, Sakai S, et al. Resected peripheral small cell carcinoma of the lung: computed tomographic-histologic correlation. *J Thorac Imaging* 1999;14:105–108.
26. Iwasaki Y. Large cell carcinoma. *Nippon Rinsho* 2000;58:1127–1131.

4

LYMPHOPROLIFERATIVE DISORDERS AND LEUKEMIA

DEFINITION AND CLASSIFICATION

Lymphoid tissue is a normal component of the lung and includes (a) *hilar and intrapulmonary peribronchial lymph nodes,* the latter extending to the level of fourth-order bronchi; (b) *bronchus-associated lymphoid tissue* (BALT), consisting of mucosal lymphoid follicles located in distal bronchi and bronchioles, particularly at airway bifurcations (1,2); *peripheral intrapulmonary lymphoreticular aggregates and lymph nodes* that tend to be distributed along interlobular septa and the visceral pleura (c); and (d) widely scattered, *solitary lymphocytes and phagocytic cells* located in the airway epithelium and mucosa (2–4).

As can be seen from this description, pulmonary lymphoid tissue is located predominantly in the axial interstitium (i.e., the interstitial tissue associated with interlobular septa, pulmonary veins and arteries, bronchi, and the pleura) (Fig. 4.1). The various lymphoproliferative disorders and leukemias that affect the lung have a pronounced tendency to involve this interstitial compartment (5,6).

BENIGN LYMPHOPROLIFERATIVE DISORDERS

Lymphocytic Interstitial Pneumonia

Lymphocytic interstitial pneumonia (LIP) is an uncommon lymphoproliferative disorder characterized by diffuse infiltration of the pulmonary parenchymal interstitium (i.e., the alveolar walls) by lymphocytes and plasma cells (3,5). Although the term implies a benign proliferation, the histologic distinction between such a proliferation and low-grade lymphoma can be difficult and may require the use of ancillary immunohistochemical and molecular studies. The abnormality occurs most commonly in patients who have an underlying immunologic abnormality, particularly Sjögren syndrome and AIDS, and less often disorders such as multicentric Castleman's disease, chronic hepatitis, and chronic thyroiditis (5).

Histologically, the lymphoid cells are located predominantly in the interstitial tissue adjacent to intralobular vessels and airways and in the alveolar septa (Fig. 4.2). Although usually more or less diffuse within the lobule, small nodular foci may be seen as a result of localized proliferation or the formation of germinal centers. Fibrosis is usually absent or mild; rarely, it is associated with remodeling and a honeycomb appearance. Airspaces are typically unaffected.

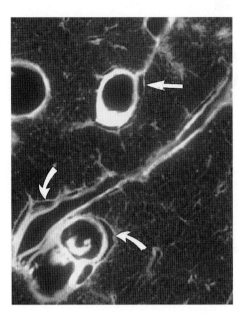

FIGURE 4.1. Pulmonary lymphatics. Contact radiograph of an autopsy lung shows dilated lymphatics adjacent to a pulmonary vein (*straight arrow*) and a bronchovascular bundle (*curved arrows*).

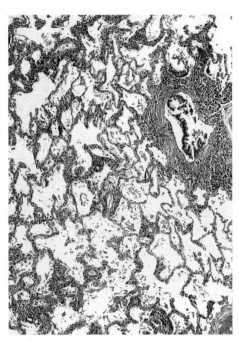

FIGURE 4.2. Lymphocytic interstitial pneumonia. Photomicrograph shows extensive infiltration of the alveolar interstitial tissue by mononuclear cells (shown at higher magnification to be predominantly lymphocytes with scattered plasma cells). The interstitium adjacent to a membranous bronchiole is expanded by the same cellular proliferation. The patient was a 26-year-old man with AIDS.

The most common radiographic findings consist of a reticular or reticulonodular pattern involving mainly the lower lung zones (Fig. 4.3) (7). Other patterns include bilateral ground-glass opacities, foci of consolidation, and small nodules (7,8). Hilar and mediastinal lymph node enlargement, pleural effusion, and honeycombing are uncommon.

The main HRCT findings consist of bilateral areas of ground-glass attenuation and cysts (Fig. 4.4) (9,10). The former reflects the infiltration of the parenchymal interstitium. The cysts tend to be few in number and have a random distribution and thin walls. It has been postulated that they result from overdistension of airspaces distal to bronchioles that are partly obstructed by the lymphocytic infiltrate (10). Other common findings include thickening of bronchovascular bundles (Fig. 4.5), poorly defined centrilobular nodules, and interlobular septal thickening (Fig. 4.3) (10). These findings reflect the involvement of perilymphatic interstitium. Less common HRCT findings include honeycombing, bronchiectasis, areas of airspace consolidation, large nodules, and pleural thickening and effusion. It should be remembered, however, that the presence of consolidation and nodules suggests a more pronounced proliferation of lymphoid cells and raises the possibility of lymphoma (11).

Follicular Bronchiolitis

Follicular bronchiolitis, also known as diffuse lymphoid hyperplasia, is characterized by the presence of more or less discrete foci of hyperplastic lymphoid tissue, often associated with germinal centers, along the bronchovascular bundles (Fig. 4.6) (3,12). Identical tissue also may be present within interlobular septa and the visceral pleura, particularly in patients who have an underlying immunodeficiency disorder (12). The hyperplastic lymphoid foci may compress the adjacent bronchiolar lumen, resulting in obstructive pneumonitis.

The chest radiograph shows a diffuse reticular or reticulonodular pattern (12). Characteristic abnormalities on HRCT include centrilobular nodules, reflecting the foci of

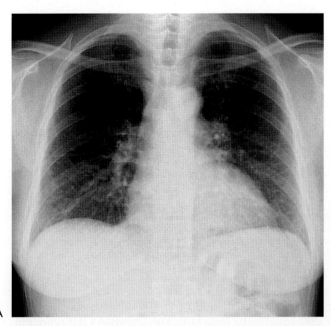

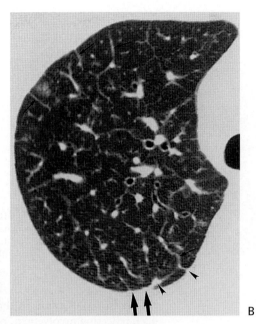

A

B

FIGURE 4.3. Lymphocytic interstitial pneumonia. **A:** Chest radiograph shows a reticulonodular pattern. **B:** HRCT image shows extensive interlobular septal thickening (*thin arrows*). The septa have smooth margins. Subpleural small nodules (arrowheads) and pleural thickening (*thick arrows*) are also seen. The patient was a 32-year-old woman. (Courtesy of Dr. Noboru Maeda, Osaka University Hospital, Suita, Japan.)

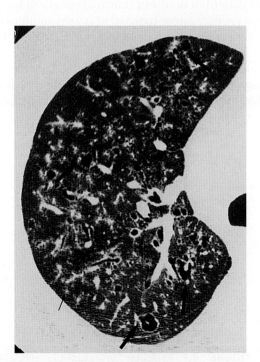

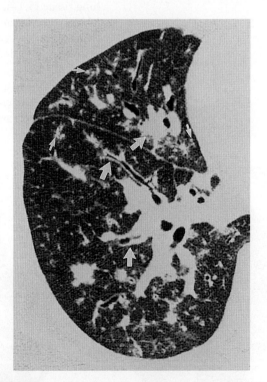

FIGURE 4.4. Lymphocytic interstitial pneumonia. HRCT image demonstrates several thin-walled cysts (*thick arrows*) and several faint centrilobular nodular opacities (*thin arrows*). The patient was a 76-year-old woman.

FIGURE 4.5. Lymphocytic interstitial pneumonia. HRCT image targeted to the right lung demonstrates diffuse thickening of bronchovascular bundles (*large arrows*), peripherally seen as central dots or faint centrilobular nodules (*small arrows*).

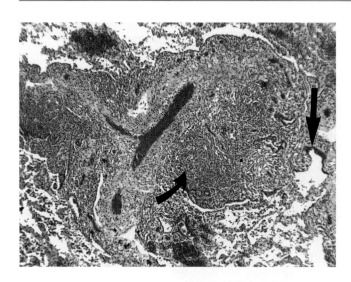

FIGURE 4.6. Follicular bronchiolitis. Photomicrograph shows marked expansion of the interstitial tissue around a membranous bronchiole (*straight arrow*) and its accompanying pulmonary artery. Follicle formation is evident focally (*curved arrow*).

lymphoid proliferation in the bronchiolar interstitium, and ground-glass opacities (Fig. 4.7), reflecting involvement of adjacent alveolar walls (13). Less common CT findings include bronchial wall thickening, bronchial dilatation, interlobular septal thickening, and peribronchovascular airspace consolidation.

MALIGNANT LYMPHOPROLIFERATIVE DISORDERS

Primary Pulmonary Lymphoma

Primary pulmonary lymphoma can be defined as lymphoma that is initially localized in lung tissue (5,14). Most are low-grade B-cell tumors. They are also called BALTomas or MALTomas because of a presumed origin from bronchus (mucosa) associated lymphoid tissue (15). The second most common primary tumor (referred to as angioimmunoproliferative lesion or lymphomatoid granulomatosis) is high grade and may have either a B- or T-cell phenotype.

Grossly, most low-grade B-cell tumors appear as a well-circumscribed nodule or a focal area of parenchymal consolidation (Fig. 4.8). Underlying lung structures such as airways and vessels are often recognizable. Histologically, the tumor consists of small, usually

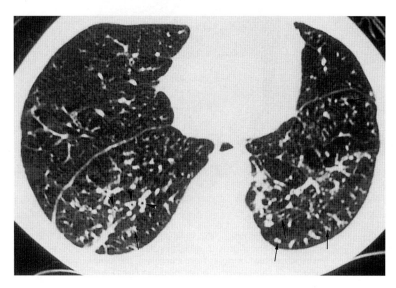

FIGURE 4.7. Follicular bronchiolitis. HRCT image demonstrates centrilobular nodules (*arrows*) and bronchial wall thickening (*arrowheads*). The margins of nodules are poorly defined. The patient was a 45-year-old woman.

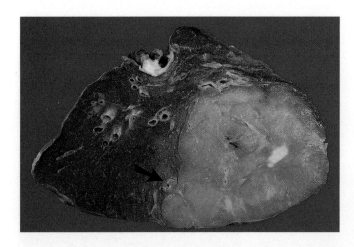

FIGURE 4.8. Low-grade B-cell lymphoma (Maltoma). Transverse slice of an upper lobe shows a well-demarcated tan-colored tumor. Unlike most low-grade B-cell tumors, patent bronchi are not visible in this example; however, focal spread in the interstitial tissue around a small vessel is evident (*arrow*).

only slightly atypical lymphocyte-like or plasmacytoid cells (Fig. 4.9). A distinct perilymphatic interstitial distribution is invariably present, although proliferation of tumor cells in some portions of the tumor may be sufficient to obscure this pattern (Fig. 4.9). Primary high-grade lymphoma consists of cells that generally show more marked cytologic atypia; foci of necrosis and vascular infiltration are common (Fig. 4.10).

The most common radiologic manifestations consist of a solitary nodule or poorly defined focal opacity measuring from 2 to 8 cm in diameter (14) (Fig. 4.11). Other patterns include a localized area of consolidation (Fig. 4.12), which may range from subsegmental areas to an entire lobe, or less commonly, multiple nodules on infiltrates (16).

Typical CT findings include solitary or multifocal nodules or masses and areas of airspace consolidation with an air bronchogram (Fig, 4.11) (17–19). The former appearance is related to proliferation of tumor cells within the interstitium such that the alveolar airspaces and transitional airways are obliterated, simulating parenchymal consolidation. Because the bronchi and membranous bronchioles tend to be unaffected, an air bron-

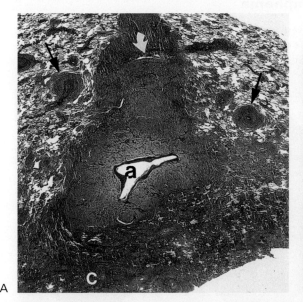
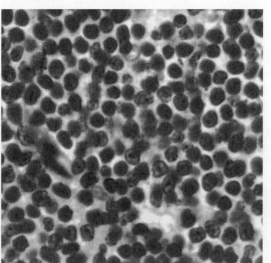

A   B

FIGURE 4.9. Low-grade B-cell lymphoma (Maltoma). **A:** Photomicrograph of a typical low-grade B-cell tumor shows prominent infiltration of the interstitial tissue adjacent to a pulmonary artery (*a*) and its accompanying airway (whose lumen has been compressed to a small slit; *white arrow*). Infiltration of the interstitial tissue around many smaller vessels can be seen (*black arrows*). Expansion of the tumor within the interstitial tissue has resulted in almost complete "consolidation" focally (*c*). **B:** Magnified view of the tumor shows it to consist of small cells that have uniform, round nuclei with small central nucleoli.

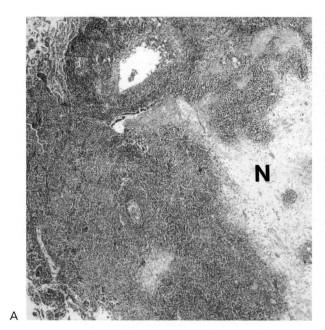
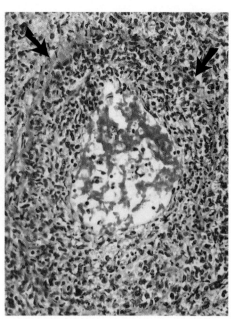

FIGURE 4.10. High-grade B-cell lymphoma. **A:** A poorly delimited focus of neoplastic cell infiltration is evident. Unlike the typical low grade B-cell lymphoma, focal necrosis (*N*) can be seen. **B:** Magnified view shows a dense lymphomatous infiltrate in the wall of a small pulmonary artery (*arrows* = media).

chogram is common. Ground-glass attenuation is seen with less severe interstitial infiltration (Fig. 4.11). Multiple bilateral lesions are common (17–19). Less common CT findings include interlobular septal thickening, centrilobular nodules, and bronchial wall thickening (all three related to perilymphatic interstitial infiltration) and pleural effusion (Fig. 4.13) (18–20).

Secondary Pulmonary Lymphoma

Secondary pulmonary lymphoma occurs more frequently than the primary form (15). It is particularly common in Hodgkin's disease but also occurs in about 5% of patients who have non-Hodgkin's lymphoma (21).

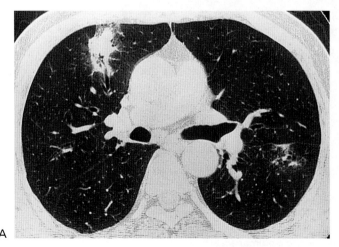
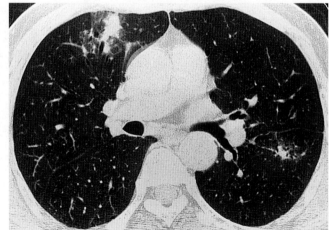

FIGURE 4.11. Low-grade B-cell lymphoma (Maltoma). **A:** HRCT image shows a focal nodular area of consolidation with air bronchograms in the right upper lobe. A small focus of consolidation is present in the left lower lobe. **B:** Image 1 cm caudad to **A** shows focal consolidation and ground-glass opacities in the right upper lobe and a more nodular appearance of the left lower lobe consolidation. Note the peribronchial distribution of both lesions.

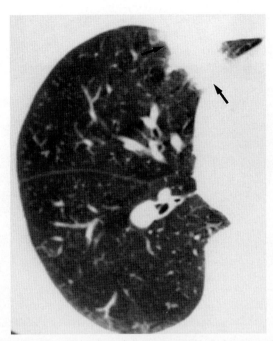

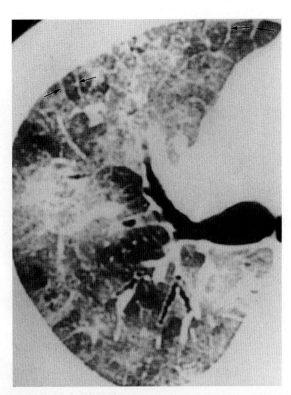

FIGURE 4.12. Low-grade B-cell lymphoma (Maltoma). An HRCT image shows focal area of consolidation in right middle lobe (*arrow*). The consolidation had increased slightly in extent over a 1-year period. The patient was a 70-year-old woman.

FIGURE 4.13. Primary pulmonary B-cell lymphoma. HRCT image demonstrates areas of airspace consolidation, extensive ground-glass attenuation, and a few thickened interlobular septa (*arrows*). The patient was a 35-year-old man.

Radiographic findings of pulmonary involvement are similar in the two forms of lymphoma (22–24), and they are thus described together. The typical radiographic pattern consists of solitary or multiple nodules or masses ranging from 0.5 to 8 cm in diameter (22,24)). They involve mainly the lower lobes (25). The nodules are round, ovoid, or polyhedral in shape and usually have poorly defined and irregular margins.

Common HRCT findings include single or multiple nodules (Fig. 4.14), a focal mass, or masslike consolidation (Fig. 4.15) (23–25). An air bronchogram and air bronchiologram are often evident on HRCT, reflecting the infiltrative but nondestructive growth of the tumor cells. Hilar and mediastinal lymph node enlargement is usually present. Less common CT findings include thickening of bronchovascular bundles, interlobular septal thickening (Fig. 4.15), pleural thickening, and ground-glass attenuation (23–25). As with primary pulmonary lymphoma, the first three are related to infiltration of the perilymphatic interstitium and the last to extension of tumor cells into the parenchymal interstitium and airspaces.

Pulmonary Lymphoma in Patients with AIDS

Most AIDS-related lymphomas can be classified as large cell (immunoblastic) or Burkitt-like (26,27). The vast majority have a B-cell phenotype and many (50% to 85%) are associated with Epstein-Barr virus genome (26). They tend to have a poor prognosis (26) and to occur at a relatively advanced stage of immunosuppression, usually in patients with CD4 level of less than 100 cells/mm^3. In contrast, Hodgkin's lymphoma tends to occur early in the course of AIDS, usually when the CD4 cell counts are greater than 200 cells/mm^3 (26).

Disease in the thorax is typically extranodal (28). The most common radiographic findings consist of single or multiple nodules (29,30). Characteristically, they are discrete

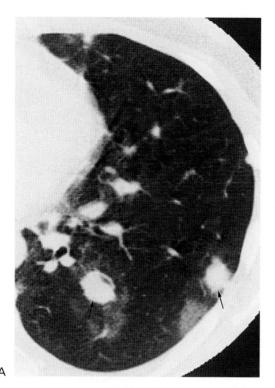
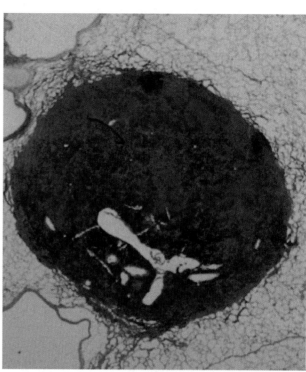

FIGURE 4.14. Secondary pulmonary lymphoma. **A:** HRCT image demonstrates nodules that have well-defined margins (*arrows*) and are surrounded by areas with ground-glass attenuation (Halo sign). **B:** Photomicrograph of one of the nodules shows it to surround several patent bronchioles. The patient was a 45-year-old man.

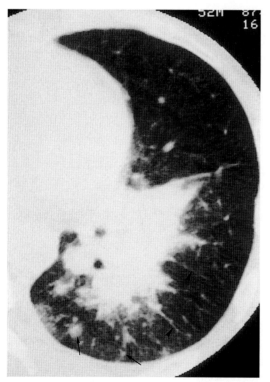

FIGURE 4.15. Secondary pulmonary Hodgkin's disease. HRCT image demonstrates focal peribronchial airspace consolidation. Faint small nodules (*arrows*), ground-glass attenuation opacities, and interlobular septal thickening (*arrowheads*) are also evident.

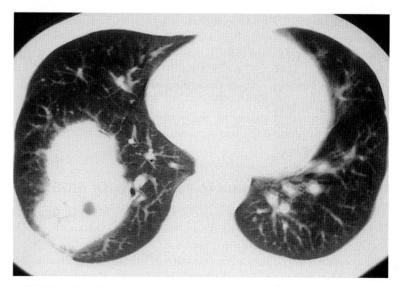

FIGURE 4.16. AIDS-related non-Hodgkin's lymphoma. CT image (10-mm collimation) demonstrates a well-defined mass with focal cavitation in the right lower lobe. The patient was a 35-year-old man with AIDS.

and usually have well-defined, smooth margins (Fig. 4.16). A solitary, well-defined nodule is particularly common and should be considered suggestive of AIDS-related lymphoma (28,31). Larger masses sometimes cavitate (31,32). Interstitial infiltrates in the absence of the masses or nodules are rare (33). Dense airspace consolidation may also be seen (26,29). Lymph node enlargement, pleural effusion, or both are present in approximately 30% of cases (30,34).

An additional rare form of AIDS-related B-cell lymphoma that presents as pleural, pericardial, or peritoneal effusions in the absence of a discrete tumor is known as body-cavity-based or primary effusion lymphoma (35).

Posttransplant Lymphoproliferative Disorders

Posttransplant lymphoproliferative disorders (PTLDs) comprise a spectrum of Epstein-Barr virus (EBV)–related B-lymphocyte proliferations occurring after exogeneous immunosuppression in organ allograft recipients (36,37). Patients receiving cyclosporin A and/or anti-T-lymphocyte monoclonal antibodies are at greatest risk and frequently develop the complication within weeks or months of initiating immunosuppressive therapy (36,37). Histologic findings are variable and range from nonspecific hyperplasia to high-grade immunoblastic lymphoma to myeloma.

The most common chest radiographic finding consists of pulmonary nodules (38,39). The characteristic HRCT findings consist of multiple well-circumscribed nodules with or without halo of ground-glass attenuation and areas of airspace consolidation (Fig. 4.17) (29,39). The nodules may be smooth or irregular and range from less than 1 to several centimeters in diameter (39). They tend to have a peribronchial or subpleural distribution (39), reflecting involvement of the interstitial tissue in these locations. In approximately 30% of cases the nodules are surrounded by a halo of ground-glass attenuation (39). This

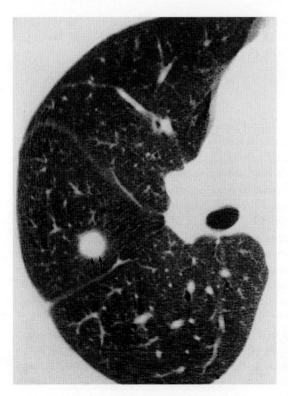

FIGURE 4.17. Posttransplant lymphoproliferative disorder. HRCT image demonstrates a nodule (*arrows*) surrounded by a thin halo of ground-glass attenuation. The patient was a 28-year-old man.

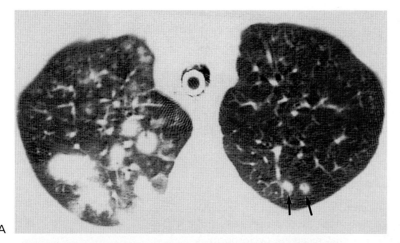

A

FIGURE 4.18. Posttransplant lymphoproliferative disorder. **A:** HRCT image shows several nodules and focal areas of consolidation and ground-glass attenuation in the right upper lobe. Note presence of a halo of ground-glass attenuation surrounding several of the right upper lobe nodules. Two small nodules are present in left upper lobe (*arrows*). **B:** Transverse slice of the right upper lobe at autopsy shows several nodules with a dark core due to hemorrhage and a surrounding lighter halo. Microscopic examination showed that the halo was due to less dense infiltration of the parenchyma by malignant cells. **C:** Photomicrograph shows high grade lymphoma that has a plasmacytoid appearance, consistent with B-cell differentiation.

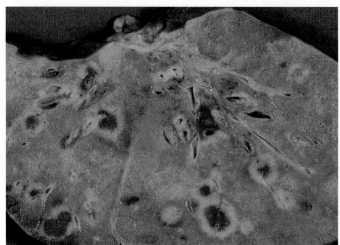

B

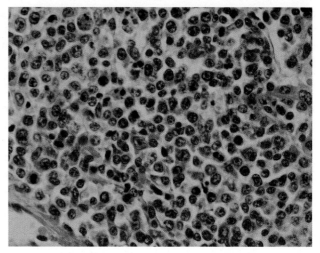

C

halo has been shown to reflect the presence of less dense infiltration of the adjacent parenchyma by malignant cells (Fig. 4.18) (40). Hilar or mediastinal lymph node enlargement is present in approximately 30% of cases (39).

LEUKEMIA

Pulmonary infiltration by leukemic cells is found at autopsy in nearly two-thirds of patients who have leukemia. However, in most cases the infiltrate is mild and unassociated with clinical or radiologic abnormalities. In fact, radiologic abnormalities in patients who have leukemia are much more likely to result from other processes than leukemic infiltration. For example, in an autopsy review of 60 patients who died from acute or chronic leukemia, radiographically demonstrable disease was related to hemorrhage in 74%, infection in 67%, edema or congestion in 57%, and leukemic infiltration in only 26% (41). Leukemic infiltrates identified during life probably occur in no more than about 5% of patients (41). In most, they are incidental findings; however, respiratory failure has been described (42,43).

Pathologically, leukemic involvement of the lung can have several patterns. As with lymphoma, the most common is localized infiltration of the perilymphatic interstitial tissue (Fig. 4.19) (44). In patients who have acute or chronic myelogenous leukemia, localized expansion of such an infiltrate can result in a mass of leukemic cells (granulocytic sarcoma) (43). Usually, this presents as one or more peripheral parenchymal nodules; occasionally, the tumor affects a bronchus (and may lead to obstruction) or involves the pleura (43,44). Large numbers of blasts in the blood (usually between 100,000 and 500,000/mm^3) may be sufficient to distend small vessels and simulate parenchymal interstitial thickening (pulmonary leukostasis).

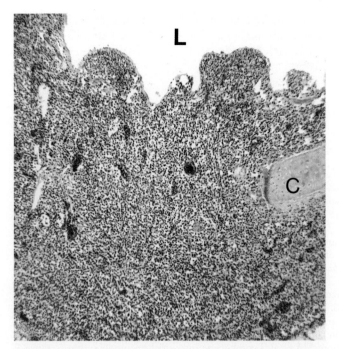

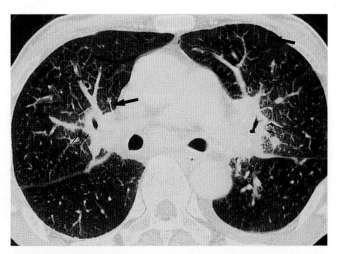

FIGURE 4.20. Acute lymphocytic leukemia. HRCT image reveals smooth thickening of interlobular septa (*thick arrows*) and bronchovascular bundles (*thin arrows*). The patient was a 27-year-old man.

FIGURE 4.19. Acute myeloblastic leukemia. Photomicrograph shows a dense neoplastic cellular infiltrate expanding the wall of a small bronchus. (Abbreviations: *C* = cartilage; *L* = airway lumen.)

The usual radiographic pattern of pulmonary parenchymal involvement consists of a diffuse bilateral reticulation or linearity that resembles interstitial edema or lymphangitic carcinomatosis (41,45). This correlates with the perilymphatic localization of the infiltrate demonstrable histologically. The corresponding HRCT findings consist of thickening of interlobular septa, small nodules (Fig. 4.20), and thickening of bronchovascular bundles (46). Areas of ground-glass attenuation and consolidation (Fig. 4.21) are also common. The

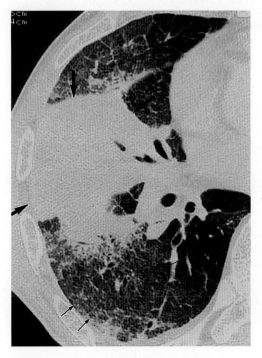

FIGURE 4.21. Adult T-cell leukemia. HRCT image scan shows areas of airspace consolidation (*thick arrows*) and ground-glass attenuation (*thin arrows*). The patient was a 45-year-old woman.

former may reflect infiltration of the alveolar interstitium by leukemic cells or alveolar capillary leukostasis. The consolidation tends to have a peribronchial distribution and may be the result of direct extension of tumor cells from the peribronchial interstitium into the adjacent airspaces.

REFERENCES

1. Okada Y, Magari S, Ito Y, Nagaishi C. Anatomical study of the pulmonary lymphatics. *Lymphology* 1979;12:118–125.
2. Bienestock J, ed. Bronchus-associated lymphoid tissue. In *Immunology of the lung and upper respiratory tract.* New York: McGraw-Hill, 1984:96–118.
3. Kradin R, Mark E. Benign lymphoid disorders of the lung. *Hum Pathol* 1983;14:857–867.
4. Berman J, Beer D, Theodore A, et al. Lymphocyte recruitment to the lung. *Am Rev Respir Dis* 1990;142:238–257.
5. Koss MN. Pulmonary lymphoid disorders. *Semin Diagn Pathol* 1995;12:158–171.
6. Colby TV, Swensen SJ. Anatomic distribution and histopathologic patterns in diffuse lung disease: correlation with HRCT. *J Thorac Imag* 1996;11:1–26.
7. Julsrud PR, Brown LR, Li CY, et al. Pulmonary process of mature-appearing lymphocytes: pseudolymphoma, well-differentiated lymphocytic lymphoma, and lymphocytic interstitial pneumonia. *Radiology* 1978;127:289–296.
8. Feigin DS, Siegelman SS, Theros EG, et al. Nonmalignant lymphoid disorders of the chest. *Am J Roentgenol* 1977;129:221–228.
9. Johkoh T, Müller NL, Pickford HA et al. Lymphocytic interstitial pneumonia: thin-section CT findings in 22 patients. *Radiology* 1999;212:567–572.
10. Ichikawa Y, Kinoshita M, Tog T, et al. Lung cyst formation in lymphocytic interstitial pneumonia: CT features. *J Comput Assist Tomogr* 1994;18:745–748.
11. Honda O, Johkoh T, Ichikado K, et al. Differential diagnosis of lymphocytic interstitial pneumonia and malignant lymphoma on high-resolution CT. *Am J Roentgenol* 1999;173:71–74.
12. Yousem SA, Colby TV, Carrington CB. Follicular bronchitis/bronchiolitis. *Hum Pathol* 1985;16:700–706.
13. Howling SJ, Hansell DM, Wells AU, et al. Follicular bronchiolitis: thin-section CT and histologic findings. *Radiology* 1999;212:637–642.
14. Addis BJ, Hyek E, Isaacson PG. Primary pulmonary lymphoma: a reappraisal of its histogenesis and its relationship to pseudolymphoma and lymphoid interstitial pneumonia. *Histopathology* 1988;13:1–17.
15. Harris NL, Jaffe ES, Stein H, et al. A revised European-American classification of lymphoid neoplasms: a proposal from the International Lymphoma Study group. *Blood* 1994;84:1361–1392.
16. O'Donnel PG, Jackson SA, Tung KT, et al. Radiological appearance of lymphoma arising from mucosa-associated lymphoid tissue (MALT) in the lung. *Clin Radiol* 1998;53:258–263.
17. Wislez M, Cadranel J, Antoine M, et al. Lymphoma of pulmonary mucosa-associated lymphoid tissues: CT scan findings and pathological correlations. *Eur Respir J* 1999;14:423–429.
18. Lee DK, Im J-G, Lee KS, et al. B-cell lymphoma of bronchus-associated lymphoid tissue (BALT): CT features in 10 patients. *J Comput Assist Tomogr* 2000;24:30–34.
19. King LJ, Padley SPG, Worhterspoon AC, et al. Pulmonary MALT lymphoma: imaging findings in 24 cases. *Eur Radiol* 2000;10:1932–1938.
20. Ooi GC, Chim CS, Lee AKW, et al. Computed tomography features of primary pulmonary non-Hodgkin's lymphoma. *Clin Radiol* 1999;54:438–443.
21. Mentzer S, Reilly J, Skarin A, et al. Patterns of lung involvement by malignant lymphoma. *Surgery* 1993;113:507–514.
22. Filly R, Blank N, Castellino RA. Radiographic distribution of intrathoracic disease in previously untreated patients with Hodgkin's disease and non-Hodgkin's lymphoma. *Radiology* 1976;120:277–281.
23. Au V, Lung AN. Radiologic manifestations of lymphoma in the thorax. *Am J Roentgenol* 1997;168:93–98.
24. Lee KS, Kim Y, Primack SL. Imaging of pulmonary lymphomas. *Am J Roentgenol* 1997;168:339–345.
25. Castellino RA, Hilton S, O'Brien JP, et al. Non-Hodgkin lymphoma: contribution of chest CT in the initial staging evaluation. *Radiology* 1996;199:129–132.
26. Wang CY, Snow JL, Su WPD. Lymphoma associated with human immunodeficiency virus infection. *Mayo Clin Proc* 1995;70:665–672.
27. Ioachin HL, Dorsett B, Cronin W, et al. Acquired immunodeficiency syndrome-associated lymphoma: clinical, pathologic, immunology, and viral characteristics in 111 cases. *Hum Pathol* 1991;22:659–673.

28. Sider LN, Weiss AJ, Smith M.D., et al. Varied appearance of AIDS-related lymphoma in the chest. *Radiology* 1989;171:629–632.
29. Carrignan S, Staples CA, Müller NL. Intrathoracic lymphoproliferative disorders in the immuno-compromised patients: CT findings. *Radiology* 1995;197:53–58.
30. Eisner MD, Kaplan LD, Herndier B et al. The pulmonary manifestations of AIDS-related non-Hodgkin's lymphoma. *Chest* 1996;110:729–736.
31. Blunt DM, Padley SPG. Radiographic manifestations of AIDS related lymphoma in the thorax. *Clin Radiol* 1995;50:607–612.
32. Ray P, Antoine M, Mary-Kraus M, et al. AIDS-related primary pulmonary lymphoma. *Am J Respir Crit Care Med* 1998;158:1221–1229.
33. Polish LB, Coh DL, Myers AM, et al. Pulmonary non-Hodgkin's lymphoma in AIDS. *Chest* 1989;86:1321–1326.
34. Huang L, Stansell JD. AIDS and the lung. *Med Clin North Am* 1996;80:755–800.
35. Arsani MQ, Dawson DB, Nador R, et al. Primary body cavity-based AIDS-related lymphomas. *Am J Clin Pathol* 1996;105:221–229.
36. Craig F, Gulley M, Banks P. Posttransplantation lymphoproliferative disorders. *Am J Clin Pathol* 1993;99:265–276.
37. Swerdlow S. Post-transplant lymphoproliferative disorders: a morphologic, phenotypic, and geno-typic spectrum of disease. *Histopathology* 1992;20:373–385.
38. Dodd GD, Ledesma-Medina J, Baron RL, Fuhrman CR. Posttransplant lymphoproliferative disor-ders: intrathoracic manifestations. *Radiology* 1992;184:65–69.
39. Collins J, Müller NL, Leung AN, et al. Epstein-Barr-Virus-associated lymphoproliferative disease of the lung: CT and histologic findings. *Radiology* 1998;208:749–759.
40. Brown MJ, Miller RR, Müller NL. Acute lung disease in the immunocompromised host: CT and pathologic examination findings. *Radiology* 1994;190:247–254
41. Maile CW, Moore AV, Ulreich S, et al. Chest radiographic-pathologic correlation in adult leukemia patients. *Invest Radiol* 1983;18:495–499.
42. Colby TV. Lymphoproliferative diseases. In: Dail DH, Hammer SA, eds. *Pulmonary pathology*, 2nd ed. New York: Springer-Verlag, 1994:1097–1122.
43. Dougdale DC, Salness TA, Knight L, et al. Endobronchial granulocytic sarcoma causing acute res-piratory failure in acute myelogenous leukemia. *Am Rev Respir Dis* 1987;136:1248–1250.
44. Myers JL, Kurtin PJ. Lymphoid proliferative disorders of the lung. In: Thurlbeck WM, Churg AM eds. *Pathology of the lung*, 2nd ed. New York: Thieme Medical , 1995:553–588.
45. Green RA, Nichols NJ. Pulmonary involvement of leukemia. *Am Rev Respir Dis* 1959:833–840.
46. Heyneman LE, Johkoh T, Ward S, et al. Pulmonary leukemic infiltrates: high-resolution CT find-ings in 10 patients. *Am J Roentgenol* 2000;174:517–521.

5

MISCELLANEOUS NEOPLASMS

MALIGNANT NEOPLASMS
Miscellaneous Primary Malignant Neoplasms
Metastatic Neoplasms

BENIGN NEOPLASMS
Tracheobronchial Papillomas
Hamartoma

TUMORS OF NONNEOPLASTIC NATURE

MALIGNANT NEOPLASMS

Miscellaneous Primary Malignant Neoplasms

Carcinoid Tumor

Carcinoid tumors are low-grade malignant neuroendocrine neoplasms that comprise about 1% to 2% of primary lung tumors (1,2). The majority (80% to 90%) arise in lobar, segmental, or proximal subsegmental bronchi (3,4), where they appear as tan-colored, well-circumscribed, polypoid masses that protrude into the airway lumen (Fig. 5.1A). A variable amount of tumor extends beyond the cartilage plates into the surrounding lung parenchyma. The remaining 10% to 20% of tumors present as well-circumscribed nodules in the lung periphery (Fig. 5.1B). Because most carcinoid tumors are low grade and relatively slow growing, they tend to compress rather than infiltrate the adjacent lung, resulting in a smooth junction between the two.

Both endobronchial and peripheral tumors can be classified histologically into typical and atypical subtypes. The neoplastic cells in both forms are grouped in small nests or trabeculae separated by a prominent vascular stroma (Fig. 5.2A). The latter may be associated with a small or large amount of fibrous tissue. Calcification or ossification of this fibrous stroma is responsible for the calcification seen radiologically in many cases (Fig. 5.2B). Individual tumor cells contain ample cytoplasm, round to oval, uniformly sized nuclei and rare mitotic figures (Fig. 5.3); necrosis is absent. Atypical carcinoid tumors have a similar overall architectural pattern but increased mitotic activity and/or foci of necrosis (Figs. 5.3 and 5.4) (5). As might be expected form this description, atypical carcinoids have a greater propensity to infiltrate the adjacent lung (Fig. 5.5) and to metastasize than typical carcinoids and are associated with a significantly poorer prognosis.

The most common radiologic presentation of carcinoid tumors consists of a nodule or mass (6,7) (Fig. 5.4). Typical carcinoids tend to be smaller (average diameter, 2 cm) than atypical carcinoids (average diameter, 4 cm) (6). As indicated earlier, most typical carcinoids have smooth margins, whereas atypical tumors usually have irregular ones (6,7). The endobronchial location of the tumor is difficult to appreciate on the radiograph but can often be seen on CT (Fig. 5.6). Segmental or lobar atelectasis and obstructive pneumonitis are present in approximately 30% of typical carcinoids (6,7). Segmental oligemia as a result of decreased ventilation and hypoxic vasoconstriction is seen in some tumors that cause partial obstruction. Both of these secondary effects on distal lung parenchyma are uncommon in atypical carcinoids. Because of their vascular stroma, most carcinoid tumors show marked enhancement following intravenous administration of contrast (6,8). Approximately 30% have foci of calcification evident on CT (9).

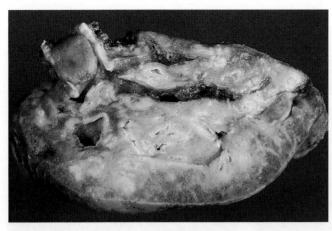
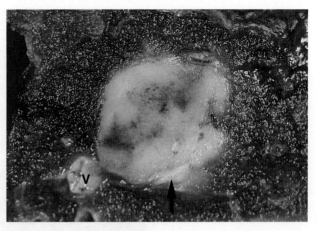

A   B

FIGURE 5.1. Carcinoid tumor—central and peripheral types. **A:** Transverse slice of right middle lobe shows a round, tan-colored tumor obstructing the lobar bronchus. There is minimal invasion of the bronchial wall. The middle lobe shows changes of obstructive pneumonitis. **B:** Magnified view of another (peripheral) tumor shows it to be well-circumscribed with a border that appears to compress rather than infiltrate the adjacent lung parenchyma. Although this tumor has arisen in a membranous bronchiole (one somewhat distorted wall is indicated by an *arrow* and its accompanying pulmonary artery by V), the distal lung shows no evidence of airway obstruction, presumably because of collateral ventilation.

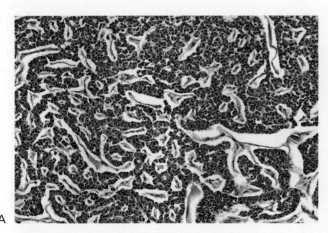
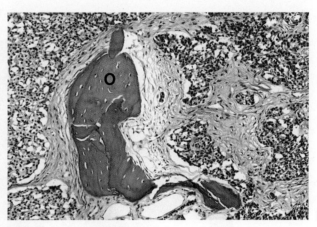

A   B

FIGURE 5.2. Carcinoid tumor. **A:** Photomicrograph of a typical carcinoid tumor shows interconnecting trabeculae of uniform cells separated by numerous thin-walled blood vessels. (The spaces between the vessels and the tumor are an artifact of tissue processing.) Connective tissue adjacent to the vessels is minimal. **B:** Section of another tumor shows much more abundant connective tissue, focally containing bone (*O*).

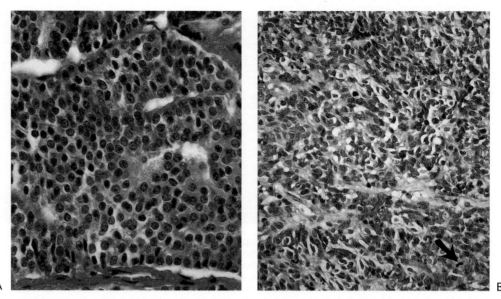

A
B

FIGURE 5.3. Carcinoid tumor. Photomicrographs show typical (**A**) and atypical (**B**) carcinoid tumors. Nuclei of tumor cells in **A** are round and similar in size and shape. Those in **B** show much more variation; a mitotic figure is evident (*arrow*).

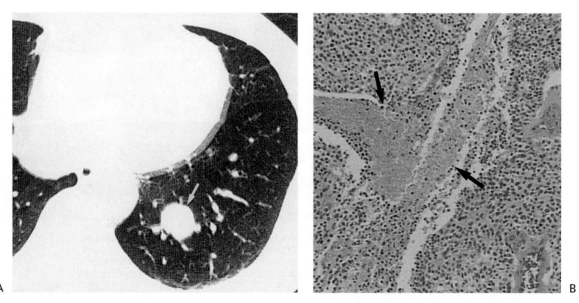

A
B

FIGURE 5.4. Atypical carcinoid tumor. **A:** CT image (1.0-mm collimation) shows a well-circumscribed nodule (*arrow*) in the left lower lobe. **B:** Photomicrograph of the tumor shows it to consist of cells that have moderately abundant cytoplasm and relatively uniform round to oval nuclei suggestive of a typical carcinoid tumor. However, focal necrosis is evident (*arrows*), indicating that the tumor should be classified as atypical.

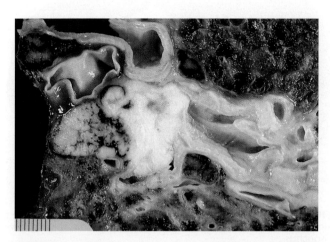

FIGURE 5.5. Atypical carcinoid tumor. Magnified view of the right lung near the hilum shows a somewhat lobulated white tumor obstructing the bronchus intermedius and the superior segmental bronchus (*arrow*) of the lower lobe. The tumor extends through the bronchial wall into adjacent lymph nodes. Although this appearance could be seen with a typical carcinoid tumor, it is more characteristic of the atypical form (confirmed on histologic examination).

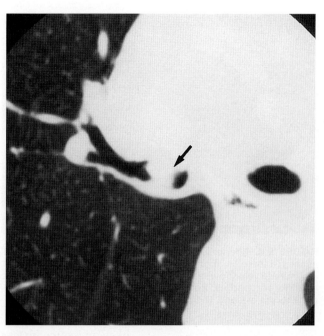

FIGURE 5.6. Carcinoid tumor. CT image (1.5-mm collimation) demonstrates a tumor (*arrow*) in the lumen of the right main bronchus. Bronchoscopy confirmed a diagnosis of carcinoid tumor.

Carcinomas of Tracheobronchial Glands

Neoplasms derived from the tracheobronchial glands account for less than 0.5% of all lung neoplasms (10). Several histologic subtypes have been described, the most common being adenoid cystic carcinoma and mucoepidermoid carcinoma (11). Because glands are normally much more common in the trachea and proximal bronchi than the distal airways, most tumors are seen in these locations. In fact, adenoid cystic carcinoma comprises approximately 40% to 50% of primary malignant tracheal neoplasms.

Adenoid cystic carcinoma consists of tubular or cribriform clusters of cells associated with relatively abundant mucoid stroma. Grossly, it usually presents as a sessile, polypoid mass (Fig. 5.7). Because the glands in which it arises are submucosal, the overlying ep-

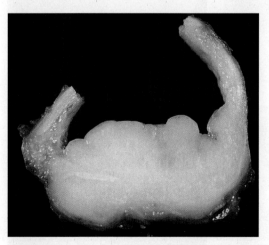

A

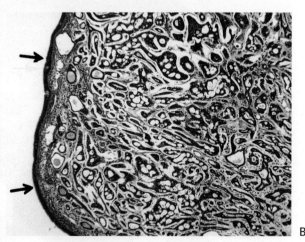

B

FIGURE 5.7. Adenoid cystic carcinoma. **A:** Cross-section of the trachea (opened anteriorly) shows a white tumor expanding the mucosa and the submucosal connective tissue. The tumor has a somewhat polypoid appearance at the luminal aspect. **B:** Section at the tracheal surface shows the epithelium overlying the tumor to be intact (*arrows*). The tumor itself consists of irregularly shaped nests of cells containing many glandlike spaces, a pattern characteristic of adenoid cystic carcinoma.

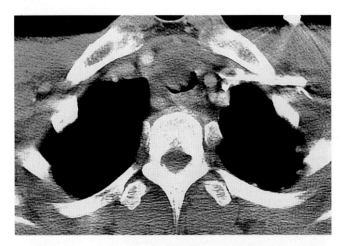

FIGURE 5.8. Adenoid cystic carcinoma. Contrast-enhanced CT image (7-mm collimation) CT scan obtained at the level of the left innominate vein shows a lesion in the right anterior aspect of the intrathoracic trachea. Both intraluminal and extraluminal components are evident. The patient was a 29-year-old man.

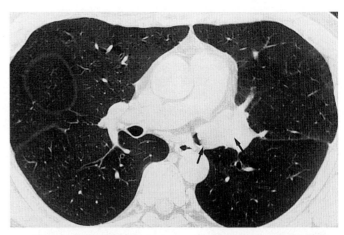

FIGURE 5.9. Adenoid cystic carcinoma. CT image (1-mm collimation) shows an intraluminal mass (*arrows*) in the distal left main bronchus.

ithelium is often intact and the luminal surface smooth. More advanced tumors may show annular or diffusely infiltrative growth, the latter sometimes resulting in extensive thickening of the tracheal (Fig. 5.8) or bronchial (Fig. 5.9) wall (8,12). Infiltration of the airway wall and adjacent tissues is well seen on CT (7).

As its name suggests, mucoepidermoid carcinoma is characterized by a mixture of mucus-secreting cells and cells that have a squamous appearance. It usually presents as a polypoid endobronchial tumor, most commonly in a segmental bronchus (Fig. 5.10), occa-

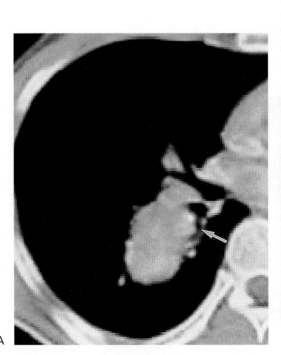

A

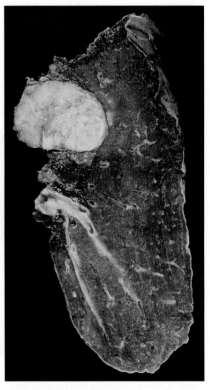

B

FIGURE 5.10. Mucoepidermoid carcinoma. **A:** CT image (10-mm collimation) shows a mass in the superior segment of the right lower lobe. The air-filled bronchial lumen (*arrow*) is displaced medial to the mass. **B:** Sagittal section of the excised specimen shows a well-circumscribed intrabronchial mass. The patient was a 27-year-old man.

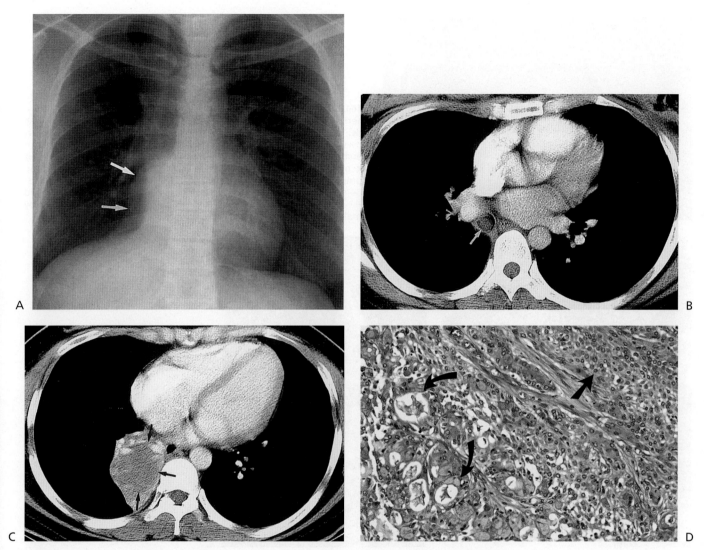

FIGURE 5.11. Mucoepidermoid carcinoma, low grade. **A:** Chest radiograph shows right lower lobe atelectasis (*arrows*). **B:** Contrast-enhanced CT image (7-mm collimation) demonstrates an endobronchial lesion (*arrow*) in the bronchus intermedius. **C:** Scan obtained 3.5 cm caudad to **B** shows the tumor (*arrows*) in the right lower lobar bronchus as well as right lower lobe atelectasis. **C:** Photomicrograph of the excised tumor shows glandular spaces containing mucus (*curved arrows*) admixed with sheets of epidermoid cells (*straight arrow*). The patient was a 26-year-old woman.

sionally in a main or lobar bronchus or the trachea, and rarely in the peripheral lung (13). Histologically, they are classified as low or high grade, depending on the degree of cytologic atypia and glandular differentiation (Fig. 5.11). The former are usually confined to the airway lumen and wall, whereas the latter frequently extend into the surrounding lung (13,14). Radiologically, the tumors can present as a solitary nodule or as parenchymal consolidation or atelectasis (13,14) (Figs. 5.10 and 5.11). CT usually demonstrates a smoothly marginated or lobulated nodule or mass within bronchi (Fig. 5.11) or trachea (8,14). Obstructive pneumonitis or atelectasis are usually present distal to the tumor (13,14).

Kaposi's Sarcoma

Kaposi's sarcoma occurs in two different conditions: (a) in elderly individuals without underlying disease (classic form) and, much more common, (b) in patients who have AIDS

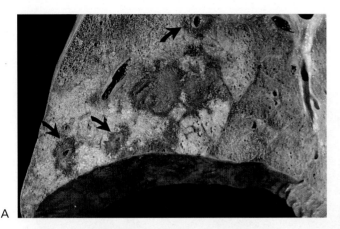

A

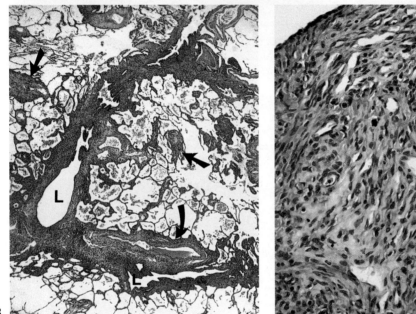

B

C

FIGURE 5.12. Kaposi's sarcoma. **A:** Magnified view of the basal segments of a lower lobe shows several irregularly shaped hemorrhagic foci, most of which are clearly centered about vessels and airways (*arrows*). **B:** Photomicrograph confirms the presence of tumor in the interstitial tissue of two membranous bronchioles (*L* = lumen) and their accompanying pulmonary arteries (*curved arrow*). Extension of the tumor into the adjacent parenchyma is evident in the interstitial tissue surrounding several small vessels (*straight arrows*). **C:** Magnified view shows the tumor to consist of spindle-shaped cells separated by small vessels and numerous red blood cells.

or receive immune-suppression therapy. Disease in the latter patients is usually much more aggressive (15,16).

Pulmonary involvement occurs initially in the interstitial tissue of the bronchovascular bundles, interlobular septa, and pleura (Fig. 5.12) (17). Infiltration into the adjacent lung parenchyma may result in nodules or poorly defined areas of "consolidation." Histologically, the tumor is composed of clusters of cytologically atypical spindle cells between which are numerous slitlike vascular spaces containing hemosiderin-laden macrophages and red blood cells (Fig. 5.12) (16). The latter are responsible for a hemorrhagic appearance on gross examination.

The most common radiographic abnormality consists of nodular opacities usually measuring 1 to 2 cm in diameter and having irregular or poorly defined margins (17–19). The abnormalities tend to be bilateral and symmetric, and in 90% of patients involve mainly the perihilar regions (20). Other common findings are bronchial wall thickening and thickening of interlobular septa (Kerley B lines) (19,20).

HRCT demonstrates bronchial wall thickening, peribronchial consolidation, and multiple bilateral nodules with irregular margins in a predominantly peribronchovascular distribution (19,21). The nodules usually have markedly irregular ("flame-shaped") or poorly defined margins (19,21,22), reflecting the extension of tumor within the peri-

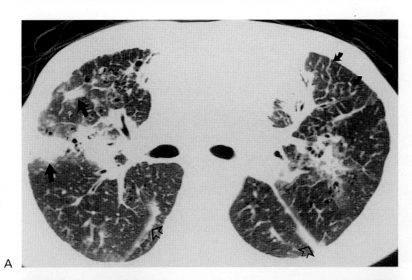

A

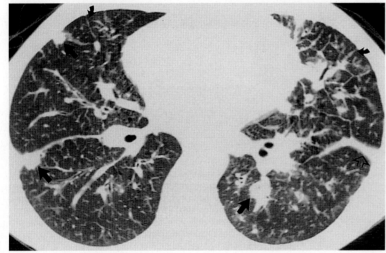

B

FIGURE 5.13. Kaposi's sarcoma. HRCT images (1.5-mm collimation) at the level of the main bronchi (**A**) and inferior pulmonary veins (**B**) demonstrate bilateral nodules with irregular margins (*large, solid arrows*) and interlobular septal thickening (*small, curved arrows*). Also note thickening of interlobar fissures (*open arrows*) due to small pleural effusions. The patient was a 36-year-old man with AIDS.

bronchovascular interstitial tissue (Fig. 5.13). Other abnormalities include interlobular septal thickening, mass lesions, and peribronchial consolidation (19,21,22). The last-named may result from tumor infiltration, hemorrhage, or pneumonitis secondary to airway obstruction. Hilar (Fig. 5.14) or mediastinal lymph node enlargement, often the result of tumor infiltration, is present in approximately 20% of patients (18,22) and pleural effusion in 40% to 50% (18,22).

Metastatic Neoplasms

Pulmonary metastases are common, being seen in 20% to 50% of patients who die of malignant disease (23,24). The most frequent sources are the breast, colon, kidney, head, and neck (25,26). All these tumors metastasize most commonly via the pulmonary arteries; however, spread via lymphatics is also important with some neoplasms, such as breast carcinoma. Less common routes include the bronchial arteries and airways (26,27). Several pathologic and radiologic patterns of pulmonary metastases can be considered. The most common are single or multiple parenchymal nodules and lymphangitic carcinomatosis. Intravascular tumor emboli and airway (endobronchial) metastases are relatively uncommon. Spiral CT is currently the imaging modality of choice for the detection of nodular metastases and HRCT for lymphangitic spread.

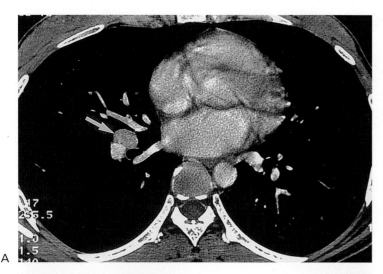

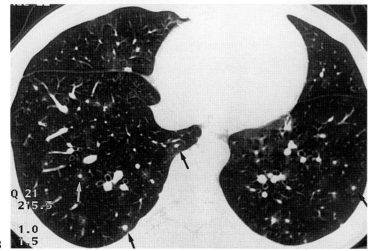

FIGURE 5.14. Kaposi's sarcoma. **A:** Contrast-enhanced HRCT image (1.5-mm collimation) shows right hilar lymph node enlargement (*arrow*). **B:** Image at a more caudad level shows small nodules with a surrounding halo of ground-glass attenuation (*arrows*). The patient was a 29-year-old woman who developed Kaposi's sarcoma following renal transplantation.

Parenchymal Nodules

The most common pattern of pulmonary metastases is multiple nodules (23). They usually involve mainly the lower lung zones (reflecting greater blood flow in these regions as a result of gravity) and the subpleural regions (23,28). Radiologically, most range from several millimeters to several centimeters in diameter. However, individual nodules can be very large or can merge with their neighbors to form a large mass (sometimes occupying an entire lobe) and, in their earliest stage, clearly are only visible microscopically. Most nodules have smooth margins (Fig. 5.15), probably because they grow relatively uniformly in all directions from their original focus; however, nodules with spiculated or poorly defined margins can be seen (28–30). One group of investigators compared the appearance of pulmonary metastases on HRCT with the histopathologic findings in lung specimens obtained at autopsy (30). They classified the margins of nodular metastases into four types according to their histologic appearance at the growing edge of the tumor: (a) expanding type (tumors that compress the surrounding normal lung), (b) alveolar space-filling type (tumors that infiltrate and fill the alveolar spaces), (c) alveolar cell type (tumors that grow along the alveolar walls similar to bronchioloalveolar carcinoma), and (d) interstitial proliferation type (tumors that infiltrate the interstitium). Nodules that had well-defined, smooth margins on HRCT scans (Fig. 5.16) corresponded to the expanding and alveolar space-filling types, nodules that had poorly defined margins (Fig. 5.17) tended to be the

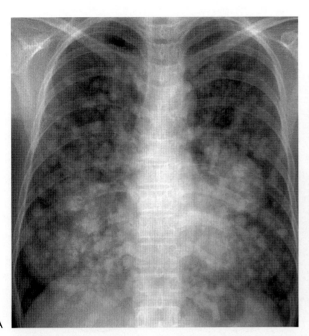

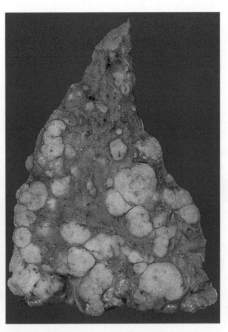

A

B

FIGURE 5.15. Pulmonary nodular metastases. **A:** Chest radiograph shows innumerable well-defined nodules and masses in both lungs. The patient was a 35-year-old woman with metastatic leiomyosarcoma. **B:** Sagittal slice of a lower lobe from another patient again shows numerous variably sized metastases, some of which are confluent. Most are well-demarcated from the adjacent parenchyma. The patient was a 56-year-old man with colonic carcinoma.

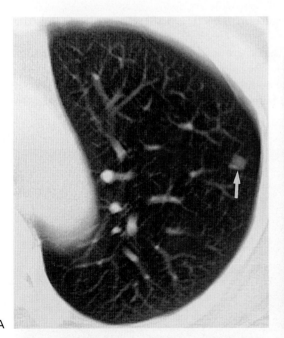

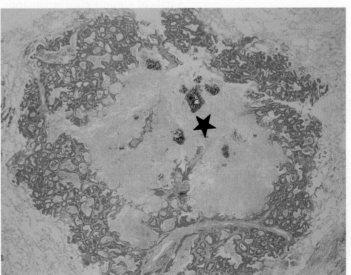

A

B

FIGURE 5.16. Pulmonary metastasis—smooth margin. **A:** CT image (7.0-mm collimation) shows 7-mm-diameter nodule in left upper lobe (*arrow*). **B:** Photomicrograph of the excised specimen shows filling of alveolar airspaces by tumor cells and prominent central necrosis (*star*). The patient was a 53-year-old woman with rectal carcinoma.

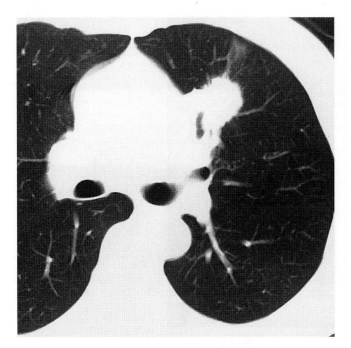

FIGURE 5.17. Pulmonary metastasis—poorly defined margin. Thin-section (1.0-mm collimation) CT scan obtained at the sub-carinal level shows a nodule with poorly defined margin in left upper lobe. Also note surrounding ground-glass opacity. The patient was a 70-year-old woman with poorly differentiated (signet-ring cell) adenocarcinoma of the stomach.

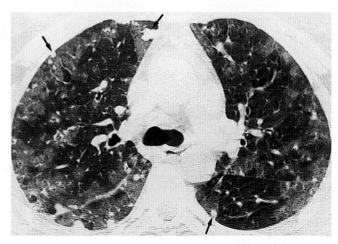

FIGURE 5.18. Pulmonary metastases—irregular margins. CT image (1.0-mm collimation) shows bilateral ground-glass opacities and multiple small nodules (*arrows*). The patient was a 52-year-old woman with metastatic angiosarcoma.

alveolar cell type, and those that had irregular margins (Fig. 5.18) were predominantly the interstitial proliferation type.

A halo of ground-glass attenuation (halo sign) is sometimes seen surrounding a nodular metastasis on HRCT (31) (Fig. 5.19). The halo usually reflects the presence of hemorrhage in the parenchyma adjacent to the nodule. Such nodules often have poorly defined margins on the radiograph; however, hemorrhage is sometimes well demarcated on

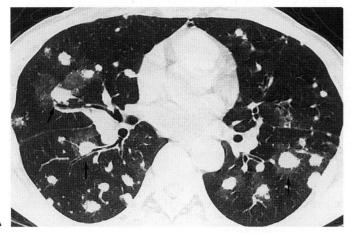

A

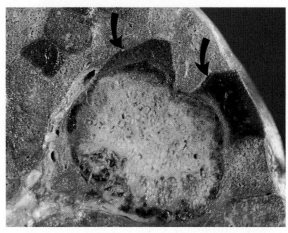

B

FIGURE 5.19. Hemorrhagic metastases. **A:** CT image (1.0-mm collimation) shows multiple nodules in both lungs, some of which are surrounded by a halo of ground-glass attenuation (*arrows*). The patient was a 51-year-old man with metastatic renal cell carcinoma. **B:** Magnified view of a slice of lung from another patient shows a well-demarcated nodule. Two adjacent secondary lobules are consolidated by blood (*arrows*). The patient was a 28-year-old woman with metastatic choriocarcinoma.

HRCT because of its isolation by interlobular septa. As might be expected, highly vascular tumors, such as angiosarcoma and choriocarcinoma, are the most common underlying cause (31,32). Occasionally, the halo is associated with spread of tumor cells along the alveolar walls in a fashion similar to bronchioloalveolar carcinoma (32,33). This is seen most commonly in metastases from adenocarcinoma of the gastrointestinal tract.

Calcification in nodular metastases is very uncommon. It is seen most frequently in sarcomas that are associated with bone formation such as osteogenic sarcoma and chondrosarcoma, and in synovial sarcoma (32,34). Dystrophic calcification also can occur in necrotic tumor and in mucin secreted by some carcinomas. Nodular metastases in which there is an abundance of either of these, such as adenocarcinoma of the colon, may show sufficient calcium deposition to be identifiable radiologically (Fig. 5.20). Cavitation occurs in approximately 4% of nodular metastases (35) (Fig. 5.21), most commonly derived from squamous cell carcinomas originating in the head and neck and genitourinary tract.

Lymphangitic Carcinomatosis

Pulmonary lymphangitic carcinomatosis (PLC) refers to spread of tumor within the pulmonary lymphatics and/or their adjacent interstitial tissue. Because the lymphatic vessels are normally located adjacent to airways and pulmonary arteries and in the interlobular septa, the process results in thickening of the bronchovascular bundles and the septa (Fig. 5.22). The thickening can be related to one or more processes (Fig. 5.23), including proliferation of the neoplastic cells themselves, the interstitial inflammation and fibrosis (desmoplastic reaction) that they engender, and lymphatic dilatation by edema fluid or tumor secretions (such as mucin). Tumors particularly likely to have this pattern of spread are carcinomas of the breast, stomach, lung, and prostate (36).

PLC can develop in two ways. The more common begins as tumor emboli located in small pulmonary arteries and arterioles (Fig. 5.24). Tumor cells from these emboli invade the interstitium adjacent to the vessels and, instead of extending into the adjacent parenchyma and causing a nodular metastasis, spread within the perivascular tissue and its lymphatic vessels. Such spread tends to be bilateral and more prominent in the lower lobes,

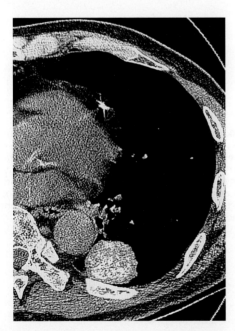

FIGURE 5.20. Calcifying metastasis. CT image (1.0-mm collimation) shows a calcified mass in left lower lobe. The patient was a 55-year-old woman with metastatic adenocarcinoma of the colon.

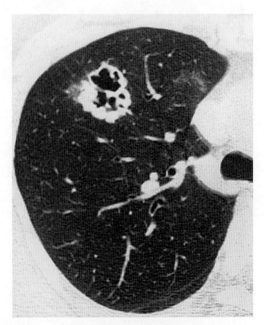

FIGURE 5.21. Cavitated metastasis. CT image (1.0-mm collimation) shows a 2.7-cm-diameter cavitated nodule in right upper lobe. The patient was a 53-year-old man with metastatic urothelial carcinoma.

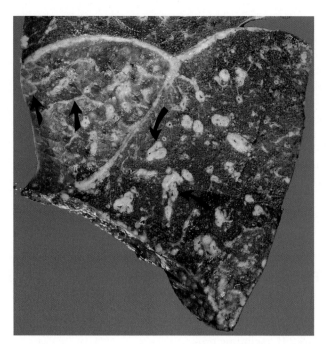

FIGURE 5.22. Pulmonary lymphangitic carcinomatosis. Sagittal slice of the lower portion of the right lung shows thickening of the interstitial tissue around many bronchi and accompanying pulmonary arteries (*curved arrows*). Mild thickening of interlobular septa in the middle lobe (*straight arrows*) and moderate thickening of the major and minor fissures can also be seen. The patient was a 48-year-old woman with metastatic carcinoma of the breast.

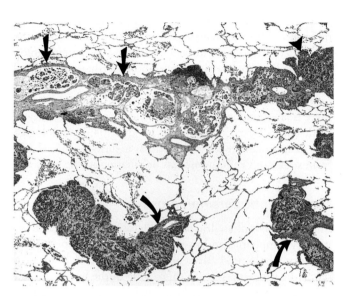

FIGURE 5.23. Pulmonary lymphangitic carcinomatosis. Photomicrograph shows thickening of an interlobular septum and the interstitial tissue around several intralobular vessels (*curved arrows*) by metastatic breast carcinoma. The thickening of the septum is partly the result of lymphatic dilatation by edema fluid and tumor (*straight arrows*). Additional thickening (*arrowhead*), as well as the thickening of the perivascular region, is the result of tumor directly infiltrating the interstitial tissue.

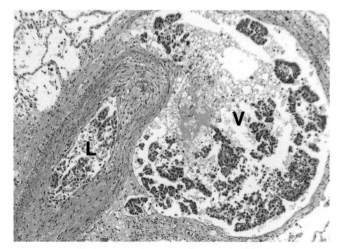

FIGURE 5.24. Pulmonary lymphangitic carcinomatosis. Photomicrograph shows marked dilatation of a lymphatic vessel (*V*) by clusters of neoplastic cells (focally necrotic). The lumen of the adjacent pulmonary artery (*L*) contains similar clusters. Such a distribution of tumor is commonly seen in lymphangitic carcinomatosis and suggests that the process begins by tumor microemboli to small pulmonary arteries and arterioles followed by invasion into the adjacent interstitial tissue and lymphatic lumen.

reflecting gravity-related increased blood flow to these regions. PLC may also occur by direct extension of tumor from hilar lymph nodes into the peribronchovascular interstitium (a pattern of spread seen most commonly with carcinoma of the breast), from the pleura into the adjacent interlobular septa (seen, for example, in carcinoma derived from the ovary) or from a primary carcinoma of the lung into adjacent peribronchovascular interstitium and/or interlobular septa. As might be expected, tumor spreading by these three mechanisms tends to be relatively localized, sometimes to only a lobe or portion thereof (Fig. 5.25).

The radiographic findings of PLC consist of a reticular network (Fig. 5.26) with septal (Kerley B) lines (36). The lower lobes are more frequently involved. Associated lymph node enlargement and pleural effusions are seen in approximately 30% of patients. It should be noted, however, that 50% of the chest radiographs in patients with histologically proved PLC are normal (37,38).

HRCT findings include smooth or nodular thickening of the bronchovascular bundles and interlobular septa, and parenchymal nodules (39,40) (Figs. 5.25 and 5.26). Smooth septal thickening is predominant in the early stage of PLC (Fig. 5.26); it tends to evolve into beaded thickening with progression of disease (41) (Fig. 5.27). The nodular (beaded) pattern is related to irregular growth of the neoplasm within the interstitium, with some foci being large enough to bulge into the adjacent parenchyma and others be-

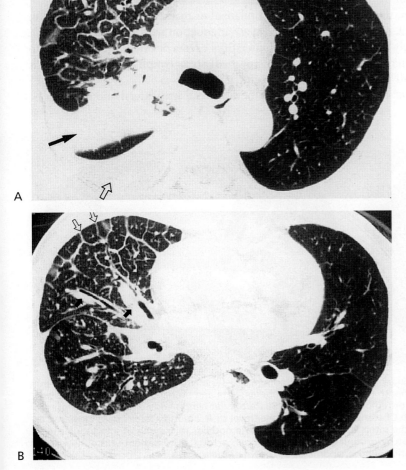

FIGURE 5.25. Pulmonary lymphangitic carcinomatosis—unilateral spread. **A:** HRCT image (1.0-mm collimation) at the level of the tracheal carina shows thickening of interlobular septa and bronchial walls in the right upper lobe. A mass is present in the posterior segment of the right upper lobe (*solid arrow*) and there is a right pleural effusion (*open arrow*). **B:** Image at the level of the lower lobar bronchi shows thickening of interlobular septa (*open arrows*) and bronchial walls (*solid arrows*) and with right pleural effusion. The patient was 67-year-old man with adenocarcinoma of the lung.

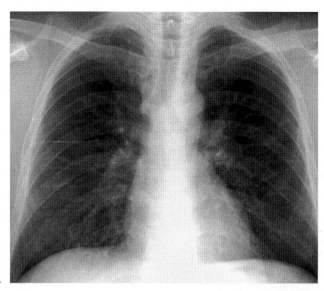
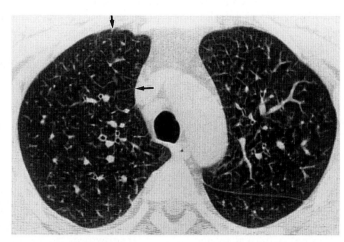

FIGURE 5.26. Pulmonary lymphangitic carcinomatosis. **A:** Chest radiograph shows a mild reticular pattern more particularly in the right lung. **B:** HRCT image (1.0-mm collimation) demonstrates smooth thickening of interlobular septa (*arrows*) and bronchial walls. The patient was a 36-year-old man with carcinoma of the stomach.

ing relatively flat (Fig. 5.28) (39,42). Smooth septal thickening may also be caused predominantly by tumor growth but is more often associated with edema of the interstitial tissue or lymphatic distension (Fig. 5.28), both of which tend to be more diffuse within the interstitium than the tumor cells themselves.

At presentation, the HRCT findings are unilateral or markedly asymmetric in up to 50% of patients (39,40) (Fig. 5.25). Ground-glass attenuation may also be present (41). The latter most likely reflects the presence of interstitial edema or extension of tumor into the parenchymal interstitium (Fig. 5.28). Hilar or mediastinal lymph node enlargement is present in 20% to 40% of patients and pleural effusion in 30% to 50% (37,39) (Figs. 5.25 and 5.27). The hilar nodal enlargement may be unilateral or bilateral and tends to be asymmetric.

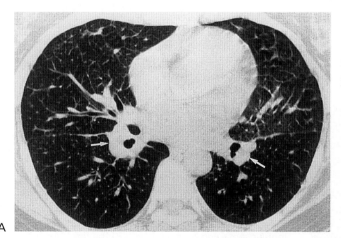
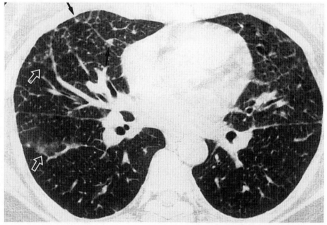

FIGURE 5.27. Pulmonary lymphangitic carcinomatosis—serial change. **A:** HRCT image (1.0-mm collimation) shows smooth thickening of interlobular septa and bronchovascular bundles, involving mainly the anterior regions of both lungs. Bilateral hilar lymph node enlargement is present (*arrows*). **B:** Follow-up CT scan obtained at a similar level to **A** 2 months later shows increased extent and severity of the interstitial abnormalities. Note nodular thickening of interlobular septa (*solid arrows*) and patchy ground-glass opacities (*open arrows*). The patient was a 40-year-old woman with metastatic adenocarcinoma of unknown primary site.

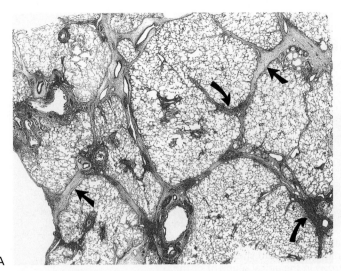
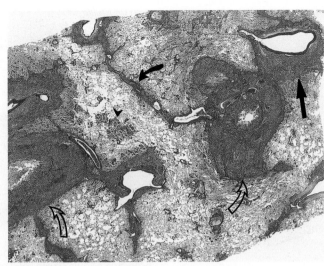

A   B

FIGURE 5.28. Pulmonary lymphangitic carcinomatosis. Photomicrographs show early (**A**) and more advanced (**B**) stages of disease. **A:** Interlobular septa are mildly thickened by a combination of edema fluid (*straight arrows*) and interstitial neoplasm (*curved arrows*). **B:** Proliferation of tumor in the perivascular interstitium (*straight arrow*) and the walls of two bronchi (*curved open arrows*) has resulted in a more nodular appearance. Mild thickening of an interlobular septum (*curved solid arrow*) and focal infiltration of the parenchymal interstitium (*arrowhead*) are also evident.

Endotracheal and Endobronchial Metastases

Endotracheal and endobronchial metastases are uncommon (27,43). The main primary tumors are carcinomas of the kidney, breast, and colon, and melanoma. The intraluminal tumor may be an extension of carcinoma from an adjacent lymph node (Fig. 5.29A) or parenchyma, or (less commonly) may originate in the bronchial wall itself (Fig. 5.29B). The radiologic manifestations include endotracheal and endobronchial polyps and pulmonary, lobar, or segmental atelectasis (8,44) (Fig. 5.30).

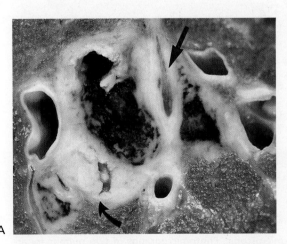
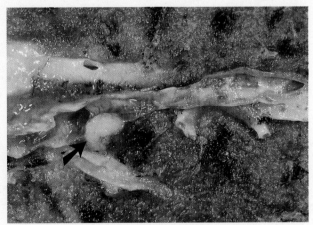

A   B

Figure 5.29. Endobronchial metastases. **A:** Magnified slice of an upper lobe shows several lymph nodes containing metastatic breast carcinoma located predominantly in their periphery. The carcinoma has extended outside the nodes causing obstruction of a small bronchus (*curved arrow*) and thrombosis of a pulmonary artery (*straight arrow*). **B:** Slice of another lung shows a small tumor nodule (*arrow*) that almost completely obstructs the bronchial lumen. The fact that only a small amount of tumor is present in the adjacent parenchyma and the absence of a lymph node suggests that the nodule originated in the airway wall itself. Metastatic urothelial carcinoma.

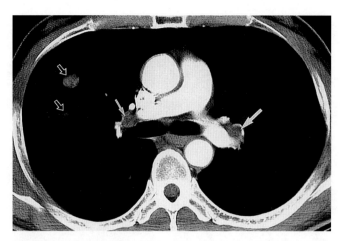

FIGURE 5.30. Endobronchial and pulmonary metastases. Contrast-enhanced CT image (7.0-mm collimation) shows an endobronchial nodule (*large solid arrow*) in the apical segment of the left upper lobe. Right hilar lymph node enlargement (*small solid arrow*) and pulmonary metastases (*open arrows*) are also evident. The patient was a 57-year-old man with hepatocellular carcinoma.

Tumor Emboli

Intravascular tumor emboli are commonly seen at autopsy but are seldom recognized radiologically. They are most frequently identified histologically in small arteries and arterioles (Fig. 5.31), where, as discussed previously, they may be associated with lymphangitic spread. Rarely, tumor emboli can be seen in segmental or larger arteries (Fig. 5.32). Such emboli are most likely to be derived from tumors that have a propensity to invade the systemic veins, such as renal cell carcinoma and hepatoma (24). Tumor emboli can result in

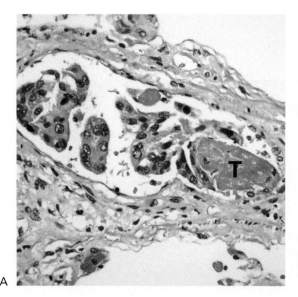

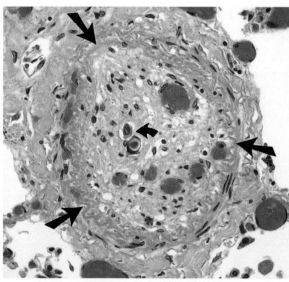

A   B

FIGURE 5.31. Endovascular metastases—microscopic. Photomicrographs of two pulmonary arteries show one (**A**) to be partly occluded by small clusters of tumor cells and thrombus (*T*) and the other (**B**) to be completely occluded by fibrous tissue (*large arrows* in **B** indicate the internal elastic lamina). Only a few viable tumor cells are present (*small arrow* in **B**). The fibrous tissue is the result of organization of thrombus associated with the tumor. The patient was a 49-year-old man who presented with clinical evidence of pulmonary hypertension and was found at autopsy to have a poorly differentiated carcinoma of the colon. Numerous small pulmonary arteries were occluded by metastatic tumor/thrombus/fibrous tissue; minimal lymphangitic carcinomatosis and no parenchymal nodules were evident.

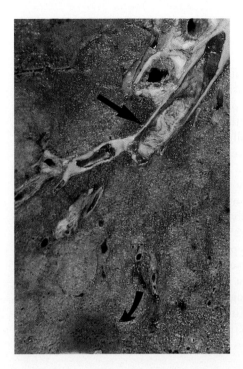

FIGURE 5.32. Endovascular metastases—macroscopic. Magnified view of a lower lobe shows complete occlusion of a segmental artery (*straight arrow*). Microscopic examination of the endovascular material showed it to consist of large fragments of carcinoma admixed with thrombus. A small infarct is evident in the basal parenchyma (*curved arrow*). The patient was a 66-year-old man with renal cell carcinoma.

any form of disease caused by thromboemboli, including pulmonary hypertension (when the emboli are numerous and small) and infarction or sudden death (when they are larger).

The chest radiograph may be normal or show findings of pulmonary arterial hypertension (45,46). Large tumor emboli can be seen on CT as filling defects within central pulmonary arteries (44,47) (Fig. 5.33) and may result in pleura-based, wedge-shaped areas of consolidation due to infarction (48,49). Tumor emboli located entirely within small pulmonary arteries occasionally grow large enough to result in nodular or beaded thickening of these vessels on CT (50); rarely, centrilobular nodules and branching linear opacities (tree-in-bud pattern) can be seen (51) (Fig. 5.34).

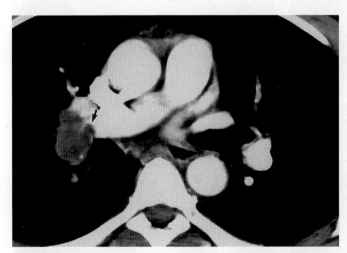

FIGURE 5.33. Endovascular metastasis. Contrast-enhanced CT image (3-mm collimation) shows a filling defect (*arrow*) in the right interlobar pulmonary artery. The distal artery is expanded and has a lobular contour. The patient was a 62-year-old man with metastatic renal cell carcinoma.

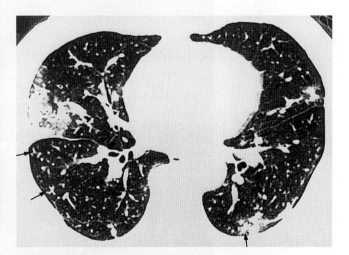

FIGURE 5.34. Endovascular metastases. HRCT image (1.5-mm collimation) shows bilateral subpleural consolidation and small branching linear and nodular opacities in a centrilobular location (*arrows*) resulting in a tree-in-bud appearance. Histologic examination showed the centrilobular nodules and linear opacities to correspond to intralobular vessels distended by carcinoma and mucin; the areas of consolidation reflected the presence of pulmonary infarction. The patient was a 60-year-old man with cholangiocarcinoma. (Case courtesy of Dr. Eun-Young Kang, Korea University Guro Hospital, Seoul, Korea.)

BENIGN NEOPLASMS

Tracheobronchial Papillomas

A papilloma is a tumor composed of epithelium-lined fibrovascular papillae that arise from and project above an epithelial surface. Those arising in the trachea or bronchi can be multiple or solitary. The former (tracheobronchial papillomatosis) are caused by the human papillomavirus, which is usually acquired at birth from an infected mother. The papillomas appear in infancy or early childhood, usually first in the larynx and subsequently in the trachea. Exceptionally, the infection spreads into distal bronchi and the lung parenchyma (see Chapter 15).

Solitary papillomas occur most commonly in middle-aged or older adults and are unassociated with a history of laryngeal involvement (52,53). Most are also caused by human papillomavirus (54). The papillomas usually measure less than 2 cm in diameter and appear as finely lobulated fleshy tumors (Fig. 5.35) that may be sessile or have a thin stalk connecting them to the underlying mucosa. Typically, they consist of mature squamous epithelium lining thin fibrovascular cores. However, cytologic atypia, carcinoma *in situ,* and, occasionally, invasive squamous carcinoma may be seen (52). The radiologic manifestations usually consist of a polypoid mass projecting into the airway lumen (Fig. 5.36) (8,55). Partial bronchial obstruction may result in decreased vascularity and hyperlucency of the affected lung or lobe. Complete obstruction results in atelectasis and obstructive pneumonitis.

Hamartoma

The term *hamartoma* implies a nonneoplastic, presumably developmental abnormality consisting of a mixture of mature but architecturally disorganized tissues. When used with respect to a pulmonary lesion, however, it is considered by some to represent a benign neoplasm that consists predominantly of cartilage. These tumors are uncommon, accounting for approximately 5% of solitary lung tumors (56,57). Most occur in adults, with the peak incidence being in the sixties (58).

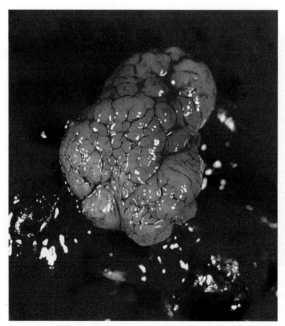
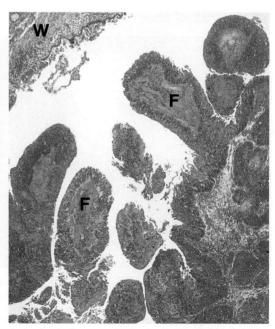

A

B

FIGURE 5.35. Intrabronchial papilloma. **A:** Magnified view of a tumor projecting from an upper lobe bronchus shows it to have a finely lobulated ("cerebriform") surface. **B:** Photomicrograph shows the tumor to consist of papillae of fibrovascular tissue (*F*) lined by squamous epithelium. (*W* = normal bronchial wall.)

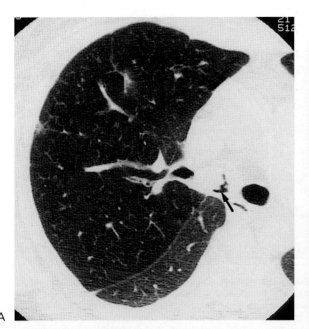 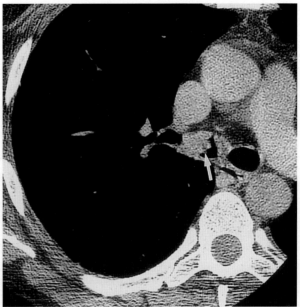

A   B

FIGURE 5.36. Intrabronchial papilloma. **A:** HRCT image (1.5-mm collimation) shows a somewhat lobulated lesion (*arrow*) in the right main and upper lobe bronchi. The right upper lobe shows decreased attenuation and vascularity as a result of reflex vasoconstriction. **B:** Soft-tissue windows (1.5-mm collimation) show soft-tissue nodule (*arrow*) with homogeneous attenuation and irregular margins. The patient was a 51-year-old woman.

Hamartomas are typically well-circumscribed, slightly lobulated tumors from 1 to 6 cm in diameter (58). Cut sections show the lobules to consist predominantly of firm or hard, pearly white tissue; softer, yellowish tissue is often present between the lobules (Fig. 5.37). Histologic examination shows the firm tissue to be composed of mature cartilage and the yellow of fat. The cartilage is often surrounded by a thin layer of loose (myxomatous) mesenchymal tissue (Fig. 5.38). It has been hypothesized that the cells in this tissue originate in the perichondrium and subsequently proliferate and differentiate into the mature cartilage that forms the bulk of most tumors. Calcification and/or ossification are fre-

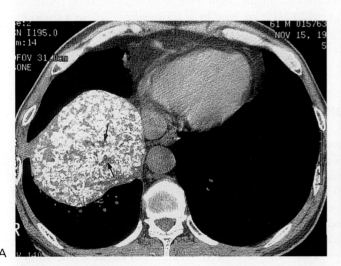 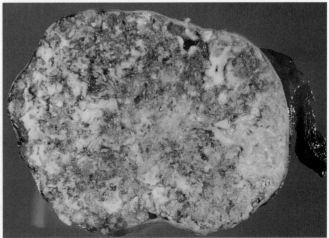

A   B

FIGURE 5.37. Hamartoma. **A:** CT image (1.0-mm collimation) shows a large mass in the right lower lobe. The mass shows extensive calcification and small foci of soft tissue and fat attenuation (*arrows*). **B:** Sagittal section of the excised specimen shows the tumor to consist of irregularly shaped pearly white lobules of cartilage and yellowish areas of adipose tissue. The patient was a 61-year-old man.

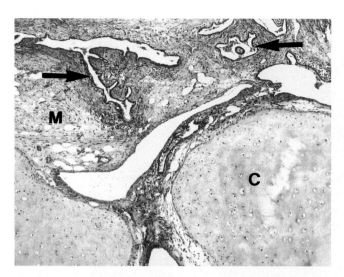

FIGURE 5.38. Hamartoma. Photomicrograph of a typical hamartoma shows two lobules of mature cartilage (*C*) adjacent to which are foci of loose (myxomatous) connective tissue containing spindle-shaped cells (*M*). Several irregular epithelium-lined clefts are present at the periphery of the tumor (*arrows*).

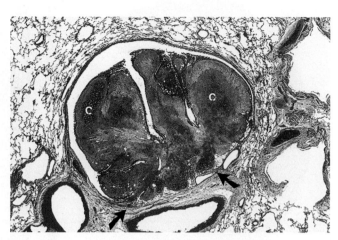

FIGURE 5.39. Hamartoma. The photomicrograph shows an intrabronchial tumor found incidentally in a lobectomy specimen for carcinoma. It is composed of lobules of cartilage (*c*) and appears to arise in the airway wall (*arrows*). Its surface and the clefts within it are lined by epithelium that is continuous with that of the adjacent bronchial wall, suggesting that it has been entrapped by the cartilaginous tissue as it has increased in size.

quently present in the cartilaginous tissue, often predominantly in the central portion. Thin, slitlike clefts lined by ciliated columnar or cuboidal epithelium are typically seen between the lobules (Fig. 5.38). The presence of these clefts was a major reason for the original conception of the hamartomatous nature of the tumor. However, examination of minute tumors suggests that the epithelium is entrapped within the expanding mesenchymal tissue rather than being an integral part of it (Fig. 5.39).

The typical radiologic presentation consists of a well-circumscribed, smoothly marginated solitary nodule (Fig. 5.40). Calcification is evident on the chest radiograph in 5% to 10% of cases (59,60). The radiographic pattern of calcification may be popcornlike, reflecting the presence of calcium or bone in the central portions of the cartilaginous lobules. Although considered virtually diagnostic, this appearance is uncommon (Fig. 5.41). The CT findings can be considered diagnostic when focal collections of fat (CT attenuation values between −40 and −120 HU) are seen in at least eight voxels in a smoothly marginated nodule measuring 2.5 cm or less in diameter (57) (Fig. 5.41). These findings are present in 30% to 50% of hamartomas (57,61). Foci of calcification are seen on CT in approximately 30% of cases.

TUMORS OF NONNEOPLASTIC NATURE

The term *plasma cell granuloma* (inflammatory pseudotumor) refers to an unusual inflammatory reaction with a variable histologic appearance. Pathologically, these lesions are usually well-demarcated parenchymal "tumors" that range from 2 to 5 cm in diameter (62) (Fig. 5.42). Endobronchial (63) or endotracheal (64) lesions occur occasionally. Extension across the pleura into the mediastinum or chest wall can occur. Histologically, they are characterized by a parenchymal interstitial and airspace infiltrate of plasma cells intermingled with lesser numbers of histiocytes, lymphocytes, and multinucleated giant cells (Fig. 5.43); mast cells and neutrophils also may be present (65). Foci of calcification, ossification, and organizing pneumonia (airspace fibroblastic tissue) are frequent (66).

Radiologic manifestations consist of either a solitary pulmonary nodule (Fig. 5.43) or a focal area of consolidation (67,68). Calcification is seen occasionally (67,68). Endobronchial lesions can cause obstructive pneumonitis. In a review of 60 patients from the Armed Forces Institute of Pathology (AFIP), 52 (87%) were found to have solitary

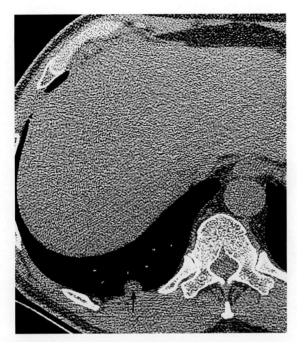

FIGURE 5.40. Hamartoma. HRCT image (1-mm collimation) shows a 12-mm-diameter nodule in the posterior basal segment of right lower lobe. Note small central calcification (*arrow*).

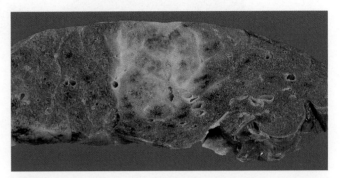

FIGURE 5.42. Plasma cell granuloma (inflammatory pseudotumor). Transverse section of an upper lobe shows a well-demarcated tumorlike focus of consolidation. Histologic examination showed it to consist of fibrous tissue and a mononuclear inflammatory cell infiltrate containing numerous plasma cells.

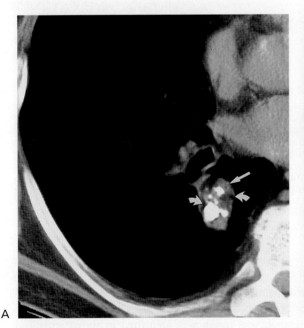
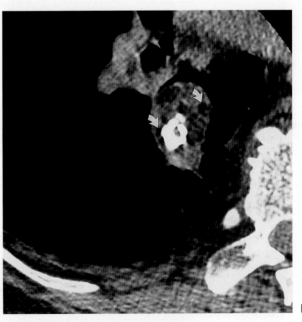

A   B

FIGURE 5.41. Hamartoma. **A:** CT image (7-mm collimation) shows a right lower lobe nodule with coarse foci of calcification (popcorn calcification) and focal areas of soft tissue (*straight arrow*) and fat (*curved arrows*) attenuation. **B:** HRCT image (1-mm collimation) better demonstrates the foci of fat attenuation (*arrows*).

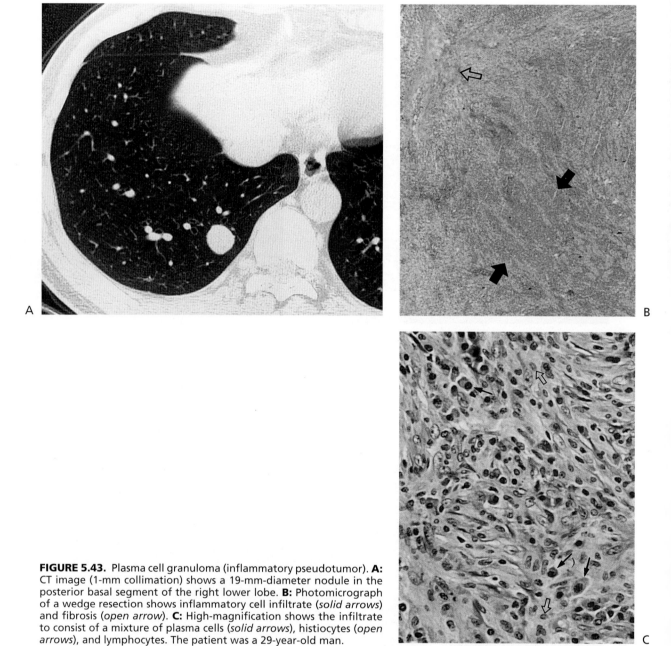

FIGURE 5.43. Plasma cell granuloma (inflammatory pseudotumor). **A:** CT image (1-mm collimation) shows a 19-mm-diameter nodule in the posterior basal segment of the right lower lobe. **B:** Photomicrograph of a wedge resection shows inflammatory cell infiltrate (*solid arrows*) and fibrosis (*open arrow*). **C:** High-magnification shows the infiltrate to consist of a mixture of plasma cells (*solid arrows*), histiocytes (*open arrows*), and lymphocytes. The patient was a 29-year-old man.

peripheral nodules or masses; three (5%), multiple nodules; two, mediastinal masses; one each, an endotracheal or endobronchial tumor; and one, a sharply defined circumscribed pleural mass (69). Tumors were larger than 3 cm in diameter in 31 patients. Secondary airway luminal involvement by a parenchymal lesion was identified in six patients and lobar atelectasis was found in five. Hilar or mediastinal lymphadenopathy and pleural effusion occurred in a small number of cases.

On CT, inflammatory pseudotumors have smooth (Fig. 5.43), lobulated, or, less commonly, spiculated (Fig. 5.44) margins, homogeneous or heterogeneous attenuation, and either no enhancement or homogeneous, heterogeneous, or peripheral rim enhancement following intravenous administration of contrast medium (69).

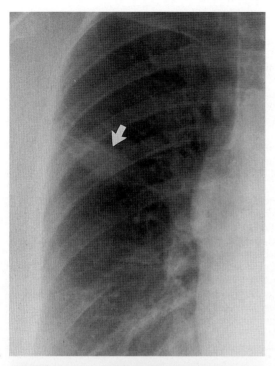

A

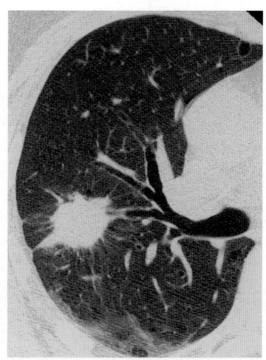

B

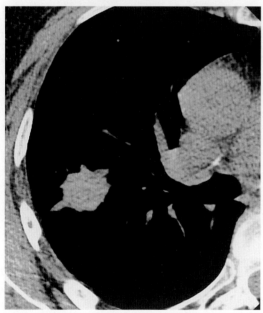

C

FIGURE 5.44. Plasma cell granuloma (inflammatory pseudotumor). **A:** View of the right lung shows a right upper lobe nodule (*arrow*) with speculated margins. **B:** HRCT image (1-mm collimation) shows the nodule to be markedly spiculated. **C:** Soft-tissue windows show the nodule to have slightly inhomogeneous attenuation. The patient was a 69-year-old woman.

REFERENCES

1. Carter D, Yesner R. Carcinomas of the lung with neuroendocrine differentiation. *Semin Diagn Pathol* 1985;2;235–254.
2. McCaughan BC, Martini N, Bains MS. Bronchial carcinoids: review of 124 cases. *J Thorac Cardiovasc Surg* 1985;89:8–17.
3. Okike N, Bernatz PE, Woolner LB. Carcinoid tumors of the lung. *Ann Thorac Surg* 1976;22: 270–277.
4. Zwiebel BR, Austin JHM, Grimes MM. Bronchial carcinoid tumors: assessment with CT of location and intratumoral calcification in 31 patients. *Radiology* 1991;179:483–486.

5. Arrigoni MG, Woolner LB, Bernatz PE. Atypical carcinoid tumors of the lung. *J Thorac Cardiovasc Surg* 1972;64:413–421.

6. Forster BB, Müller NL, Miller RR, et al. Neuroendocrine carcinomas of the lung: clinical, radiologic, and pathologic correlation. *Radiology* 1989;170:441–445.

7. Nessi R, Ricci PB, Ricci SB, et al. Bronchial carcinoid tumors: radiologic observations in 49 cases. *J Thorac Imaging* 1991;6:47–53.

8. Kwong JS, Müller NL, Miller RR. Diseases of the trachea and main-stem bronchi: correlation of CT with pathologic findings. *Radiographics* 1992;12:645–657.

9. Magid D, Siegelman SS, Eggleston JC, et al. Pulmonary carcinoid tumors: CT assessment. *J Comput Assist Tomogr* 1989;13:244–247.

10. Spencer H. Bronchial mucous gland tumors. *Virchows Arch* 1979;383:101–115.

11. Moran CA. Primary salivary gland-type tumors of the lung. *Semin Diagn Pathol* 1995;12:106–122.

12. Grillo HC. Tracheal tumors. In: Choi NC, Grillo HC, eds. *Thoracic oncology.* New York: Raven Press, 1983:271–278.

13. Yousem SA, Hochholzer L. Mucoepidermoid tumors of the lung. *Cancer* 1987;60:1346–1352.

14. Kim TS, Lee KS, Han J, et al. Mucoepidermoid carcinoma of the tracheobronchial tree: radiologic findings in 12 patients. *Radiology* 1999;212:643–648.

15. Ognibene FP, Steis RG, Macher AM, et al. Kaposi's sarcoma causing pulmonary infiltrates and respiratory failure in the acquired immunodeficiency syndrome. *Ann Intern Med* 1985;102:471–475.

16. Safai B, Johson KG, Myskowski PL, et al. The natural history of Kaposi's sarcoma in the acquired immunodeficiency syndrome. *Ann Intern Med* 1985;103:744–750.

17. Davis SD, Henschke CI, Chamides BK, et al. Intrathoracic Kaposi sarcoma in AIDS patients: radiographic-pathologic correlation. *Radiology* 1987;163:495–500.

18. Sivit CJ, Schwartz AM, Rockoff SD. Kaposi's sarcoma of the lung in AIDS: radiologic-pathologic analysis. *Am J Roentgenol* 1987;148:25–28.

19. Naidich DP, Tarras M, Garay SM, et al. Kaposi's sarcoma: CT-radiographic correlation. *Chest* 1989;96:723–728.

20. Conces DJ Jr. Noninfectious lung disease in immunocompromised patients. *J Thorac Imaging* 1999;14:9–24.

21. Wolff SD, Kuhlman JE, Fishman EK. Thoracic Kaposi sarcoma in AIDS: CT findings. *J Comput Assist Tomogr* 1993;17:60–62.

22. Khalil AM, Carette MF, Cadranel JL, et al. Intrathoracic Kaposi's sarcoma: CT findings. *Chest* 1995;108:1622–1626.

23. Crow J, Slavin G, Kreel L. Pulmonary metastasis: a pathologic and radiologic study. *Cancer* 1981;47:2595–2602.

24. Libshitz HI, North LB. Pulmonary metastases. *Radiol Clin North Am* 1982;20:437–451.

25. Johnson RM, Lindskog GE. 100 cases of tumor metastatic to the lung and mediastinum: treatment and results. *JAMA* 1967;202:94–98.

26. Coppage L, Shaw C, Curtis AM. Metastatic disease to the chest in patients with extrathoracic malignancy. *J Thorac Imag* 1987;2:24–37.

27. Albertini RE, Ekberg NL. Endobronchial metastasis in the breast cancer. *Thorax* 1980;35:435–440.

28. Meziane MA, Hruban RH, Zerhouni EA, et al. High-resolution CT of the lung parenchyma with pathologic correlation. *Radiographics* 1988;8:27–54.

29. Zwirewich CV, Vedal S, Miller RR, et al. Solitary pulmonary nodule: high-resolution CT and radiologic-pathologic correlation. *Radiology* 1991;179:469–476.

30. Hirakata K, Nakata H, Haratake J. Appearance of pulmonary metastases on high-resolution CT scans: comparison with histopathologic findings from autopsy specimens. *Am J Roentgenol* 1993;161:37–43.

31. Primack SL, Hartman TE, Lee KS, et al. Pulmonary nodules and the CT halo sign. *Radiology* 1994;190:513–515.

32. Hirakata K, Nakata H, Nakagawa T. CT of pulmonary metastases with pathological correlation. *Semin Ultrasound CT MR* 1995;16:379–394.

33. Gaeta M, Blandino A, Scribano E, et al. Computed tomography halo sign of pulmonary nodules: frequency and diagnostic value. *J Thorac Imag* 1999;14:109–113.

34. Zoillkofer C, Castaneda-Zuniga W, Stenlund R, et al. Lung metastases from synovial sarcoma simulating granulomas. *Am J Roentgenol* 1980;135:161–163.

35. Chaudhuri MR. Cavitary pulmonary metastases. *Thorax* 1970;25:375–381.

36. Janower ML, Blennerhassett JB. Lymphangitic spread of metastatic cancer to the lung: a radiologic-pathologic classification. *Radiology* 1971;101:267–273.

37. Yang S-P, Lin C-C. Lymphangitic carcinomatosis of the lungs: the clinical significance of its roentgenologic classification. *Chest* 1972;62:179–187.

38. Goldsmith HS, Bailey HD, Callahan EL, et al. Pulmonary metastases from breast carcinoma. *Arch Surg* 1967;94:483–488.

39. Munk PL, Müller NL, Miller RR, et al. Pulmonary lymphangitic carcinomatosis: CT and pathologic findings. *Radiology* 1988;166:705–709.

40. Johkoh T, Ikezoe J, Tomiyama N, et al. CT findings in lymphangitic carcinomatosis of the lung: correlation with histologic findings and pulmonary function tests. *Am J Roentgenol* 1992;158: 1217–1222.

41. Hwang JW, Kim YK, Hwang JH, et al. Lymphangitic carcinomatosis of the lung: serial changes on high-resolution CT. *J Korean Radiol Soc* 1997;37:1051–1057.

42. Ren H, Hruban RH, Kuhlman JE, et al. Computed tomography of inflation-fixed lungs: the beaded septum sign of pulmonary metastases. *J Comput Assist Tomogr* 1989;13:411–416.

43. Braman SS, Whitcomb ME. Endobronchial metastasis. *Arch Intern Med* 1975;135:543–547.

44. Fraser RS, Müller NL, Colman N, et al. *Diagnosis of diseases of the chest.* Philadelphia: WB Saunders, 1999:1381–1417.

45. Shirakusa T, Tsutsui M, Motonaga R, et al. Resection of metastatic lung tumor: the evaluation of histologic appearance in the lung. *Am Surg* 1988;54:655–658.

46. Winterbauer RH, Elfenbein IB, Ball WC Jr. Incidence and clinical significance of tumor embolization to the lungs. *Am J Med* 1968;45:271–290.

47. Seo JB, Im JG, Goo JM, et al. Atypical pulmonary metastases: spectrum of radiologic findings. *Radiographics* 2001;21:403–417.

48. Kim AE, Haramati LB, Janus D, et al. Pulmonary tumor embolism presenting as infarct on computed tomography. *J Thorac Imaging* 1999;14:135–137.

49. Kang CH, Choi J-A, Kim HR, et al. Lung metastases manifesting as pulmonary infarction by mucin and tumor embolization: radiographic, high-resolution CT, and pathologic findings. *J Comput Assist Tomogr* 1999;23:644–646.

50. Shepard JO, Moore EH, Templeton PA, et al. Pulmonary intravascular tumor emboli: dilated and beaded peripheral pulmonary arteries at CT. *Radiology* 1993;187:797–801.

51. Tack D, Nollevaux MC, Gevenois PA. Tree-in-bud pattern in neoplastic pulmonary emboli. *Am J Roentgenol* 2001;176:1421–1422.

52. Spencer H, Dail DH, Arneaud J. Noninvasive bronchial epithelial papillary tumors. *Cancer* 1980;45:1486–1497.

53. Maxwell RJ, Gibbons JR, O'Hara MD. Solitary squamous papilloma of the bronchus. *Thorax* 1985;40:68–71.

54. Popper HH, el-Shabrawi Y, Wockel W, et al. Prognostic importance of human papillomavirus typing in squamous cell papilloma of the bronchus: comparison of *in situ* hybridization and the polymerase chain reaction. *Hum Pathol* 1994;25:1191–1197.

55. McCarthy MJ, Rosado-de-Christenson ML. Tumors of the trachea. *J Thorac Imaging* 1995;10: 180–198.

56. Swensen SJ, Brown LR, Colby TV, et al. Pulmonary nodules: CT evaluation of enhancement with iodinated contrast material. *Radiology* 1995;194:393–398.

57. Siegelman SS, Khouri NF, Scott WW, et al. Pulmonary hamartoma: CT findings. *Radiology* 1986;160:313–317.

58. Gjevre JA, Myers JL, Prakash UBS. Pulmonary hamartomas. *Mayo Clin Proc* 1996;71:14–20.

59. Poirier TJ, Van Ordstrand HS. Pulmonary chondromatous hamartomas: report of seventeen cases and review of the literature. *Chest* 1971;59:50–55.

60. Shah JP, Choudhry KU, Huvos AG, et al. Hamartomas of the lung. *Surg Gynecol Obstet* 1973;136: 406–408.

61. Potente G, Macori F, Caimi M, et al. Noncalcified pulmonary hamartomas: computed tomography enhancement patterns with histologic correlation. *J Thorac Imaging* 1999;14:101–104.

62. Bahadori M, Liebow AA. Plasma cell granulomas of the lung. *Cancer* 1973;31:191–208.

63. Aisner SC, Albin RJ, Templeton PA, et al. Endobronchial fibrous histiocytoma. *Ann Thorac Surg* 1995;60:710–712.

64. Sandstrom RE, Proppe KH, Trelstad RL. Fibrous histiocytoma of the trachea. *Am J Clin Pathol* 1978;70:429–433.

65. Harjula A, Mattila S, Kyosola K, et al. Plasma cell granuloma of lung and pleura. *Scand J Thorac Cardiovasc Surg* 1986;20:119–121.

66. Matsubara O, Tan-Liu NS, Kenney RM, et al. Inflammatory pseudotumors of the lung: progression from organizing pneumonia to fibrous histiocytoma or to plasma cell granuloma in 32 cases. *Hum Pathol* 1988;19:807–814.

67. Strutynsky N, Balthazar EJ, Klein RM. Inflammatory pseudotumours of the lung. *Br J Radiol* 1974;47:94–96.

68. Schwartz EE, Katz SM, Mandell GA. Postinflammatory pseudotumors of the lung: fibrous histiocytoma and related lesions. *Radiology* 1980;136:609–613.

69. Agrons GA, Rosado-de-Christenson ML, Kirejczyk WM, et al. Pulmonary inflammatory pseudotumor: radiologic features. *Radiology* 1998;206:511–518.

6

CONNECTIVE TISSUE DISEASES

SYSTEMIC LUPUS ERYTHEMATOSUS

RHEUMATOID ARTHRITIS
Parenchymal Disease
Airway Disease
Pleural Disease

PROGRESSIVE SYSTEMIC SCLEROSIS

POLYMYOSITIS AND DERMATOMYOSITIS

SJÖGREN'S SYNDROME

MIXED CONNECTIVE TISSUE DISEASE

ANKYLOSING SPONDYLITIS

The connective tissue diseases constitute a group of autoimmune disorders whose common denominator is damage to components of connective tissue at a variety of sites in the body. Specific entities include systemic lupus erythematosus, rheumatoid disease, progressive systemic sclerosis, polymyositis and dermatomyositis, Sjögren's syndrome, mixed connective tissue disease, and ankylosing spondylitis.

SYSTEMIC LUPUS ERYTHEMATOSUS

Systemic lupus erythematosus (SLE) is characterized immunologically by the presence of autoantibodies against various nuclear antigens (1). It is seen most commonly in young women. Pleuropulmonary involvement occurs in approximately 50% to 60% of patients (1). In one series of 1,000 patients studied prospectively, lung involvement was identified in 3% and pleural involvement in 17% at the onset of the disease (2); an additional 7% developed lung disease and 36% developed pleural disease over the period of observation.

The most common pulmonary abnormalities are infectious pneumonia (usually bacterial), pulmonary hemorrhage, and noninfectious (lupus) pneumonitis (1,2). The last-named occurs in 1% to 4% of patients (1,3). It is characterized clinically by fever, dyspnea, and hypoxemia, and radiographically by patchy or diffuse opacities; by definition, an infectious etiology is excluded. The radiologic manifestations of drug-induced SLE are similar to those of the idiopathic form (4).

A wide variety of histologic abnormalities are seen in the lungs of patients who have SLE, including pleuritis and pleural fibrosis (with or without effusion), interstitial pneumonia, bronchiolitis obliterans organizing pneumonia (BOOP), vasculitis, plexogenic arteriopathy (related to pulmonary hypertension), hemorrhage, thromboembolism (related to the procoagulant effect of antiphospholipid antibodies), and follicular bronchiolitis (5).

Pleural fibrosis is the most common finding at autopsy (2,6). Fibrinous pleuritis is seen in some patients who have pleural effusion during life and is presumably the precursor of the autopsy finding (7). Diffuse interstitial pneumonia and fibrosis is uncommon; in one series of 120 patients, only five (4%) had the complication (8). Pathologic findings in these cases may be those of usual interstitial pneumonia (UIP) or nonspecific interstitial pneumonia (NSIP) (5). Two major histologic abnormalities are seen in patients who have lupus pneumonitis (Fig. 6.1): diffuse alveolar damage (intraalveolar proteinaceous exudate, hyaline membranes, and interstitial edema and mononuclear inflammatory cell infiltration) (6), and capillaritis and alveolar hemorrhage (1,9).

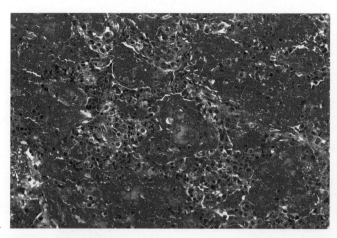 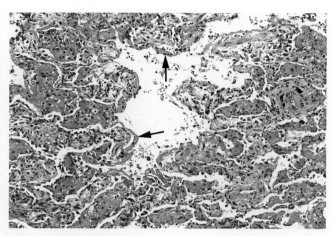

A   B

FIGURE 6.1. Acute lupus pneumonitis—histologic appearance. **A:** Photomicrograph shows airspace hemorrhage associated with an infiltrate of neutrophils in the vicinity of the alveolar septa (capillaritis). **B:** Photomicrograph from another patient shows a proteinaceous exudate in alveolar airspaces associated with hyaline membrane formation in an alveolar duct (*arrows*) (diffuse alveolar damage). The alveolar interstitium also shows mild fibrosis and inflammation, consistent with chronic pneumonitis.

Clinically important pulmonary hypertension is rare in SLE. An underlying mechanism responsible for the hypertension, such as interstitial fibrosis or thromboembolism, can be found in some patients. In others the histologic findings resemble those of primary pulmonary hypertension, including intimal fibrosis, medial hypertrophy, and plexiform lesions (10).

Radiologic abnormalities may be seen in the lungs, pleura, and heart, alone or in combination. In one investigation of 275 patients, 46% had normal chest radiographs, 35% had pleural effusion or thickening, 13% had pulmonary abnormalities, and 37% had cardiomegaly or pericardial effusion (11).

Pleural effusion is the most common thoracic manifestation (12). It is frequently bilateral. Although usually small, it may be massive (13). It may resolve completely with no residual abnormality; however, residual pleural thickening (usually mild) is evident in some patients.

The most common radiographic abnormalities in the lungs consist of poorly defined, patchy areas of parenchymal consolidation involving mainly the bases (13). In most patients, these are the result of infection (13); occasionally, they correspond to idiopathic BOOP (14). The radiographic findings in acute lupus pneumonitis consist of patchy, unilateral or bilateral areas of ground-glass opacity or air-space consolidation, often associated with elevation of the diaphragm and small bilateral pleural effusions (Fig. 6.2) (3,13). The ground-glass opacities reflect the presence of capillaritis with early hemorrhage (Fig. 6.3) or the early exudative stage of diffuse alveolar damage (Fig. 6.2); consolidation reflects more severe parenchymal involvement by either process (13,15).

Horizontal line shadows are relatively common. They are usually present in the lung bases, are sometimes migratory, and are probably the result of subsegmental atelectasis. In some patients, sequential radiographs show progressive loss of lung volume that may be associated with an elevated diaphragm as a result of muscle weakness (3,13).

Radiographic evidence of interstitial fibrosis, consisting of a reticular pattern involving mainly the lower lung zones, is seen in only about 3% of patients who have SLE (12). By contrast, interstitial abnormalities are seen in approximately 30% of patients on HRCT (12,16,17). These include interlobular septal thickening (33%), intralobular interstitial thickening (33%), and architectural distortion (22%). Such abnormalities are usually mild and focal; diffuse disease occurs in only 4% of patients (8). Honeycombing is uncommon.

Ground-glass opacity and consolidation on the radiograph or HRCT may reflect the presence of pneumonia, lupus pneumonitis, or, occasionally, BOOP (12). Findings of air-

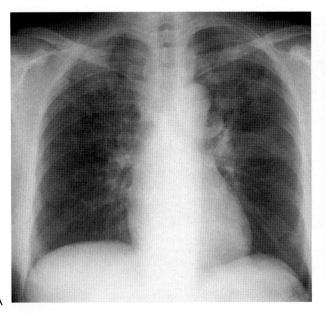

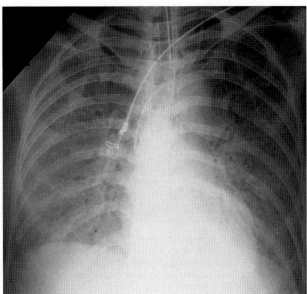

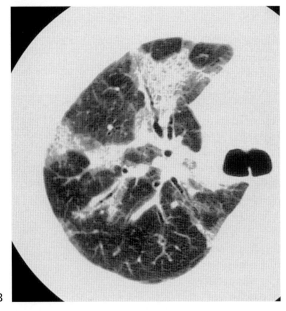

FIGURE 6.2. Acute lupus pneumonitis. **A:** Chest radiograph shows poorly defined areas of airspace consolidation in the upper lung zones. **B:** HRCT image of the right upper lobe demonstrates extensive ground-glass attenuation and patchy areas of airspace consolidation. **C:** Chest radiograph made 7 days after **A** shows diffuse bilateral airspace consolidation. Pathologic examination showed the exudative phase of diffuse alveolar damage. The patient was a 45-year-old woman.

way disease such as bronchial wall thickening and bronchiectasis have been reported in approximately 20% of patients (16,17).

Cardiovascular changes frequently occur in association with pulmonary and pleural manifestations. An increase in the size of the cardiac silhouette is usually the result of pericardial effusion. Both cardiomegaly and pulmonary edema may be caused by lupus myocardiopathy.

RHEUMATOID ARTHRITIS

Rheumatoid arthritis (RA) is characterized by the presence of symmetric arthritis, morning stiffness, and rheumatoid factor in the blood. Pleuropulmonary complications are common and include interstitial pneumonitis and fibrosis, rheumatoid (necrobiotic) nodules, BOOP, bronchiectasis, obliterative bronchiolitis, follicular bronchiolitis, and pleural effusion or thickening (18,19).

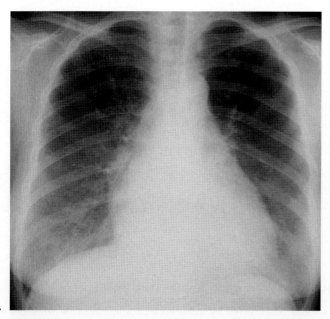
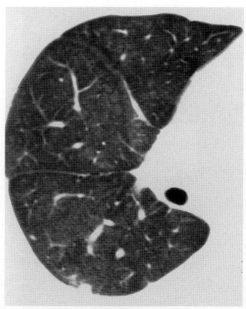

A   B

FIGURE 6.3. Acute lupus pneumonitis. **A:** Chest radiograph shows poorly defined ground-glass opacities in the middle and lower lung zones. **B:** HRCT image of the right lung demonstrates diffuse ground-glass attenuation and a small focus of consolidation in the right lower lobe. Pathologic examination showed diffuse alveolar hemorrhage. The patient was a 37-year-old woman with systemic lupus erythematosus.

Parenchymal Disease

Interstitial Pneumonitis and Fibrosis

Interstitial pneumonitis and fibrosis is the most common pulmonary manifestation of RA (18). In fact, pulmonary function abnormalities consistent with interstitial fibrosis have been reported in as many as 40% of patients who have RA (20,21); however, in more than half of these patients, the chest radiograph is normal (22). Evidence of interstitial fibrosis is seen on chest radiographs in approximately 5% of patients with RA (18,20) and on HRCT in 30% to 40% (19,23). The complication is seen most frequently in men between 50 and 60 years of age (24).

Most patients who have interstitial fibrosis associated with RA have usual interstitial pneumonia (UIP); a small percentage has histologic findings of NSIP (25). Histologic changes in the early stages of UIP consist of an interstitial infiltrate of lymphocytes, histiocytes, and plasma cells (26); the last of these are often more frequent than in idiopathic pulmonary fibrosis. Nodular aggregates of lymphocytes may be prominent in both the parenchymal interstitium (27) and the interstitial tissue in bronchiolar walls and interlobular septa (follicular bronchiolitis) (28). Progression of disease is associated with increasing fibrosis, which eventually may result in an appearance of "honeycomb" lung (Fig. 6.4).

The pattern and distribution of fibrosis in RA on both the chest radiograph and HRCT are indistinguishable from those of idiopathic pulmonary fibrosis (Fig. 6.5) (29,30). In the early stage, the radiographic appearance consists of irregular linear opacities causing a fine reticular pattern. The abnormality usually involves mainly the lower lung zones. With progression of disease, the reticular pattern becomes more coarse and diffuse, and honeycombing may be seen.

Similar to the radiograph, the predominant abnormality on HRCT consists of a reticular pattern caused by a combination of intralobular lines and irregular thickening of interlobular septa (Fig. 6.5) (19,30). These are present mainly in the subpleural parenchyma and the lower lung zones. Although irregular linear opacities representing fibrosis can be seen on HRCT at any level, honeycombing is usually most marked near the diaphragm (30).

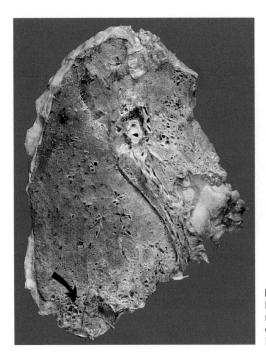

FIGURE 6.4. Rheumatoid disease—usual interstitial pneumonia. Parasagittal slice of the left lung shows extensive (albeit mild) pleural fibrosis (manifested by adherence of adipose tissue from the chest wall) and patchy, predominantly subpleural interstitial fibrosis. Honeycomb change can be seen in some areas (*arrow*).

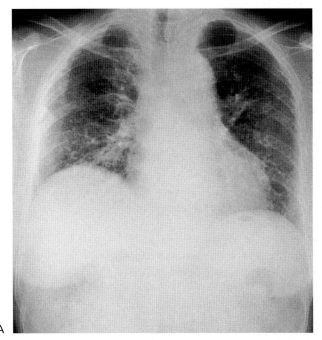

A

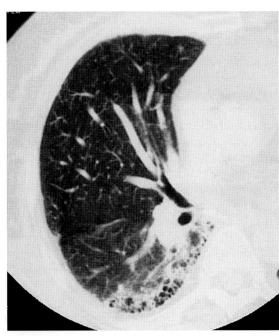

B

FIGURE 6.5. Rheumatoid disease—usual interstitial pneumonia. **A:** Chest radiograph shows a reticular pattern and ground-glass opacities involving mainly the middle and lower lung zones. **B:** HRCT image of the right lung demonstrates subpleural honeycombing and ground glass opacities in the superior segment of the right lower lobe.

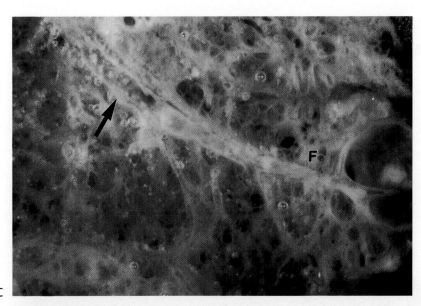

C

FIGURE 6.5. *(continued)* **C:** Stereomicroscopic view shows areas of normal parenchyma admixed with foci of fibrosis (*F*) and cyst formation within the same secondary pulmonary lobule. (*Arrow* indicates a bronchiole.) The patient was a 68-year-old woman.

Rheumatoid Nodules

Pulmonary rheumatoid (necrobiotic) nodules are rare and almost always associated with multiple subcutaneous rheumatoid nodules (12). They may be solitary or multiple and are usually situated peripherally in relation to the pleura or interlobular septa (31,32). Histologically, the nodule is composed of a central region of necrotic material that is surrounded by a layer of palisaded epithelioid histiocytes (Fig. 6.6). The adjacent tissue shows fibrosis and a variably intense plasma cell and lymphocyte infiltrate.

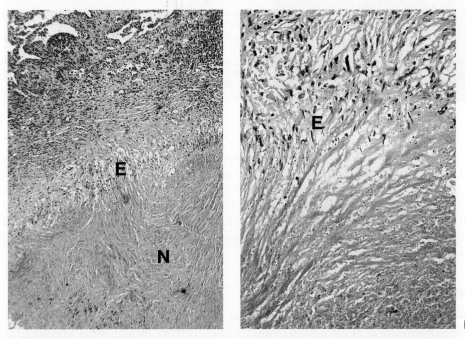

A   B

FIGURE 6.6. Rheumatoid disease—rheumatoid nodules. Photomicrographs (**A** and **B**) of a subpleural nodule show a focus of necrosis (*N*) bordered by a rim of epithelioid histiocytes (*E*) and fibrous tissue. Culture and special stains revealed no organisms. The patient was a 56-year-old man with rheumatoid arthritis. The nodule was an incidental finding in a lobe resected for carcinoma.

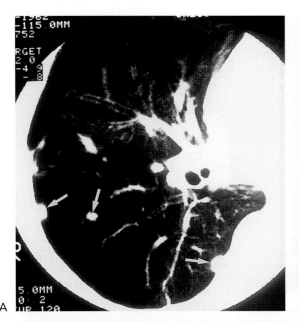

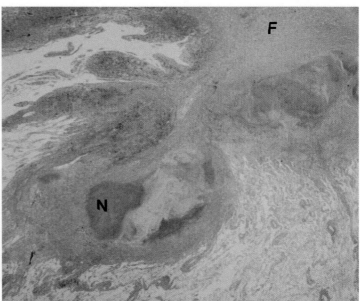

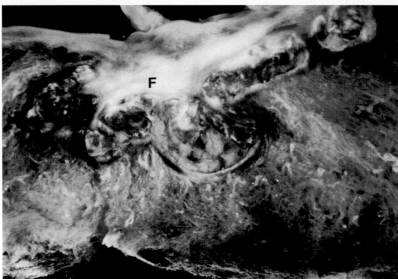

FIGURE 6.7. Rheumatoid disease—rheumatoid nodules. **A:** CT image of the right lung shows several nodules (*arrows*). **B:** Magnified view of a slice of the specimen shows pleural fibrosis (*F*) and several well-demarcated subpleural nodules. **C:** Photomicrograph shows the pleural fibrosis (*F*) and a portion of the nodule consisting of a central region of necrotic material (*N*) surrounded by a fibrous capsule. (Courtesy of Dr. Harumi Itoh, Fukui Medical University, Fukui, Japan.)

Necrobiotic nodules can be detected radiographically in the lung in approximately two per 1,000 patients who have RA (33). As might be expected, they are seen more commonly with CT, being observed in three of 77 (4%) patients in one series (19). Typically, they present as well-circumscribed nodules or masses, usually multiple, ranging from 5 mm to 7 cm in diameter. They are commonly located in the periphery of the lung next to the pleura (Fig. 6.7) (19). Cavitation is frequent; the cavity walls tend to be thick and to have a smooth inner lining.

Airway Disease

Airway abnormalities are frequently evident on HRCT in patients who have RA (34,35). In one investigation of 50 patients who had no evidence of interstitial fibrosis (35), bronchial or pulmonary abnormalities, or both, were seen on HRCT in 35 (70%). These consisted of air trapping in 16 (32%), cylindrical bronchiectasis in 15 (30%), and mild heterogeneity in lung attenuation (i.e., mosaic perfusion) in 10 (20%). Evidence of airway

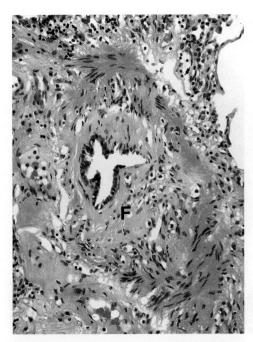

FIGURE 6.8. Rheumatoid disease—obliterative bronchiolitis. Photomicrograph shows infiltration of the wall of a small membranous bronchiole by scattered lymphocytes. The lamina propria (between the muscularis mucosa and the epithelium) is moderately thickened by mature fibrous tissue (*F*).

obstruction on pulmonary function test was present in only nine patients (18%). Airway complications of RA include bronchiectasis, obliterative bronchiolitis, BOOP, and follicular bronchitis/bronchiolitis.

Obliterative Bronchiolitis

Histologically, obliterative bronchiolitis is characterized by fibrosis and a variably intense inflammatory infiltrate of lymphocytes and plasma cells in and around the walls of bronchioles and (occasionally) small bronchi (36). Usually, the fibroblastic proliferation occurs between the airway muscle and the airway epithelium ("constrictive" bronchiolitis) (Fig. 6.8). In the late stages, there may be complete fibrous obliteration of airway lumina (36).

The chest radiograph is usually normal or shows only hyperinflation (34). The characteristic HRCT findings consist of areas of decreased attenuation and vascularity adjacent to areas of increased attenuation and vascularity (mosaic perfusion pattern) and, commonly, bronchiectasis (Fig. 6.9) (34,37). The mosaic perfusion pattern is related to the presence of localized areas of decreased blood flow secondary to hypoxic vasoconstriction. The latter is the result of decreased ventilation associated with airway obstruction. Because not all bronchioles are affected to the same degree, there is a variation in the severity of perfusion abnormality, and hence a variable HRCT appearance. Expiratory HRCT demonstrates focal areas of air trapping (34).

Follicular Bronchiolitis

Follicular bronchiolitis is characterized histologically by the presence of abundant lymphoid tissue, frequently with prominent germinal centers, in the walls of bronchioles and, to a lesser extent, bronchi (Fig. 6.10) (38). Although the alveolar interstitium may contain a similar lymphocytic infiltrate, this is usually minimal.

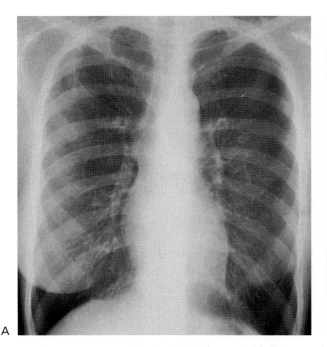
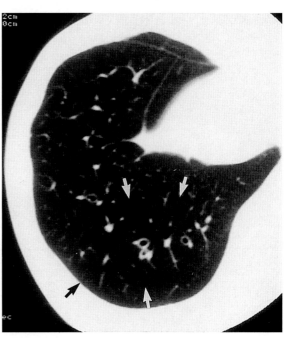

FIGURE 6.9. Rheumatoid disease—obliterative bronchiolitis. **A:** Chest radiograph shows increased lung volumes. **B:** HRCT image demonstrates decreased attenuation and vascularity (*arrows*) as well as mild bronchial dilatation. The patient was a 25-year-old woman.

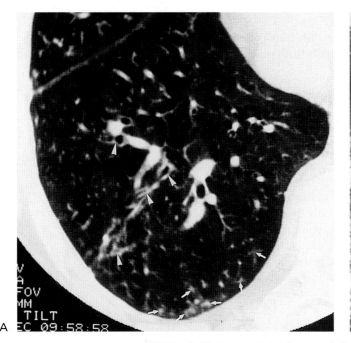
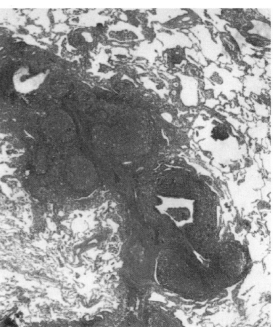

FIGURE 6.10. Rheumatoid disease—follicular bronchiolitis. **A:** HRCT image demonstrates centrilobular nodules (*arrows*) and bronchial wall thickening (*arrowheads*). **B:** Photomicrograph shows marked thickening of the wall of a membranous bronchiole by an infiltrate of lymphocytes, focally with germinal center formation (*arrows*). (Courtesy of Dr. Kingo Chida, Hamamtsu Medical University, Hamamatsu, Japan.)

The chest radiograph shows a reticulonodular pattern (38). HRCT demonstrates nodules, mainly in a centrilobular, subpleural, and peribronchial distribution (39,40). These usually measure 1 to 4 mm in diameter (Fig. 6.10). Other findings include bronchial wall thickening and centrilobular branching linear opacities (40).

Pleural Disease

The most frequent manifestation of RA in the thorax is probably pleuritis with or without pleural effusion (12,18). Pleural effusion or thickening is evident radiographically at some stage in 5% to 20% of patients (29,33) and on HRCT in approximately 30% of patients (41). Effusions are usually small and unilateral. Although they usually resolve over a period of weeks or months, they may recur or persist for many months or even years (42). Histologic examination of the pleura usually shows nonspecific chronic inflammation; occasionally, there is fibrinous pleuritis.

PROGRESSIVE SYSTEMIC SCLEROSIS

Progressive systemic sclerosis (PSS, scleroderma) is a disorder of connective tissue characterized by deposition of excessive extracellular matrix and vascular obliteration (43). It is an uncommon condition, with an estimated incidence of approximately 10 cases per million population per year (43). It has a female predominance of approximately 3:1.

The most common pulmonary manifestations are interstitial fibrosis, which occurs in approximately 80% of patients, and pulmonary arterial hypertension, which occurs in approximately 50% (43).

At autopsy, some degree of parenchymal interstitial fibrosis is frequent (44). It is typically bilateral and most marked in the subpleural regions of the lower lobes. Occasionally, it is severe (Fig. 6.11). The histologic features are those of nonspecific interstitial pneumonia (NSIP) or usual interstitial pneumonia (UIP). Local or diffuse pleural fibrosis is seen in approximately 25% of cases.

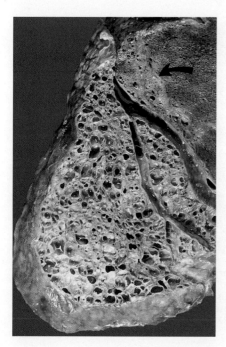

FIGURE 6.11. Progressive systemic sclerosis—usual interstitial pneumonia. Magnified view of a parasagittal slice of the right lung shows marked interstitial fibrosis with extensive honeycomb change in the lower and middle lobes. Somewhat less severe disease is evident in the subpleural region of the upper lobe (*arrow*).

Histologic evidence of pulmonary arterial hypertension may be seen in association with diffuse interstitial fibrosis or, occasionally, as an isolated finding (44). The most prominent findings are in the small muscular arteries and arterioles that show intimal thickening by fibroblastic connective tissue and medial muscle hypertrophy (Fig. 6.12) (43). Plexiform lesions are uncommon.

Evidence of interstitial fibrosis has been reported on the chest radiograph in 20% to 65% of patients (43). The initial radiographic abnormalities may be subtle and typically consist of a fine reticulation involving predominantly or exclusively the lower lung zones; as the disease progresses, the reticulation becomes coarser and more extensive (Fig. 6.13). Serial radiographs over several years may show progressive loss of lung volume in addition to a worsening of the interstitial disease.

HRCT frequently demonstrates evidence of interstitial pneumonitis and fibrosis in patients who have normal or questionable radiographic findings (45,46). For example, in one prospective study of 23 patients, a definitive reticular pattern consistent with fibrosis was seen on the chest radiograph in nine (39%) and minimal or equivocal findings in six (26%); by contrast, evidence of fibrosis was seen on HRCT in 21 patients (91%) (47).

The HRCT findings include intralobular linear opacities, giving a reticular pattern; subpleural lines; areas of ground-glass attenuation; and honeycombing (47,48) (Figs. 6.13 and 6.14). The abnormalities involve mainly the lower lobes and have a predominantly peripheral and posterior distribution (48).

There is evidence that the pattern of abnormality on HRCT reflects the relative proportions of fibrosis and inflammation. In one study of 12 patients, comparison was made between the CT findings and open lung biopsy specimens obtained from 20 different lobes (49). In 13 of the lobes, HRCT demonstrated a predominant reticular pattern; in the other seven lobes there was an equivalent extent of reticulation and ground-glass attenuation. On histologic examination, the predominant reticular pattern was associated with a predominantly fibrotic appearance in 12 of 13 lobes. In the lobes that had an equivalent extent of reticulation and ground-glass attenuation, there was an inflammatory ap-

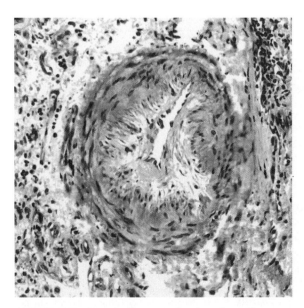

FIGURE 6.12. Progressive systemic sclerosis—pulmonary arterial hypertension. Photomicrograph of a small pulmonary artery shows a moderate degree of medial muscle hypertrophy and marked intimal thickening by loose (fibroblastic) connective tissue. The patient was a 32-year-old woman.

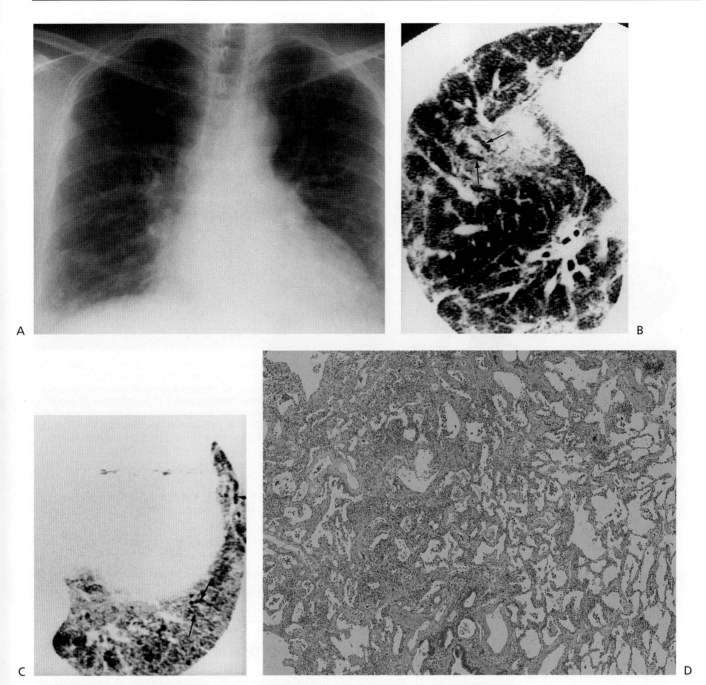

FIGURE 6.13. Progressive systemic sclerosis—nonspecific interstitial pneumonia. **A:** Chest radiograph shows poorly defined ground glass opacities and mild reticulation involving the middle and lower lung zones. **B** and **C.** HRCT images demonstrate areas with ground-glass attenuation, intralobular reticular opacities, and traction bronchiectasis (*arrows*). **D:** Photomicrograph shows diffuse thickening of alveolar septa by mature collagen and a mild infiltrate of lymphocytes. The patient was a 42-year-old woman.

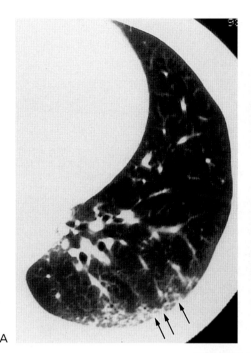
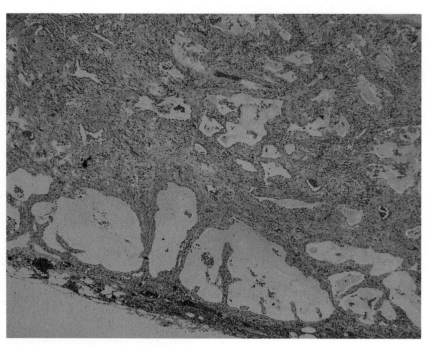

A   B

FIGURE 6.14. Progressive systemic sclerosis—usual interstitial pneumonia. **A:** HRCT image of the left lung demonstrates subpleural intralobular reticular opacities and ground-glass opacities in the posterior and lateral segments of left lower lobe. **B:** Photomicrograph demonstrates subpleural honeycomb change, variably severe interstitial fibrosis, and a mild infiltrate of lymphocytes. Findings characteristic of usual interstitial pneumonia were present in other regions of the specimen. The patient was a 35-year-old woman. (Courtesy of Dr. Kazuya Ichikado, The First Department of Internal Medicine, Kumamoto University School of Medicine, Kumamoto, Japan)

pearance in four lobes and a fibrotic appearance in three lobes. CT thus allowed correct discrimination between inflammatory and fibrotic histologic findings in 16 (80%) of 20 biopsy specimens.

Radiographic evidence of pleural effusion or thickening is less common in PSS than in other connective tissue diseases, being seen in approximately 10% to 15% of patients (50,51). Pleural thickening is seen more commonly on CT: In one series of 55 patients evaluated with HRCT, diffuse pleural thickening was seen in one-third, all of whom also had pulmonary abnormalities (48).

POLYMYOSITIS AND DERMATOMYOSITIS

Polymyositis is an autoimmune inflammatory myopathy characterized by symmetric weakness of limb girdle and anterior neck muscles (52). Dermatomyositis is similar to polymyositis except for the presence of a characteristic skin rash. Polymyositis/dermatomyositis has an incidence of approximately five to 10 per million individuals in the population per year (52); it occurs twice as often in women as in men.

The thorax is commonly affected, generally in one or more of three forms (52,53): (a) hypoventilation and respiratory failure as a result of involvement of the respiratory muscles; (b) interstitial pneumonitis (usually with a histologic pattern of UIP or, less commonly, NSIP (Fig. 6.15); and (c) aspiration pneumonia secondary to pharyngeal muscle weakness (probably the most common pulmonary complication).

The frequency of radiographic parenchymal abnormalities is low (about 5%) (54). The most common is a symmetric, predominantly basal reticular pattern indistinguishable from that of idiopathic pulmonary fibrosis (52). This pattern can become diffuse over time and progress to honeycombing (52). Some patients develop bilateral areas of consolidation

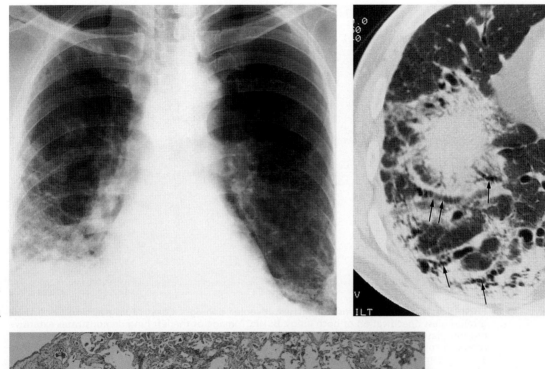

A

B

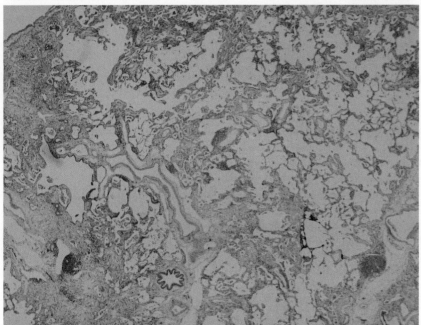

C

FIGURE 6.15. Polymyositis—nonspecific interstitial pneumonia. **A:** Chest radiograph shows ground-glass opacities and mild reticulation involving mainly the lower lung zones. **B:** HRCT image of the right lung demonstrates ground glass attenuation, mild reticulation, and traction bronchiectasis (*arrows*). **C:** Photomicrograph demonstrates patchy, mild to moderate interstitial fibrosis, and chronic inflammation. The patient was a 65-year-old man.

developing over a 2- to 3-week period (Fig. 6.16). This abnormality usually corresponds histologically to diffuse alveolar damage or BOOP (52,53). In patients with BOOP, the consolidation tends to involve mainly the middle and lower lung zones and often has a predominantly peribronchoarterial or subpleural distribution on HRCT (55,56). In patients with diffuse alveolar damage the consolidation tends to be diffuse or to involve mainly the dependent lung regions (Fig. 6.16).

When the respiratory muscles are affected, diaphragmatic elevation and small-volume lungs may be apparent, often in conjunction with basal linear opacities related to subsegmental atelectasis (57). When pharyngeal muscle paralysis is present, unilateral or bilateral segmental pneumonia may result from aspiration of food and oral secretions (52).

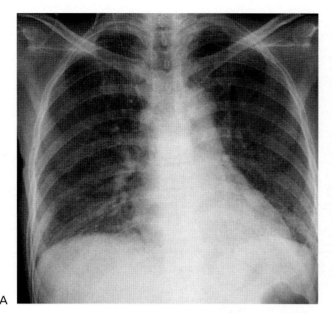
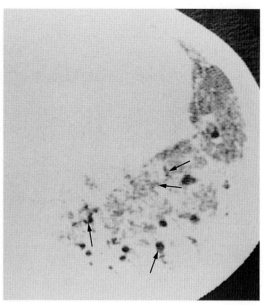

A   B

FIGURE 6.16. Dermatomyositis—diffuse alveolar damage. Chest radiograph shows diffuse ground-glass opacification of both lungs. **B:** HRCT image of the left lung demonstrates extensive ground-glass attenuation, dependent airspace consolidation, and traction bronchiectasis (*arrows*). Histologic examination showed changes consistent with the organizing phase of diffuse alveolar damage. The patient was a 63-year-old woman.

SJÖGREN'S SYNDROME

Sjögren's syndrome is characterized clinically by a triad of dry eyes (keratoconjunctivitis sicca), dry mouth (xerostomia), and arthritis (58). It is relatively common, affecting 0.1% of the general population and 3% of older adults (58). It may be primary, without features of other connective tissue disease, or secondary, when associated with other connective tissue disease, most commonly rheumatoid arthritis.

The most common thoracic complications are lymphocytic interstitial pneumonia (LIP) and airway abnormalities such as follicular bronchitis, bronchiectasis, and bronchiolitis (58). Less common complications include interstitial pneumonitis, BOOP, lymphoma, pulmonary hypertension, and pleural effusion or fibrosis (58).

Pathologic findings in the trachea and bronchi include atrophy of mucous glands associated with a diffuse lymphoplasmacytic cellular infiltrate, abnormalities that are believed to responsible for chronic cough. Aggregates of lymphoid cells (follicular bronchitis) are present on endobronchial biopsy specimens in as many as 20% to 30% of patients (58). LIP is characterized by a diffuse, usually bilateral, interstitial infiltrate of lymphocytes and plasma cells (Fig. 6.17) (5,59). It is usually most prominent in relation to bronchioles and their accompanying vessels, but also is seen in the alveolar interstitium. Fibrosis is usually mild (59). The distinction between LIP and well-differentiated (small lymphocyte) lymphoma can be difficult on routine histologic sections.

Parenchymal abnormalities are evident on the chest radiograph in 10% to 30% of patients (60,61). The most common finding is a reticulonodular pattern involving mainly the lower lung zones. It may reflect the presence of LIP, interstitial fibrosis, or, less commonly, lymphoma (61). The HRCT findings were assessed in a prospective study of 50 patients in whom the onset of SS had occurred a mean of 12 years (range, 2 to 37 years) before the scans (62); 37 (74%) of the 50 patients had no respiratory symptoms at the time of the scan. Abnormalities were detected in 17 patients (34%) on HRCT, compared with seven (14%) on chest radiographs. The most common findings consisted of bronchiolectasis and poorly defined centrilobular nodular or branching linear opacities (seen in 11 patients), areas of ground-glass attenuation (seen in seven), and honeycombing (seen in

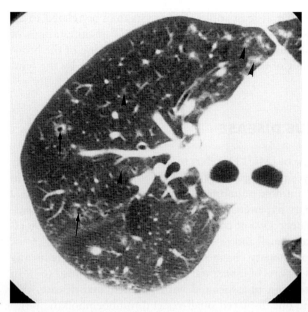
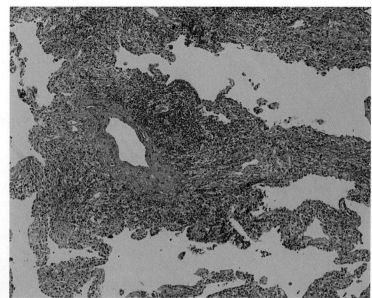

A   B

FIGURE 6.17. Sjögren syndrome—lymphocytic interstitial pneumonia. **A:** HRCT image shows small cysts (*arrows*), faint centrilobular opacities (*arrowheads*), and patchy areas of ground-glass attenuation. **B:** Photomicrograph shows a dense infiltrate of lymphocytes, plasma cells, and histiocytes in peribronchiolar and perivascular interstitium, and, to a lesser extent, alveolar walls. The patient was a 28-year-old woman.

four). The latter was bilateral and asymmetric and present almost exclusively in the periphery of the lower lobes.

A characteristic pattern of extensive areas of ground-glass attenuation with scattered thin-walled cysts has been reported in approximately 50% of patients with LIP (Fig. 6.18) (63,64). Similar findings have been described in LIP not associated with Sjögren's syndrome (64,65). A biopsy specimen in one patient showed interstitial peribronchiolar lymphoplasmacytic infiltrates associated with overinflation of the secondary pul-

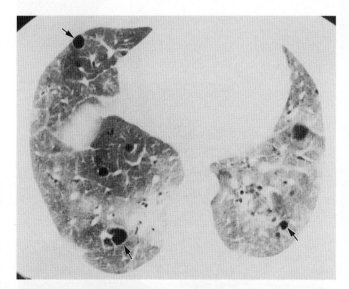

FIGURE 6.18. Sjögren syndrome—lymphocytic interstitial pneumonia. An HRCT image at the level of the dome of the right hemidiaphragm shows diffuse ground-glass opacities and several cysts (*arrows*) in both lungs. The patient was a 50-year-old woman.

monary lobule (65); this suggests that at least some of the cysts may be related to air trapping secondary to bronchiolar stenosis. Other common HRCT manifestations of LIP include poorly defined centrilobular nodular opacities and thickening of the bronchovascular bundles, both the result of expansion of the interstitial tissue by the lymphoid infiltrate (64).

MIXED CONNECTIVE TISSUE DISEASE

The term *mixed connective tissue disease* (MCTD) refers to a condition in which there are features of SLE, PSS, and polymyositis. Respiratory involvement has been described in 20% to 80% of patients (66). Common pulmonary abnormalities include interstitial pneumonitis and fibrosis, pulmonary hypertension, and pleural effusion. The last is particularly common, with approximately 35% of patients developing pleurisy and 50% effusion (66). The effusions are usually small and resolve spontaneously.

Pathologic characteristics of pulmonary changes in MCTD have been infrequently described. There have been several reports of interstitial pneumonitis and fibrosis (67). In three cases of pulmonary hypertension unassociated with parenchymal disease, two showed plexogenic arteriopathy and one displayed small-vessel thromboemboli (67,68).

The radiologic manifestations of MCTD include findings seen in patients who have SLE, progressive systemic sclerosis, and polymyositis (69). The frequency of pulmonary abnormalities varies considerably in different series. For example, in a retrospective study of 81 patients from the Mayo Clinic, an interstitial pattern was seen on the chest radiograph in 19% (70). On the other hand, careful prospective study of 34 patients in another investigation demonstrated interstitial abnormalities in 85% (71). The abnormalities consisted of irregular linear opacities having a reticular pattern and involving mainly the lung bases (71). With progression of disease, the fibrosis gradually extends superiorly; in the late stage, honeycombing may be identified. HRCT shows a predominantly subpleural distribution of fibrosis, similar to that seen in the interstitial fibrosis associated with other connective tissue diseases (Fig. 6.19) (69). Other radiographic abnormalities include areas of

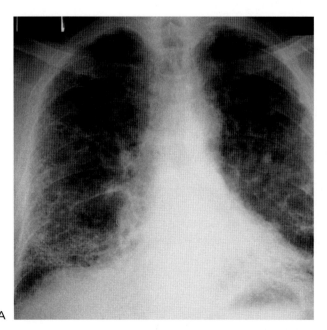
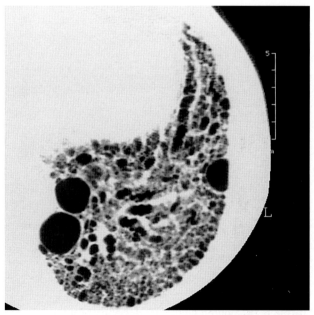

A   B

FIGURE 6.19. Mixed connective tissue disease—usual interstitial pneumonia. **A:** Chest radiograph shows reticular opacities, honeycomb cysts, and ground-glass opacities involving mainly the middle and lower lung zones. **B:** HRCT image of the left lung base demonstrates extensive honeycombing, reticulation, and traction bronchiectasis. The patient was a 74-year-old man.

parenchymal consolidation that may be related to aspiration pneumonia (69) or diffuse pulmonary hemorrhage (72).

ANKYLOSING SPONDYLITIS

Ankylosing spondylitis is a chronic inflammatory disease affecting mainly the joints of the axial skeleton (sacroiliac, costovertebral and apophyseal joints). It affects mainly men (male-to-female ratio of 10:1) (73). Approximately 1% to 2% of patients have pleuropulmonary complications (73). The most common pulmonary manifestation is upper lobe fibrobullous disease. Radiologically, the process begins as apical pleural involvement followed by an apical infiltrate that progresses to cavity and bulla formation (12). Generally, the disease begins unilaterally and becomes bilateral.

A variety of abnormalities can be seen on HRCT, including evidence of apical fibrosis, paraseptal emphysema, bronchiectasis, interstitial fibrosis, mediastinal lymph node enlargement, and tracheal dilatation (74).

REFERENCES

1. Murin S, Wiedemann HP, Matthay RA. Pulmonary manifestations of systemic lupus erythematosus. *Clin Chest Med* 1998;19:641–665.
2. Cervera R, Khamashta MA, Font J, et al. Systemic lupus erythematosus: clinical and immunologic patterns of disease expression in a cohort of 1,000 patients. *Medicine (Baltimore)* 1993;72:113–124.
3. King JS, Lee KS, Koh EM, et al. Thoracic involvement of systemic lupus erythematosus: clinical, pathologic, and radiologic findings. *J Comput Assist Tomogr* 2000;24:9–18.
4. Auerbach RC, Snyder NE, Bragg DG. The chest roentgenographic manifestations of pronestyl-induced lupus erythematosus. *Radiology* 1973;109:287–290.
5. Colby TV. Pulmonary pathology in patients with systemic autoimmune diseases. *Clin Chest Medicine* 1998;19:587–612
6. Matthay RA, Schwarz MI, Petty TL, et al. Pulmonary manifestations of systemic lupus erythematosus: review of twelve cases of acute lupus pneumonitis. *Medicine (Baltimore)* 1975;54:397–409.
7. Miller LR, Greenberg SD, McLarty JW. Lupus lung. *Chest* 1985;88:265–269.
8. Haupt HM, Moore GW, Hutchins GM. The lung in systemic lupus erythematosus: analysis of the pathologic changes in 120 patients. *Am J Med* 1981;71:791–798.
9. Myers JL, Katzenstein A-LA. Microangiitis in lupus-induced pulmonary hemorrhage. *Am J Clin Pathol* 1986;85:552–556.
10. Asherson RA, Oakley CM. Pulmonary hypertension and systemic lupus erythematosus. *J Rheumatol* 1986;13:1–5.
11. Bulgrin JG, Dubois EL, Jacobson G. Chest roentgenographic changes in systemic lupus erythematosus. *Radiology* 1960;74:42–49.
12. Primack SL, Müller NL. Radiologic manifestations of the systemic autoimmune diseases. *Clin Chest Med* 1998;19:573–586.
13. Wiedemann HP, Matthay RA. Pulmonary manifestations of systemic lupus erythematosus. *J Thorac Imaging* 1992;7:1–18.
14. Gammon RB, Bridges TA, Al-Nezir H, et al. Bronchiolitis obliterans organizing pneumonia associated with systemic lupus erythematosus. *Chest* 1992;102:1171–1174.
15. Onomura K, Nakata H, Tanaka Y, et al. Pulmonary hemorrhage in patients with systemic lupus erythematosus. *J Thorac Imaging* 1991;6:57–61.
16. Bankier AA, Kiener HP, Wiesmayr MN, et al. Discrete lung involvement in systemic lupus erythematosus. CT assessment. *Radiology* 1995;196:835–840.
17. Fenlon HM, Doran M, Sant SM, et al. High-resolution chest CT in systemic lupus erythematosus. *Am J Roentgenol* 1996;166:301–307.
18. Tanoue LT. Pulmonary manifestations of rheumatoid arthritis. *Clin Chest Med* 1998;19:667–685.
19. Remy-Jardin M, Remy J, Cortet B, et al. Lung changes in rheumatoid arthritis: CT findings. *Radiology* 1994;193:375–382.
20. Jurik AG, Davidsen D, Graudal H. Prevalence of pulmonary involvement in rheumatoid arthritis and its relationship to some characteristics of the patients—a radiological and clinical study. *Scand J Rheumatol* 1982;11:217–224.
21. Laitinen O, Nissila M, Salorinne Y, et al. Pulmonary involvement in patients who have rheumatoid arthritis. *Scand J Respir Dis* 1975;56:297.

22. Frank ST, Weg JG, Harkleroad LE, et al. Pulmonary dysfunction in rheumatoid disease. *Chest* 1973; 63:27–34.
23. Gabbay E, Tarala R, Will R, et al. Interstitial lung disease in recent-onset rheumatoid arthritis. *Am J Respir Crit Care Med* 1997;156:528–535.
24. Anaya JM, Diethelm L, Ortiz LA, et al. Pulmonary involvement in rheumatoid arthritis. *Semin Arthritis Rheum* 1995;24:242–254.
25. Katzenstein AL, Fiorelli RF. Nonspecific interstitial pneumonia/fibrosis: histologic features and clinical significance. *Am J Surg Pathol* 1994;18:136–147.
26. Hakala M, Paakko P, Huhti E, et al. Open lung biopsy of patients with rheumatoid arthritis. *Clin Rheumatol* 1990;9:452–460.
27. DeHoratius RJ, Abruzzo JL, Williams RC Jr. Immunofluorescent and immunologic studies of rheumatoid lung. *Arch Intern Med* 1972;129:441–446.
28. Yousem SA, Colby TV, Carrington CB. Lung biopsy in rheumatoid arthritis. *Am Rev Respir Dis* 1985;131:770–777.
29. Gamsu G. Radiographic manifestations of thoracic involvement by collagen vascular diseases. *J Thorac Imaging* 1992;7:1–12.
30. Staples CA, Müller NL, Vedal S, et al. Usual interstitial pneumonia: correlation of CT with clinical, functional, and radiologic findings. *Radiology* 1987;162:377–381.
31. Nusslein HG, Rodl W, Giedel J, et al. Multiple peripheral pulmonary nodules preceding rheumatoid arthritis. *Rheumatol Int* 1987;7:89–91.
32. Walters MN, Ojeda VJ. Pleuropulmonary necrobiotic rheumatoid nodules: A review and clinico-pathological study of six patients. *Med J Aust* 1986;144:648–651.
33. Shannon TM, Gale ME. Noncardiac manifestations of rheumatoid arthritis in the thorax. *J Thorac Imaging* 1992;7:19–29.
34. Aquino SL, Webb RW, Golden J. Bronchiolitis obliterans associated with rheumatoid arthritis: findings on HRCT and dynamic expiratory CT. *J Comput Assist Tomogr* 1994;18:555–558.
35. Perez T, Remy-Jardin M, Cortet B. Airways involvement in rheumatoid arthritis: clinical, functional, and HRCT findings. *Am J Respir Crit Care Med* 1998;157:1658–1665.
36. Begin R, Masse S, Cantin A, et al. Airway disease in a subset of nonsmoking rheumatoid patients: characterization of the disease and evidence for an autoimmune pathogenesis. *Am J Med* 1982;72:743–750.
37. Padley SPG, Adler BD, Hansell DM, et al. Bronchiolitis obliterans: high-resolution CT findings and correlation with pulmonary function tests. *Clin Radiol* 1993;47:236–240.
38. Yousem SA, Colby TV, Carrington CB. Follicular bronchitis/bronchiolitis. *Hum Pathol* 1985;16: 700–706.
39. Hayakawa H, Sato A, Imokawa S, et al. Bronchiolar disease in rheumatoid arthritis. *Am J Respir Crit Care Med* 1996;154:1531–—1536.
40. Howling SJ, Hansell DM, Wells AU, et al. Follicular bronchiolitis: thin-section CT and histologic findings. *Radiology* 1999;212:637–642.
41. Fujii M, Adachi S, Shimizu T, et al. Interstitial lung disease in rheumatoid arthritis: assessment with high-resolution computed tomography. *J Thorac Imag* 1993;8:54–62.
42. Faurschou P, Francis D, Faarup P. Thoracoscopic, histological, and clinical findings in nine cases of rheumatoid pleural effusion. *Thorax* 1985;40:371–375.
43. Minai OA, Dweik RA, Arroliga AC. Manifestations of scleroderma pulmonary disease. *Clin Chest Medicine* 1998;19:713–731.
44. Young RH, Mark GJ. Pulmonary vascular changes in scleroderma. *Am J Med* 1978; 64:998–1004.
45. Arroliga AC, Podell DN, Matthay RA. Pulmonary manifestations of scleroderma. *J Thorac Imaging* 1992;7:30–45.
46. Warrick JH, Bhalla M, Schabel SI, et al. High-resolution computed tomography in early scleroderma lung disease. *J Rheumatol* 1991;18:1520–1528.
47. Schurawitzki H, Stiglbauer R, Graninger W, et al. Interstitial lung disease in progressive systemic sclerosis: high-resolution CT versus radiography. *Radiology* 1990;176:755–759.
48. Remy-Jardin M, Remy J, Wallaert B, et al. Pulmonary involvement in progressive systemic sclerosis: sequential evaluation with CT, pulmonary function tests, and bronchoalveolar lavage. *Radiology* 1993;188:499–506.
49. Wells AU, Hansell DM, Corrin B, et al. High-resolution computed tomography as a predictor of lung histology in systemic sclerosis. *Thorax* 1992;47:508–512.
50. Owens GR, Fino GJ, Herbert DL, et al. Pulmonary function in progressive systemic sclerosis: comparison of CREST syndrome variant with diffuse scleroderma. *Chest* 1983;84:546–550.
51. McCarthy DS, Baragar FD, Dhingra S, et al. The lung in systemic sclerosis (scleroderma): a review and new information. *Semin Arthritis Rheum* 1988;17:271–283.
52. Schwarz MI. The lung in polymyositis. *Clin Chest Medicine* 1998;19:701–712
53. Tazelaar HD, Viggiano RW, Pickersgill J, et al. Interstitial lung disease in polymyositis and dermatomyositis: clinical features and prognosis as correlated with histologic findings. *Am Rev Respir Dis* 1990;141:727–733.

54. Frazier AR, Miller RD. Interstitial pneumonitis in association with polymyositis and dermatomyositis. *Chest* 1974;65:403–407.
55. Ikezoe J, Johkoh T, Nohno N, et al. High-resolution CT findings of lung disease in patients with polymyositis and dermatomyositis. *J Thorac Imaging* 1996;11:250–259.
56. Mino M, Noma S, Taguchi Y, et al. Pulmonary involvement in polymyositis and dermatomyositis: segmental evaluation with CT. *Am J Roentgenol* 1997;169:83–87.
57. Schiavi EA, Roncoroni AJ, Puy RJM. Isolated bilateral diaphragmatic paresis with interstitial lung disease: an unusual presentation of dermatomyositis. *Am Rev Respir Dis* 1984;129:337–339.
58. Cain HC, Noble PW, Matthay RA. Pulmonary manifestations of Sjögren's syndrome. *Clin Chest Medicine* 1998;19:687–699
59. Deheinzelin D, Capelozzi VL, Kairalla RA, et al. Interstitial lung disease in primary Sjögren's syndrome. *Am J Respir Crit Care Med* 1996;154:794–799.
60. Silbiger ML, Peterson CC Jr. Sjögren's syndrome: its roentgenographic features. *Am J Roentgenol Radium Ther Nucl Med* 1967;100:554–558.
61. Strimlan CV, Rosenow EC III, Divertie MB, et al. Pulmonary manifestations of Sjögren's syndrome. *Chest* 1976;70:354–361.
62. Franquet T, Gimenez A, Monill JM, et al. Primary Sjögren's syndrome and associated lung disease: CT findings in 50 patients. *Am J Roentgenol* 1997;169:655–658.
63. Meyer CA, Pina JS, Taillon D, et al. Inspiratory and expiratory high-resolution CT findings in a patient with Sjögren's syndrome and cystic lung disease. *Am J Roentgenol* 1997;168:101–103.
64. Johkoh T, Müller NL, Pickford M, et al. Lymphocytic interstitial pneumonia: thin-section CT findings in 22 patients. *Radiology* 1999;212:567–572.
65. Ichikawa Y, Kinoshita M, Koga T, et al. Lung cyst formation in lymphocytic interstitial pneumonia: CT features. *J Comput Assist Tomogr* 1994;18:745–748.
66. Prakash UBS. Respiratory complications in mixed connective tissue disease. *Clin Chest Medicine* 1998;19:733–746.
67. Wiener-Kronish JP, Solinger AM, Warnock ML, et al. Severe pulmonary involvement in mixed connective tissue disease. *Am Rev Respir Dis* 1981;124:499–503.
68. Jones MB, Osterholm RK, Wilson RB, et al. Fatal pulmonary hypertension and resolving immune-complex glomerulonephritis in mixed connective tissue disease: a case report and review of the literature. *Am J Med* 1978;65:855–863.
69. Prakash UBS. Lungs in mixed connective tissue disease. *J Thorac Imaging* 1992;7:55–61.
70. Prakash UBS, Luthra HS, Divertie MB. Intrathoracic manifestations in mixed connective tissue disease. *Mayo Clin Proc* 1985;60:813–821.
71. Sullivan WD, Hurst DJ, Harmon CE, et al. A prospective evaluation emphasizing pulmonary involvement in patients with mixed connective tissue disease. *Medicine (Baltimore)* 1984;63:92–107.
72. Müller NL, Miller RR. Diffuse pulmonary hemorrhage. *Radiol Clin North Am* 1991;29:965–971.
73. Lee-Chiong TL. Pulmonary manifestations of ankylosing spondylitis and relapsing polychondritis. *Clin Chest Med* 1998;19:747–757
74. Fenlon HM, Casserly I, Sant SM, et al. Plain radiographs and thoracic high-resolution CT in patients who have ankylosing spondylitis. *Am J Roentgenol* 1997;168:1067–1072.

EOSINOPHILIC LUNG DISEASE

The term *eosinophilic lung disease* encompasses a group of entities characterized pathologically by the accumulation of eosinophils in alveolar airspaces and the adjacent interstitial tissue (1,2). They can be classified into groups with and without known cause; those of unknown origin are distinguished from one another largely by their clinical features.

IDIOPATHIC EOSINOPHILIC LUNG DISEASE

Simple Pulmonary Eosinophilia

Simple pulmonary eosinophilia (Loeffler's syndrome) is an uncommon disorder characterized by nonsegmental areas of parenchymal consolidation, usually transient, on chest radiographs and blood eosinophilia. Apart from a background of asthma and atopy (1), patients have few or no symptoms, and the diagnosis often is suspected initially by the finding of characteristic opacities on a chest radiograph. Transbronchial biopsy specimens show edema and accumulation of eosinophils in alveolar septa and interstitium (1,3).

The radiographic manifestations consist of transient and migratory areas of consolidation that typically clear spontaneously within 1 month (2). These are nonsegmental, may be single or multiple, usually have ill-defined margins, and often have a predominantly peripheral distribution (1,2). The main findings on high-resolution computed tomography (HRCT) consist of ground-glass opacities or airspace consolidation, again usually transient and migratory, involving mainly the peripheral regions of the middle and upper lung zones (4). Airspace nodules may also be present within the areas of ground-glass attenuation (4,5).

Acute Eosinophilic Pneumonia

Acute eosinophilic pneumonia is an acute febrile illness associated with rapidly increasing shortness of breath and hypoxemic respiratory failure (1,6). Eosinophils are characteristically markedly increased in number in bronchoalveolar lavage (BAL) fluid (6), whereas blood eosinophilia is usually absent. The principal histologic finding is diffuse alveolar damage (airspace exudate and edema with hyaline membrane formation) associated with numerous eosinophils (Fig. 7.1) (7).

The radiographic manifestations are similar to those of hydrostatic pulmonary edema (1,8). The earliest manifestation consists of reticular opacities, frequently with septal (Kerley B) lines (Fig. 7.2). This progresses over a few hours or days to bilateral airspace con-

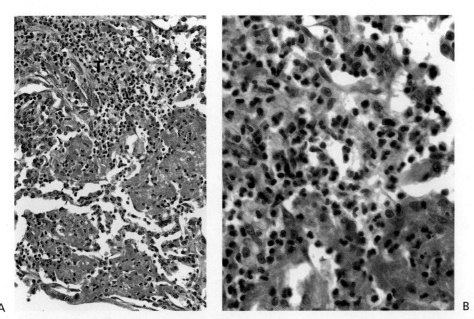

FIGURE 7.1. Acute eosinophilic pneumonia. Low- (**A**) and high- (**B**) magnification photomicrographs show filling of several alveolar airspaces by a proteinaceous exudate. Numerous eosinophils are present in the interstitial tissue (*T*) and the airspaces.

solidation involving mainly the lower lung zones (1). Small bilateral pleural effusions are present in the majority of patients (8).

The HRCT findings include bilateral areas of ground-glass attenuation, smooth interlobular septal thickening, small pleural effusions, and, occasionally, areas of consolidation (Figs. 7.2 and 7.3) (4,9). The parenchymal abnormalities have a random distribution in both cephalocaudal and cross-sectional planes (4). In contrast to chronic eosinophilic pneumonia, a peripheral distribution is seldom seen (1,4).

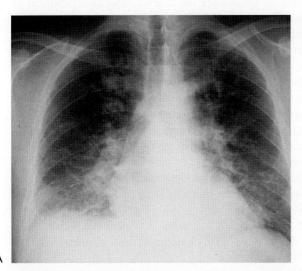
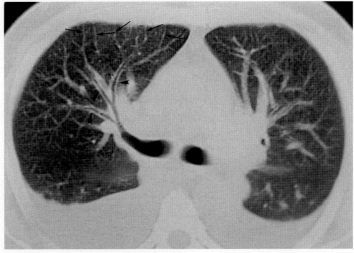

FIGURE 7.2. Acute eosinophilic pneumonia. **A:** Chest radiograph shows enlargement of the hilar and lower lobe pulmonary vascular markings, poorly defined ground-glass opacities in the lower lung zones, and small pleural effusions. The findings are similar to those of hydrostatic pulmonary edema. **B:** CT image demonstrates diffusely distributed thickening of interlobular septa (*arrows*), areas of ground-glass attenuation and thickened bronchovascular bundles (*arrowheads*). The patient was a 28-year-old man.

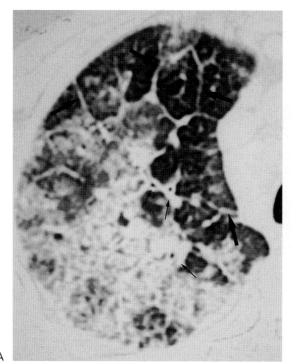
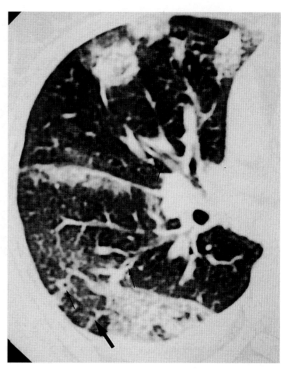

A   B

FIGURE 7.3. Acute eosinophilic pneumonia. **A:** HRCT image of the right upper lobe shows smooth thickening of interlobular septa (*large arrows*) and bronchovascular bundles (*small arrows*) and extensive areas of ground-glass attenuation and consolidation. **B:** Image of the right middle and lower lobes shows less extensive septal thickening (*large arrow*) and bronchovascular bundles (*small arrows*) and patchy ground-glass opacities. The patient was a 58-year-old woman. (Courtesy of Dr. Yasuhiro Kondo, Tosei Municipal Hospital, Seto, Japan.)

Chronic Eosinophilic Pneumonia

Patients with chronic eosinophilic pneumonia usually present with a history of fever, cough, and shortness of breath. These symptoms are often severe and last 3 months or longer (10). Blood eosinophilia is usually present.

The predominant histologic finding is filling of alveolar airspaces by an inflammatory infiltrate containing a high proportion of eosinophils (Fig. 7.4) (1,11). Aggregates of necrotic eosinophils surrounded by a rim of palisaded histiocytes are often present. The interstitium usually contains a similar, albeit often less pronounced, cellular infiltrate and may show fibrosis (11). Pulmonary vessels frequently contain eosinophils and other inflammatory cells in their walls; however, necrosis or thrombosis is not seen.

Approximately 60% of patients have homogeneous peripheral airspace consolidation, "the photographic negative of pulmonary edema," involving mainly the upper lobes (Fig. 7.5) (10). This pattern can remain unchanged for weeks or months unless steroid therapy is given. A review of the radiographic manifestations of 119 patients revealed that consolidation involved mainly the outer two-thirds of the lungs in 74 (62%) and was limited to the lung periphery in 30 (25%) (10).

On HRCT, bilateral areas of consolidation are seen in 100% of patients and ground-glass opacities in 90% (4). In 85% to 95% of patients these abnormalities involve predominantly or exclusively the subpleural lung regions (Fig. 7. 5) (4,12,13). In one review of the findings in 40 patients, upper lung zone predominance was evident in approximately 40%; lower zone predominance, in 20%; and a random distribution, in 40% (4). Less common findings include airspace nodules, bronchial wall thickening, and bandlike opacities (4,13). The latter usually occur with clearing of disease and likely reflect atelectasis.

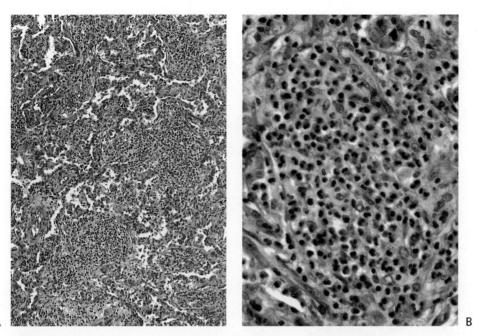

FIGURE 7.4. A, B: Chronic eosinophilic pneumonia. Photomicrographs show interstitial thickening and airspace filling by macrophages and numerous eosinophils.

Hypereosinophilic Syndrome

Hypereosinophilic syndrome (HES) is considered to be present in patients who have blood eosinophilia for at least 6 months and multiorgan tissue infiltration by eosinophils (1,14). The heart and central nervous system are affected most commonly (14). Pulmonary and pleural involvement is seen in approximately 40% of cases.

The syndrome may occur in association with a clear-cut cause or may be idiopathic. Three criteria have been established for the diagnosis of idiopathic HES (15): (a) persis-

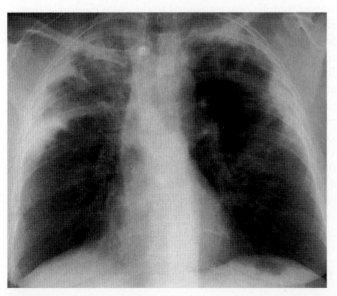

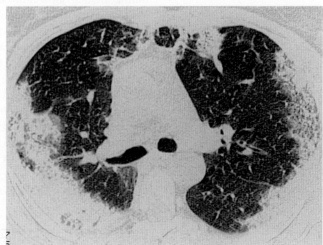

FIGURE 7.5. Chronic eosinophilic pneumonia. **A:** Chest radiograph shows nonsegmental airspace consolidation involving mainly the subpleural regions of the upper lobes. **B:** HRCT image demonstrates subpleural consolidation and ground-glass opacities. (Case courtesy of Dr. Maura Brown, Surrey Memorial Hospital, Vancouver, BC.)

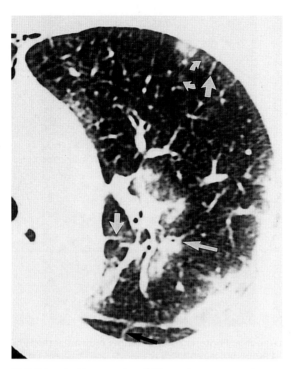

FIGURE 7.6. Hypereosinophilic syndrome. HRCT image of the left upper lobe demonstrates bronchial wall thickening (*long arrow*), interlobular septal thickening (*short arrows*), poorly defined centrilobular nodules (*small, curved arrows*), and patchy areas of ground-glass attenuation and consolidation. Also noted is mild thickening of interlobar fissure. The patient was a 59-year-woman.

tent eosinophilia of $1,500/mm^3$ for at least 6 months, or death before 6 months in individuals with appropriate signs and symptoms; (b) lack of evidence for parasitic, allergic, or other recognized cause of the syndrome; and (c) signs and symptoms of organ involvement, either directly related to eosinophilia or unexplained in the given clinical setting.

Pathologic features of pulmonary disease have rarely been documented. Histologic examination may show infiltration of the walls of small pulmonary arteries by eosinophils (16); associated luminal obliteration may be associated with parenchymal infarction. Pulmonary fibrosis may be present, usually in patients who also have HES-related heart disease (15).

Initially, chest radiographs may reveal transient hazy opacities or areas of consolidation that can resolve spontaneously (14). When other organs are involved, an interstitial pattern has been described, presumably related to perivascular eosinophilic infiltration or fibrosis (1,16). Cardiac decompensation is manifested by cardiomegaly, pulmonary edema, and pleural effusion (17).

In one investigation of the HRCT findings in five patients, the predominant abnormality in all five was bilateral pulmonary nodules 1 cm or less in diameter (Fig. 7.6) (18). Most nodules had a halo of ground-glass attenuation and involved the peripheral lung regions. The pathologic correlate of these abnormalities is uncertain. Three patients had focal ground-glass opacities and two had small pleural effusions.

EOSINOPHILIC LUNG DISEASE OF SPECIFIC ETIOLOGY

Drugs

A large number of drugs have been reported to be associated with eosinophilic lung disease, including antibiotics, nonsteroidal antiinflammatory agents, drugs used for inflam-

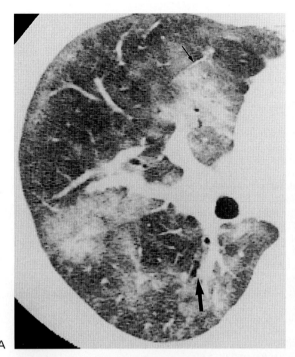
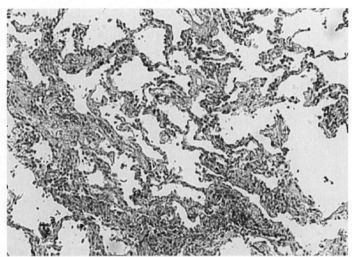

A

B

FIGURE 7.7. Drug-induced eosinophilic pneumonia. **A:** HRCT image of the right lung shows extensive ground-glass opacities and patchy airspace consolidation. Similar findings were present throughout both lungs. Mild thickening of bronchovascular bundles (*small arrow*) and interlobular septa (*large arrow*) is also evident. **B:** Photomicrograph of a biopsy specimen shows a moderate degree of interstitial pneumonitis, which, at higher magnification, was seen to be related predominantly to an infiltrate of eosinophils. The patient was a 56-year-old man with reaction to busulfan.

matory bowel disease, and illicit drugs such as cocaine and heroin (1,2). Reactions range from those similar to simple pulmonary eosinophilia to those imitating acute eosinophilic pneumonia (Fig. 7.7). These reactions are discussed in greater detail in Chapter 10.

Parasitic Infestation

Parasitic infestation most commonly results in findings similar to simple pulmonary eosinophilia (5). Most cases are due to roundworms such as *Ascaris lumbricoides, Toxocara* species, *Ancylostoma,* and *Strongyloides stercoralis* (1,2,5). Tropical pulmonary eosinophilia is caused by the worms *Wuchereria bancrofti* and *Brugia malayi,* with most cases being reported in India, Africa, South America, and Southeast Asia (19). In the Far East, the lung fluke *Paragonimus westermani* is typically responsible.

Fungal Infection

The primary fungal disease associated with pulmonary eosinophilia is allergic bronchopulmonary aspergillosis, characterized clinically by asthma and peripheral eosinophilia, and radiologically by central bronchiectasis and mucous plugging (see Chapter 2). Uncommonly, various other mycotic organisms cause a similar hypersensitivity reaction.

Connective Tissue Disease and Vasculitis

Connective tissue disease and vasculitis are characterized by their multisystemic nature and, in most instances, immunopathogenesis. The most common of these that are associated with blood or tissue eosinophilia are allergic granulomatosis (Churg-Strauss syndrome; see Chapter 19) (20) and rheumatoid arthritis (21).

REFERENCES

1. Allen JN, Davis WB. Eosinophilic lung diseases. *Am J Respir Crit Care Med* 1994;150:1423–1438.
2. Bain GA, Flower CD. Pulmonary eosinophilia. *Eur J Radiol* 1996;23:3–8.
3. Ford RM. Transient pulmonary eosinophilia and asthma: a review of 20 cases occurring in 5,702 asthma sufferers. *Am Rev Respir Dis* 1966;93:797–803.
4. Johkoh T, Müller NL, Akira M, et al. Eosinophilic lung diseases: diagnostic accuracy of thin-section CT in 111 patients. *Radiology* 2000;216:773–780.
5. Kim Y, Lee KS, Choi DC, et al. The spectrum of eosinophilic lung disease: radiologic findings. *J Comput Assist Tomogr* 1997;21:920–930.
6. Allen JN, Pacht ER, Gadek JE, et al. Acute eosinophilic pneumonia as a reversible cause of noninfectious respiratory failure. *N Engl J Med* 1989;321:569–574.
7. Tazelaar HD, Linz LJ, Colby TV, et al. Acute eosinophilic pneumonia: histopathologic findings in nine patients. *Am J Respir Crit Care Med* 1997;155:296–302.
8. Cheon JE, Lee KS, Jung GS, et al. Acute eosinophilic pneumonia: radiographic and CT findings in six patients. *Am J Roentgenol* 1996;167:1195–1199.
9. King MA, Pope-Harman AL, Allen JN, et al. Acute eosinophilic pneumonia: radiologic and clinical features. *Radiology* 1997;203:715–719.
10. Jederlinic PJ, Sicilian L, Gaensler EA. Chronic eosinophilic pneumonia: a report of 19 cases and a review of the literature. *Medicine* 1988;67:154–162.
11. Carrington CB, Addington WW, Goff AM, et al. Chronic eosinophilic pneumonia. *N Engl J Med* 1969;280:787–798.
12. Mayo JR, Müller NL, Road J, et al. Chronic eosinophilic pneumonia: CT findings in six cases. *Am J Roentgenol* 1989;153:727–730.
13. Ebara H, Ikezoe J, Johkoh T, et al. Chronic eosinophilic pneumonia: evolution of chest radiograms and CT features. *J Comput Assist Tomogr* 1994;18:737–744.
14. Winn RE, Kollef MH, Meyer JI. Pulmonary involvement in the hypereosinophilic syndrome. *Chest* 1994;105:656–660.
15. Fauci AS, Harley JB, Roberts WC, et al. The idiopathic hypereosinophilic syndrome. *Ann Intern Med* 1982;97:78–92.
16. Hill R, Wang NS, Berry G. Hypereosinophilic syndrome with pulmonary vascular involvement. *Angiology* 1984;35:238.
17. Epstein DM, Taormina V, Gefter WB, et al. The hypereosinophilic syndrome. *Radiology* 1981;140:59–62.
18. Kang EY, Shim JJ, Kim JS, et al. Pulmonary involvement of idiopathic hypereosinophilic syndrome: CT findings in five patients. *J Comput Assist Tomogr* 1997;21:612–615.
19. Ottesen EA, Nutman TB. Tropical pulmonary eosinophilia. *Annu Rev Med* 1992;43:417–424.
20. Masi AT, Hunder GG, Lie JT, et al. The American College of Rheumatology 1990 criteria for the classification of Churg-Strauss syndrome (allergic granulomatosis and angiitis). *Arthritis Rheum* 1990;33:1094–1100.
21. Cooney TP. Interrelationship of chronic eosinophilic pneumonia, bronchiolitis obliterans, and rheumatoid disease: a hypothesis. *J Clin Pathol* 1981;34:129–137.

8

INTERSTITIAL PNEUMONIA

USUAL INTERSTITIAL PNEUMONIA/IDIOPATHIC
  PULMONARY FIBROSIS

DESQUAMATIVE INTERSTITIAL PNEUMONIA

RESPIRATORY BRONCHIOLITIS–INTERSTITIAL LUNG
  DISEASE

BRONCHIOLITIS OBLITERANS ORGANIZING
  PNEUMONIA

ACUTE INTERSTITIAL PNEUMONIA

NONSPECIFIC INTERSTITIAL PNEUMONIA

The conditions discussed in this chapter are a heterogeneous group of diseases characterized histologically by inflammation and fibrosis of the parenchymal interstitial tissue. Some degree of airspace disease commonly accompanies the interstitial abnormality in all these conditions; however, because of the prominence of the interstitial involvement in many cases they are often grouped together for the purposes of discussion. The abnormalities include usual interstitial pneumonia (UIP), desquamative interstitial pneumonia (DIP), respiratory bronchiolitis–associated interstitial lung disease (RBILD), bronchiolitis obliterans organizing pneumonia (BOOP), acute interstitial pneumonia (AIP), and nonspecific interstitial pneumonia (NSIP) (1,2). Although the cause of disease is unknown in many patients, the histologic patterns characteristic of these disorders can be seen in association with a variety of etiologies and the term *idiopathic* should only be applied after careful review of the clinical history.

USUAL INTERSTITIAL PNEUMONIA/IDIOPATHIC PULMONARY FIBROSIS

As the name implies, usual interstitial pneumonia (UIP) is the most common type of interstitial pneumonia. It is idiopathic in most patients, in which case it corresponds to the clinical diagnosis of idiopathic pulmonary fibrosis (IPF). IPF occurs most commonly in patients between 50 and 70 years of age (2,3). It has a poor prognosis, with a mean survival of approximately 4 years from the onset of symptoms (4,5). When considering a diagnosis of IPF, it should be remembered that the histologic pattern of UIP also can be seen in association with specific etiologies, such as drugs (e.g., bleomycin), and connective tissue diseases (e.g., rheumatoid disease) (6).

Histologically, UIP is typically variable in appearance, with foci of normal lung alternating with areas that show a variable degree of interstitial inflammation and fibrosis ("spatial heterogeneity") (Fig. 8.1) (1–3). The inflammation is composed predominantly of lymphocytes, with variable numbers of plasma cells and eosinophils; granulomas are not seen. Alveolar airspaces commonly contain an increased number of macrophages; however, unlike DIP, this increase is quite variable in severity, with some regions containing many cells and others few. Airspace fibrosis is minimal or absent. Although most of the interstitial fibrous tissue is composed of mature collagen, small foci of loose (fibroblastic) connective tissue are invariably present (Fig. 8.2). This combination of old and active disease has been termed *temporal heterogeneity* and is generally considered to be necessary for the diagnosis (2–4).

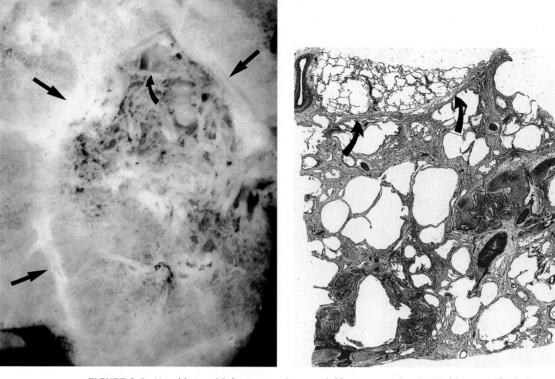

FIGURE 8.1. Usual interstitial pneumonia—spatial heterogeneity. **A:** Highly magnified view of a pulmonary lobule shows fibrosis and honeycomb change (*curved arrow*) in one region and normal parenchyma in another. (*Straight arrows* indicate interlobular septa.) **B:** Low-magnification photomicrograph of lung from another patient shows severe fibrosis and early honeycomb change in one lobule and virtually normal lung in the adjacent one. (*Arrows* indicate interlobular septum.)

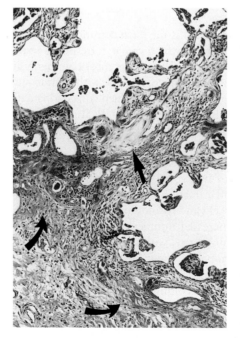

FIGURE 8.2. Usual interstitial pneumonia—temporal heterogeneity. Photomicrograph shows severe fibrosis and mild chronic inflammation associated with obliteration of alveolar airspaces. Foci of dense (mature) fibrous tissue (*curved arrows*) and loose fibroblastic tissue (*straight arrow*) are evident. (HPS stain.)

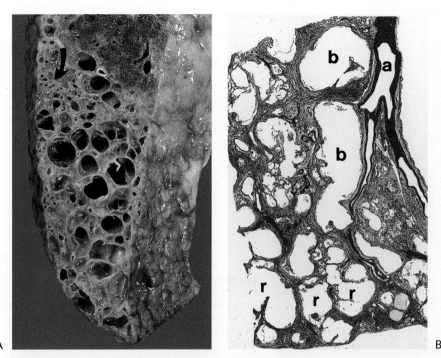

A   B

FIGURE 8.3. Usual interstitial pneumonia—honeycomb change. **A:** Magnified view of a transverse slice of lung shows severe fibrosis and the presence of multiple cystic spaces 0.5 to 1 cm in diameter. **B:** Photomicrograph of tissue taken from a focus of relatively mild cystic change (*arrow* in **A**) shows the central lobular bronchiole (*b*) and artery (*a*). The distal respiratory bronchioles (*r*) are mildly dilated; an increase in this dilatation and in the intervening fibrous tissue leads to the larger cystic spaces seen in **A.**

As might be expected, mild involvement is manifested as a slight degree of alveolar interstitial thickening with preservation of the parenchymal architecture. As disease becomes more severe, alveoli are replaced by fibrous tissue. Contraction of this tissue results in dilatation of residual respiratory bronchioles and alveolar ducts, leading to the formation of cystic spaces (honeycombing) (Fig. 8.3). The same process can occur adjacent to membranous bronchioles and bronchi, resulting in bronchiolectasis and bronchiectasis, respectively (Fig. 8.4). Disease tends to be more prominent in the subpleural than in the central

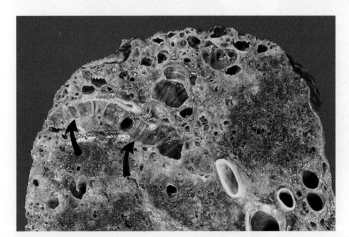

FIGURE 8.4. Usual interstitial pneumonia—traction bronchiectasis. Magnified view of a transverse slice of an upper lobe shows subpleural fibrosis and focal honeycomb change. A moderately dilated bronchus surrounded by fibrous tissue can be seen extending almost to the pleura (*arrows*).

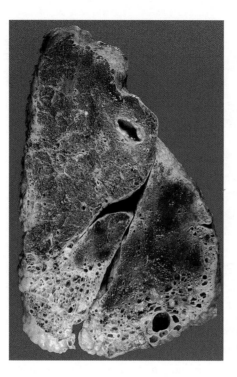

FIGURE 8.5. Usual interstitial pneumonia. Sagittal slice of the right lung shows severe fibrosis and honeycomb change in the basal aspects of the lower and middle lobes. Less marked disease can be seen in the subpleural region of the anterior portion of the upper lobe and the posterior portion of the lower.

parenchyma, and is usually more severe in the basal region of the lower lobes (Fig. 8.5) (7–9).

The radiographic findings of UIP consist of bilateral irregular linear opacities, causing a reticular pattern (Fig. 8.6) (10,11). In approximately 70% of patients, this pattern is most severe in the lower lung zones; in approximately 25%, all zones are involved to a similar degree; and in approximately 5%, the abnormalities involve mainly the middle or up-

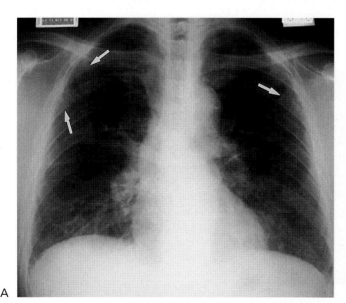

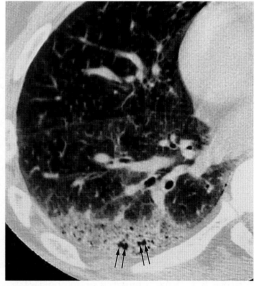

A   B

FIGURE 8.6. Usual interstitial pneumonia. **A:** Chest radiograph shows mild ground-glass opacities and reticulation in the lower lung zones. Focal peripheral reticulation (*arrows*) is also evident in the upper lobes. **B:** HRCT image of the right lung demonstrates subpleural ground-glass opacities, intralobular reticular opacities and mild honeycombing (*arrows*).

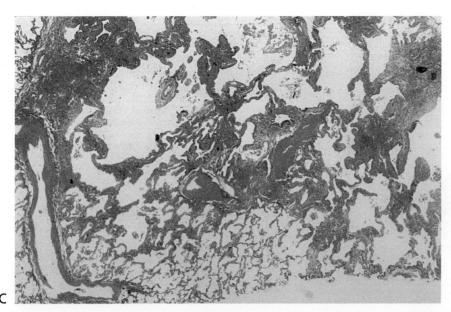

C

FIGURE 8.6. *(continued)* **C:** Photomicrograph shows areas of normal lung, foci of chronic inflammation and fibrosis, and honeycombing cysts. The patient was a 50-year-old man. (Courtesy of Dr. Kazuya Ichikado, Kumamoto University School of Medicine, Kumamoto, Japan.)

per lung zones (12,13). The reticular pattern is initially fine; as fibrosis progresses, it becomes coarser and is associated with progressive loss of lung volume. In the end stage there is diffuse honeycombing.

The characteristic HRCT findings consist of intralobular linear opacities and honeycombing involving mainly the subpleural regions and lung bases (Figs. 8.6 and 8.7) (1,2,8). This subpleural predominance is evident on HRCT in 80% to 95% of patients (7,12). The intralobular linear opacities reflect the presence of interstitial fibrosis. The bronchioles and bronchi in areas of fibrosis are often dilated and tortuous (traction bronchiolectasis and bronchiectasis). Thickening of the intralobular interstitium also results in the presence of irregular interfaces between the lung and pulmonary vessels, bronchi, and pleural surfaces (9). As is seen histologically, parenchymal involvement is typically patchy on HRCT, with areas of normal and markedly abnormal lung often present in the same lobe, and sometimes even in the same lobule (1–3).

Honeycombing is seen on HRCT in most cases and typically involves the subpleural regions and lung bases (1,9,14). It is identified as clustered cystic airspaces usually measuring 2 to 10 mm in diameter and having well-defined walls (Figs. 8.6 and 8.7). The cysts typically appear to share walls on HRCT and usually occur in several layers. The presence of predominantly subpleural and basal reticulation and honeycombing on HRCT is virtually diagnostic of UIP. In a multicenter prospective study of 91 patients suspected of having IPF, 54 were proven to have UIP pathologically (14). The presence of both reticulation and honeycombing in a predominantly subpleural and basal distribution on HRCT had a positive predictive value of 96% in the diagnosis of IPF (14).

Irregular thickening of interlobular septa is sometimes seen on HRCT but is a less conspicuous finding than intralobular interstitial thickening or honeycombing (Fig. 8.7). This septal thickening reflects the presence of fibrosis in the periphery of the secondary lobule (15,16). Patchy areas of ground-glass attenuation are also commonly present, albeit usually less extensive than the reticular pattern (1,7). They correspond to areas of inflammation or, less commonly, fibrosis below the resolution of HRCT (17). Ground-glass opacity should be considered to represent inflammation only when there are no associated HRCT findings of fibrosis such as intralobular reticular opacities, honeycombing, and traction bronchiectasis in the same area (18).

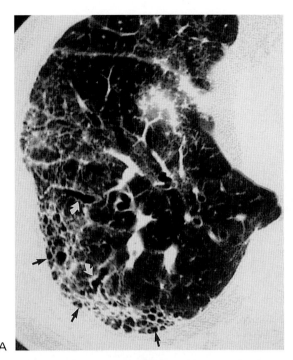

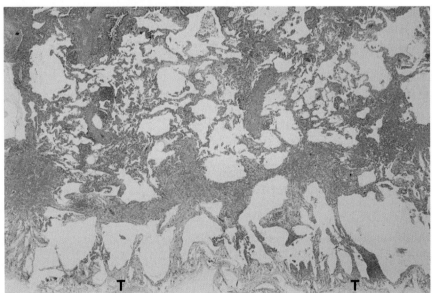

FIGURE 8.7. Usual interstitial pneumonia. **A:** HRCT image demonstrates irregular linear opacities and honeycombing (*black arrows*) involving mainly the subpleural regions of the right lower lobe. Traction bronchiectasis (*white arrows*) is evident in the regions of fibrosis. Patchy ground-glass opacities are present in the right lower and middle lobes. **B:** Photomicrograph of the pathologic specimen shows patchy interstitial fibrosis and chronic inflammation and a row of cystic spaces (honeycomb cysts) in the subpleural region (*T* = pleura). The patient was a 73-year-old man.

Occasionally, patients with IPF develop a fulminant and often fatal acute exacerbation (Fig. 8.8) (19). The HRCT findings consist of extensive multifocal, diffuse or (less commonly) peripheral ground-glass attenuation superimposed on a background of interstitial fibrosis (20,21). The histologic appearance is that of acute interstitial pneumonia (i.e., diffuse alveolar damage). Multifocal and diffuse ground-glass attenuation corresponds to the exudative phase of this abnormality, whereas peripheral ground-glass attenuation relates to the proliferative (fibroblastic) phase (20,21).

DESQUAMATIVE INTERSTITIAL PNEUMONIA

DIP is an uncommon from of interstitial pneumonia that occurs most frequently in patients between 30 and 50 years of age (10). Approximately 90% are cigarette smokers

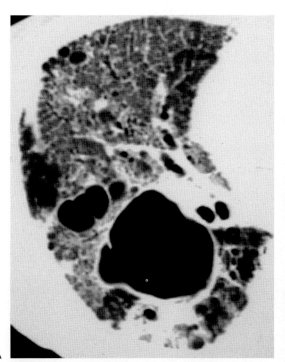

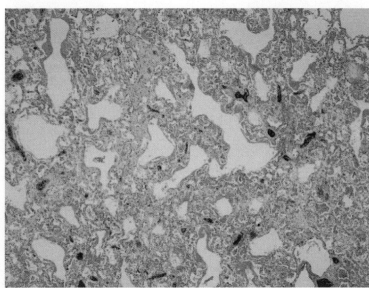

A

B

FIGURE 8.8. Usual interstitial pneumonia—acute exacerbation. **A:** HRCT image of the right lung demonstrates extensive areas of ground-glass attenuation superimposed on a background of reticulation and honeycombing. Similar findings were present in the left lung. **B:** Photomicrograph of tissue sampled at autopsy shows a pattern of diffuse alveolar damage. The patient was a 69-year-old woman with previously diagnosed UIP.

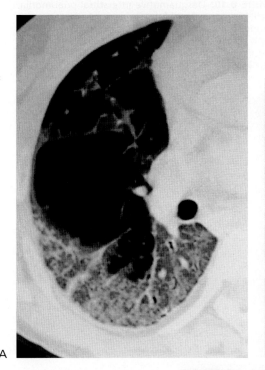

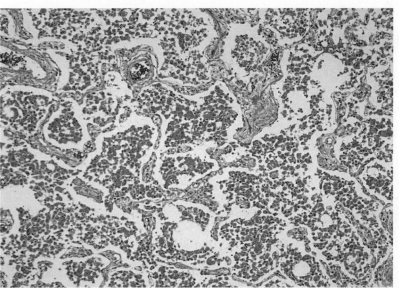

A

B

FIGURE 8.9. Desquamative interstitial pneumonia. **A:** HRCT image of the right lung demonstrates predominantly subpleural ground-glass opacities and mild reticulation. Similar changes were present in the left lung. **B:** Photomicrograph shows uniform filling of alveolar airspaces by macrophages and mild alveolar interstitial thickening by mature fibrous tissue. The patient was a 47-year-old woman.

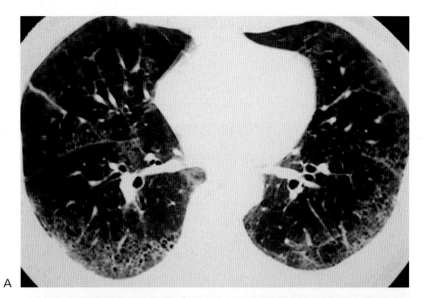

A

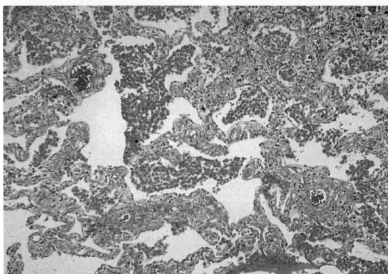

B

FIGURE 8.10. Desquamative interstitial pneumonia. **A:** HRCT image demonstrates peripheral areas with ground-glass attenuation and cysts. **B:** Photomicrograph shows filling of alveolar airspaces by macrophages and moderately severe interstitial fibrosis. The patient was a 57-year-old woman.

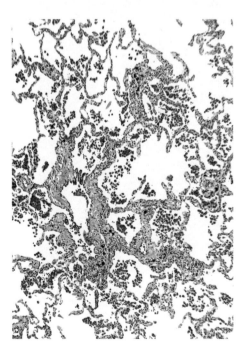

FIGURE 8.11. Respiratory bronchiolitis. Photomicrograph shows mild thickening of the walls of several respiratory bronchioles by mature fibrous tissue and an infiltrate of lymphocytes. Numerous tan-colored macrophages are present in the airway lumen and the adjacent alveolar airspaces.

(10,22); it has been speculated that an unusual reaction to such smoke is the cause in these individuals. When considering the diagnosis, it must be remembered that a DIP-like appearance can be seen focally in some drug reactions, in Langerhans cell histiocytosis, and occasionally in other forms of interstitial pneumonia such as UIP (6).

The condition is characterized histologically by the presence of numerous macrophages within alveolar airspaces (Fig. 8.9). Unlike UIP, this involvement is typically more or less uniform in severity within affected lobules. Interstitial inflammation and fibrosis are usually mild but may be moderate or (rarely) severe (Fig. 8.10) (1,10). Airspace fibrosis and exudate are not seen.

The most common finding on the chest radiograph is the presence of ground-glass opacities in the lower lung zones (10). It is important to note, however, that radiographs are normal in about 5% to 20% of patients who have biopsy-proven disease (10,23).

The predominant HRCT abnormality is also bilateral areas of ground-glass attenuation (Fig. 8.9) (22), reflecting the filling of alveolar airspaces by macrophages. A subpleural and basal predominance is often present. Although reticular opacities may be associated with the ground-glass opacity, honeycombing is uncommon (Fig. 8.10). Because of its association with cigarette smoking, centrilobular emphysema is also commonly present (Fig. 8.10).

RESPIRATORY BRONCHIOLITIS–INTERSTITIAL LUNG DISEASE

Respiratory bronchiolitis (RB) is a common incidental finding in cigarette smokers (hence the additional designation *smokers' bronchiolitis*) (24,25). It is characterized histologically by the presence of macrophages within respiratory bronchioles and adjacent alveoli (Fig. 8.11); mild chronic inflammation and fibrosis also may be apparent in the bronchiolar wall and, to a lesser extent, the walls of adjacent alveoli (24,25). The macrophages contain abundant, finely granular pigmented material derived from cigarette smoke. RB by itself is not associated with any symptoms (2). However, a small percentage of patients have more extensive disease that mimics interstitial lung disease, a condition known as respiratory bronchiolitis interstitial lung disease (RB-ILD) (2,24,25) (Fig. 8.12). Affected patients are typically 30 to 40 years of age and present with chronic cough and progressive shortness of breath (26,27).

There is some overlap between the histologic findings of RB-ILD and those of DIP; it has therefore has been suggested that the term *DIP* be replaced by *RB-ILD* (3). However, histologically RB-ILD has a bronchiolocentric distribution, whereas DIP is diffuse (2). Therefore, although RB-ILD and DIP may represent different parts of the spectrum of the same disease process (3), they are currently considered separate entities (2).

Most patients who have RB have no abnormalities on either the radiograph or HRCT (25,28). When present, HRCT findings consist of poorly defined centrilobular nodules and multifocal ground-glass opacities (28—30) (Fig. 8.13). These findings can be diffuse but tend to involve mainly the upper lung zones (28,30). Correlation with excised lungs has shown the areas of ground-glass opacity to correspond predominantly to foci of interstitial fibrosis and inflammation with or without intraalveolar macrophage accumulation (28).

About 30% of patients with RBILD have a normal chest radiograph; ground-glass opacities or a mild reticular pattern can be seen in the remaining 70% (31,32). The most common HRCT findings consist of centrilobular nodules, ground-glass opacities, and bronchial wall thickening (Figs. 8.12 and 8.14) (30,32). The abnormalities can involve all lobes but tend to have an upper lobe predominance (28,30). Centrilobular emphysema is commonly present (Fig. 8.12). A small number of patients have a reticular pattern due to interstitial fibrosis (30,33); this is usually mild and tends to involve mainly the lower lung zones (30).

One group of investigators (32) correlated HRCT findings with pathologic findings in 17 patients who had RB-ILD. All patients were current or former cigarette smokers.

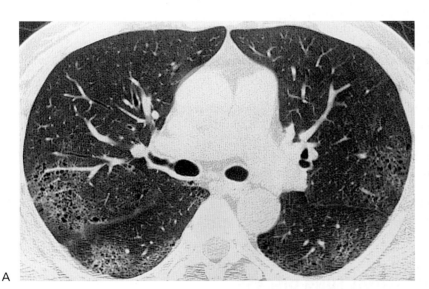

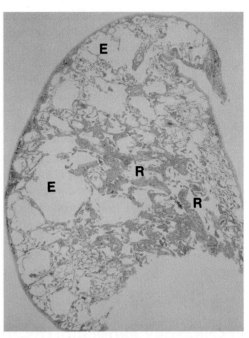

A   B

FIGURE 8.12. Respiratory bronchiolitis-interstitial lung disease. **A:** HRCT image demonstrates patchy bilateral ground-glass opacities in a predominantly peripheral distribution. Also note mild emphysema. **B:** Biopsy specimen shows a moderate degree of fibrosis in the walls of several respiratory bronchioles (*R*). Focal emphysema (*E*) is evident.

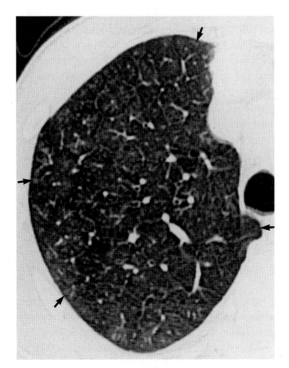

FIGURE 8.13. Respiratory bronchiolitis. HRCT image of the right upper lobe shows numerous poorly defined centrilobular nodules (*arrows*). The patient was a 49-year-old man. (Case courtesy of Dr. Martine Remy-Jardin, Hôpital Calmette, Lille, France.)

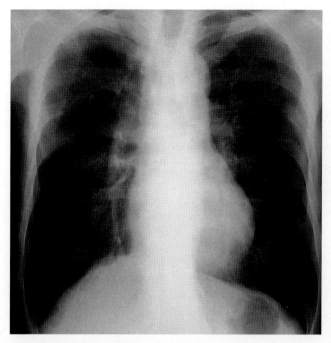
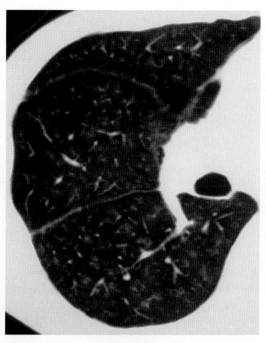

A

B

FIGURE 8.14. Respiratory bronchiolitis-interstitial lung disease. **A:** Chest radiograph shows just moderate hyperinflation due to emphysema. **B:** HRCT image demonstrates numerous poorly defined centrilobular nodular opacities. The patient was a 54-year-old man.

The predominant HRCT findings consisted of bronchial wall thickening in 16 patients (94%), centrilobular nodules in 13 (76%), ground-glass opacities in 14 (82%), and upper lobe predominant emphysema in 10 (59%). The extent of centrilobular nodules correlated with the severity of inflammation and number of macrophages in the respiratory bronchioles, whereas the ground-glass opacities correlated with macrophage accumulation in alveolar ducts and alveoli (32).

BRONCHIOLITIS OBLITERANS ORGANIZING PNEUMONIA

Bronchiolitis obliterans organizing pneumonia (BOOP) is a relatively common pulmonary abnormality characterized pathologically by the presence of fibroblastic tissue within alveolar airspaces and the lumina of respiratory bronchioles and alveolar ducts and by a variable degree of fibrosis and chronic inflammation of the parenchymal interstitium (Fig. 8.15) (34,35). The interstitial inflammation is usually most prominent in the regions of fibrosis; however, it may also be seen in areas in which the airspaces are relatively unaffected. The etiology is unknown in most cases (idiopathic BOOP); however, the histologic pattern can be caused by infection, drugs, connective tissue diseases, and toxic fume inhalation (36–38). It can also be seen focally in many other pulmonary abnormalities, including, for example, Langerhans cell histiocytosis and Wegener's granulomatosis.

Patients who have idiopathic BOOP typically present with a 1- to 6-month history of nonproductive cough, low-grade fever, malaise, and shortness of breath (39). The characteristic radiographic features consist of patchy, nonsegmental, unilateral, or bilateral areas of airspace consolidation (Fig. 8.15) (39–41). Irregular linear opacities may be present, but they are seldom a major feature. In some patients, the consolidation has a peripheral distribution similar to that seen in chronic eosinophilic pneumonia (41,42). Small nodular opacities may be seen as the only finding or, more commonly, in association with areas of airspace consolidation.

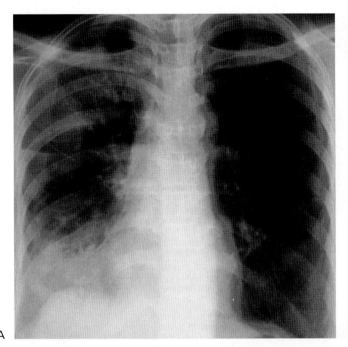

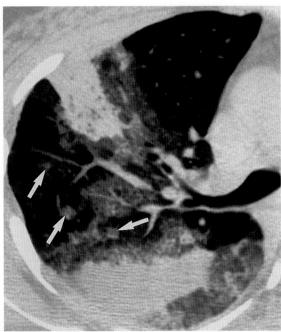

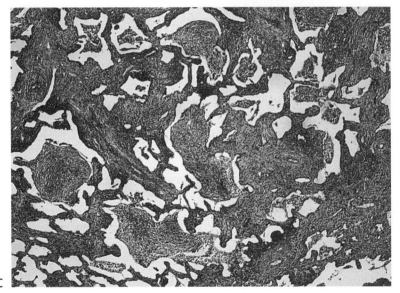

FIGURE 8.15. Idiopathic bronchiolitis obliterans organizing pneumonia. **A:** Chest radiograph shows nonsegmental airspace consolidation and ground-glass opacities in the right lung. **B:** HRCT image of the right lung demonstrates patchy airspace consolidation, areas of ground-glass attenuation and a few focal nodular areas of consolidation (*arrows*). **C:** Photomicrograph shows polyps of fibroblastic tissue within the lumens of respiratory bronchioles, alveolar ducts and occasional alveoli. The parenchymal interstitium is moderately thickened by fibrous tissue and a mononuclear inflammatory cell infiltrate. The patient was a 43-year-old woman.

The typical HRCT findings also consist of unilateral or bilateral areas of airspace consolidation (Fig. 8.15) (43–45). In approximately 60% of cases, the consolidation involves mainly the subpleural or peribronchial lung regions or both (43). Ground-glass opacities are commonly present in association with the areas of consolidation. Small, ill-defined nodules, often in a centrilobular distribution, are seen in 30% to 50% of cases (43,46) (Fig. 8.16). Bronchial wall thickening and dilatation may be seen in patients who have extensive consolidation and are usually restricted to these areas (43). Occasionally, the disease is manifested as a large nodule or masslike area of consolidation (47). The areas of consolidation correspond histologically to the regions of lung parenchyma that show airspace fibrosis (43,48). The ground-glass opacities correlate with areas of alveolar septal inflammation and minimal airspace fibrosis (48). The small nodules are related to foci of organizing pneumonia limited to the peribronchiolar region and/or to fibroblastic tissue plugs within the bronchiolar lumen (46,48) (Fig. 8.16).

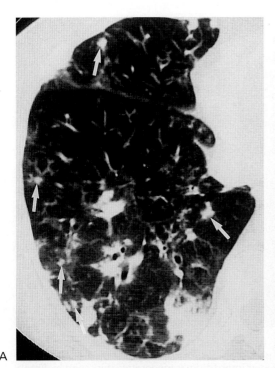
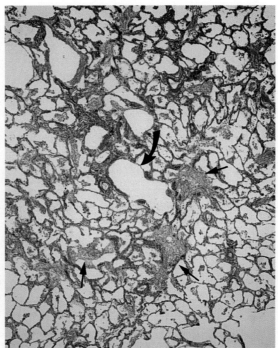

A

B

FIGURE 8.16. Idiopathic bronchiolitis obliterans organizing pneumonia. **A:** HRCT image shows centrilobular nodules (*arrows*) and peribronchial and subpleural areas of consolidation. **B:** Photomicrograph shows plugs of fibroblastic tissue in the lumens of several respiratory bronchioles (*straight arrows*) adjacent to a small membranous bronchiole (*curved arrow*) (elastica van Gieson stain). The remaining parenchyma is relatively unaffected. The patient was a 55-year-old woman.

ACUTE INTERSTITIAL PNEUMONIA

Acute interstitial pneumonia (AIP) is a clinicopathologic entity characterized histologically by the presence of diffuse alveolar damage (DAD) and clinically by respiratory failure developing over days or weeks without clear etiology (49,50). In early disease, histologic abnormalities consist of alveolar wall thickening by edema fluid and inflammatory cells, alveolar airspace filling by a proteinaceous exudate, and hyaline membranes on the surface of transitional airways (Fig. 8.17) (3,49). Fibroblastic tissue increases in amount as the disease progresses and eventually is transformed into mature collagen. Because the histologic features are similar to those of the acute respiratory distress syndrome (ARDS), AIP has also been referred to as idiopathic ARDS (51).

The radiographic manifestations consist of bilateral airspace consolidation (52). The HRCT findings consist of extensive bilateral ground-glass attenuation and patchy airspace consolidation (Figs. 8.18 and 8.19) (52,53). In one review of the HRCT findings in 36 patients extensive areas of ground-glass attenuation were present in all patients and areas of consolidation in 33 (92%) (53). Other common findings included architectural distortion, traction bronchiectasis, thickening of the bronchovascular bundles, and thickening of interlobular septa. The abnormalities involved mainly the lower lung zones in 13 patients (39%) and the upper lung zones in five (14%). In the remaining patients, there was equal involvement of all three lung zones. A predominant dependent distribution was present in nine patients (25%) and a peripheral distribution in three (8%).

The extent of ground-glass attenuation and traction bronchiectasis increase as disease evolves and fibrosis develops (53,54). One group of investigators correlated the HRCT and the histologic findings in 14 patients who had AIP (54). Areas of ground-glass attenuation and consolidation without traction bronchiectasis were present in the exudative or early proliferative phase. Traction bronchiectasis was seen in the late proliferative and fibrotic phases (54). Honeycombing is seen in a small percentage of patients; as in UIP, it

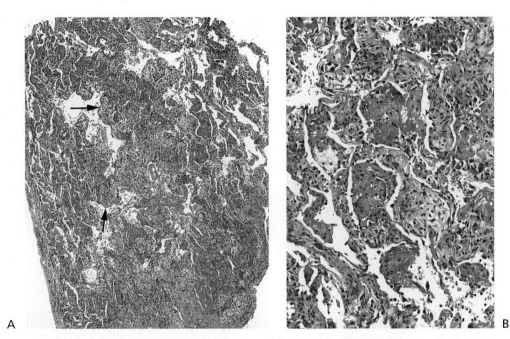

FIGURE 8.17. Acute interstitial pneumonia. Low- (**A**) and high- (**B**) magnification photomicrographs show extensive airspace filling by a proteinaceous exudate. Hyaline membranes can be seen in some alveolar ducts (*arrows*). The alveolar interstitium is moderately thickened by fibroblastic tissue and scattered lymphocytes.

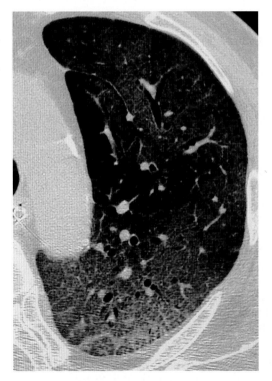

FIGURE 8.18. Acute interstitial pneumonia. HRCT image of the left upper lobe demonstrates extensive ground-glass attenuation and intralobular reticular opacities. Similar abnormalities were seen throughout both lungs. Examination of the lung at autopsy showed the exudative phase of diffuse alveolar damage. The patient was a 65-year-old man.

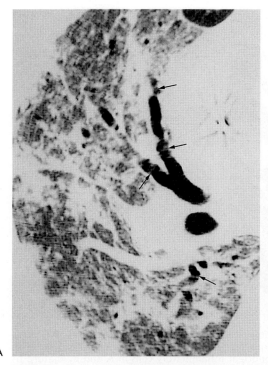

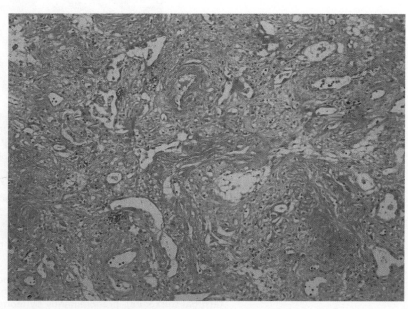

A   B

FIGURE 8.19. Acute interstitial pneumonia. **A:** HRCT image of the right lung shows extensive ground-glass attenuation, areas of airspace consolidation and focal bronchial dilatation (*arrows*). Similar changes were present in the left lung. **B:** Photomicrograph of lung taken at autopsy demonstrates marked interstitial and airspace fibrosis. The patient was a 65-year-old woman.

correlates histologically with the presence of interstitial fibrosis, alveolar destruction, and dilatation of distal airspaces (52,54).

NONSPECIFIC INTERSTITIAL PNEUMONIA

As the name suggests, *nonspecific interstitial pneumonia* (NSIP) is characterized histologically by interstitial inflammation and fibrosis without specific features that allow a diagnosis of UIP, DIP, or AIP (3,55). It is therefore largely a diagnosis of exclusion. In contrast to UIP, with which it is most likely to be confused, foci of active-appearing (fibroblastic) connective tissue are few or absent and honeycombing is uncommon. Interstitial thickening by inflammatory cells and fibrous tissue is usually greater than in DIP, and the extent and severity of airspace filling by macrophages are much less. The airspace exudate characteristic of acute lung injury is absent. Foci of intraluminal fibroblastic tissue such as seen in BOOP may accompany the interstitial disease but are relatively inconspicuous (3,55).

NSIP can be subcategorized according to the relative amounts of inflammation and fibrosis. In one scheme, three groups are defined: predominant inflammation (group 1), roughly equal inflammation and fibrosis (group 2), and predominant fibrosis (group 3) (55). In another, there are two main patterns: cellular and fibrotic (Fig. 8.20) (56,57). There is evidence that the former has a greater likelihood of response to corticosteroid therapy and a better prognosis than the fibrotic form (58,59).

Many cases of NSIP are idiopathic; however, it can be seen in association with a number of drugs, connective tissue disease, and hypersensitivity pneumonitis (3,55). Clinically, patients present with symptoms similar to IPF: dyspnea and cough with an average duration of 8 months (55). Most cases occur in adults, the average age being approximately 50 years (55,56).

The radiographic findings consist mainly of ground-glass opacities or consolidation involving predominantly the lower lung zones (Figs. 8.21 and 8.22) (56). Other manifes-

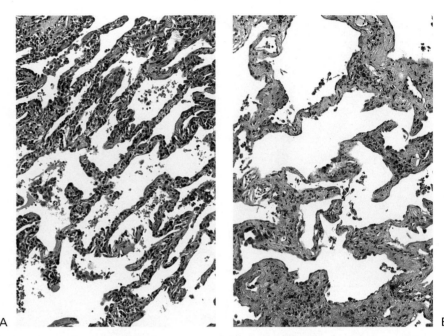

FIGURE 8.20. Nonspecific interstitial pneumonia—cellular and fibrotic patterns. High-magnification photomicrographs of biopsy specimens from two patients show mild to moderate alveolar interstitial thickening, predominantly by mononuclear inflammatory cells in **A** and by mature fibrous tissue in **B.** Alveolar airspaces are essentially unaffected. The architecture is normal in **A;** in **B,** loss of alveolar septa is evident.

tations include a reticular pattern or a combination of interstitial and airspace patterns (56). In approximately 10% of cases, the radiograph is normal (3). The most common HRCT manifestations consist of patchy or confluent areas of ground-glass attenuation, often with a peripheral predominance, patchy airspace consolidation, and irregular linear opacities (Figs. 8.21 to 8.23) (56,57). Although honeycombing may be present, it tends to be mild. It should be noted, however, that the HRCT manifestations of NSIP are quite

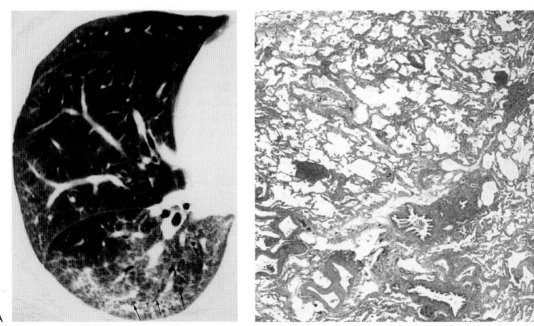

FIGURE 8.21. Nonspecific interstitial pneumonia. **A:** HRCT image of the right lung demonstrates peripheral ground-glass attenuation and mild reticulation. Also note mild traction bronchiectasis (*arrows*). **B:** Photomicrograph shows relatively uniform, mild to moderate alveolar wall thickening, consistent with type 1 NSIP. The patient was a 51-year-old woman.

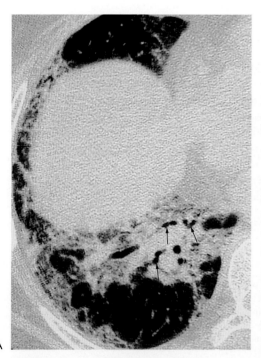
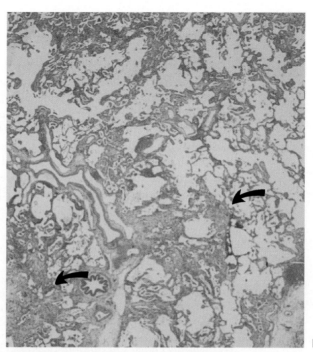

A

B

FIGURE 8.22. Nonspecific interstitial pneumonia. **A:** HRCT image of the right lung at the level of the dome of the hemidiaphragm shows extensive ground-glass opacities and mild reticulation. Also note traction bronchiectasis (*arrows*). Similar findings were present in the left lung base. **B:** Photomicrograph shows patchy interstitial thickening by inflammatory cells and focal fibrosis (*arrows*). The findings are those of type 2 NSIP. The patient was a 59-year-old woman.

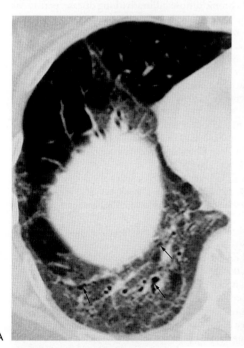
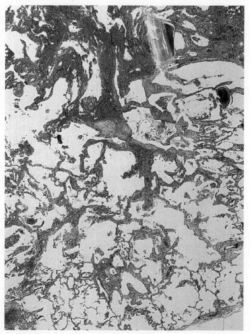

A

B

FIGURE 8.23. Nonspecific interstitial pneumonia. **A:** HRCT image at the level of the dome of the right hemidiaphragm demonstrates areas of ground-glass attenuation and reticulation in the right lower lobe. Also noted is traction bronchiectasis (*arrows*). Similar abnormalities were present in the left lower lobe. **B:** Photomicrograph shows patchy foci of interstitial fibrosis, consistent with type 3 NSIP. The patient was a 48-year-old woman.

variable (60,61). The findings in any given patient may consist mainly of ground-glass attenuation, consolidation, or reticulation (60,61). The appearance therefore can mimic DIP, UIP, AIP, and BOOP (60,61).

One group of investigators compared HRCT with the pathologic findings in 23 patients who had NSIP (62). The predominant HRCT abnormality (seen in all patients) was bilateral ground-glass opacity, with (35%) or without (65%) consolidation. Other common findings included irregular linear opacities (87%), thickening of bronchovascular bundles (65%), and bronchial dilatation (Figs. 8.22 and 8.23) (52%). The parenchymal abnormalities involved mainly the subpleural lung regions. The ground-glass opacities corresponded histologically to interstitial thickening by inflammatory cells and fibrous tissue, whereas the areas of consolidation were related to areas of BOOP or foci of honeycombing in which the cystic spaces were filled with mucus (Fig. 8.22) (62).

REFERENCES

1. Müller NL, Colby TV. Idiopathic interstitial pneumonias: high-resolution CT and histologic findings. *Radiographics* 1997;17:1016–1022.
2. ATS/ERS International Multidisciplinary Consensus Classification of Idiopathic Interstitial Pneumonias. *Am J Respir Crit Case Med* 2000; 165:277–304.
3. Katzenstein AL, Myers JL. Idiopathic pulmonary fibrosis: clinical relevance of pathologic classification. *Am J Respir Crit Care Med* 1998;157:1301–1315.
4. American Thoracic Society. Idiopathic pulmonary fibrosis: diagnosis and treatment International Consensus Statement. American Thoracic Society (ATS) and the European Respiratory Society (ERS). *Am J Respir Crit Care Med* 2000;161:646–664.
5. Bjoraker JA, Ryu JH, Edwin MK, et al. Prognostic significance of histopathologic subsets in idiopathic pulmonary fibrosis. *Am J Respir Crit Care Med* 1998;157:199–203.
6. Colby T, Carrington C. Interstitial lung disease. In: Thurlbeck WM, Churg AM, eds. *Pathology of the lung*. New York: Thieme, 1995:589–737.
7. Müller NL, Miller RR, Webb WR, et al. Fibrosing alveolitis: CT–pathologic correlation. *Radiology* 1986;160:585–588.
8. Müller NL, Miller RR. Computed tomography of chronic diffuse infiltrative lung disease: part 1. *Am Rev Respir Dis* 1990;142:1206–1215.
9. Nishimura K, Kitaichi M, Izumi T, et al. Usual interstitial pneumonia: histologic correlation with high-resolution CT. *Radiology* 1992;182:337–342.
10. Carrington CB, Gaensler EA, Coute RE, et al. Natural history and treated course of usual and desquamative interstitial pneumonia. *N Engl J Med* 1978;298:801–809.
11. Grenier P, Chevret S, Beigelman C, et al. Chronic diffuse infiltrative lung disease: determination of the diagnostic value of clinical data, chest radiography, and CT with Bayesian analysis. *Radiology* 1994;191:383–390.
12. Mathieson JR, Mayo JR, Staples CA, et al. Chronic diffuse infiltrative lung disease: comparison of diagnostic accuracy of CT and chest radiography. *Radiology* 1989;171:111–116.
13. Wells AU, Rubens MB, du Bois RM, et al. Serial CT in fibrosing alveolitis: prognostic significance of the initial pattern. *Am J Roentgenol* 1993;161:1159–1165.
14. Hunninghake G. Zimmerman M, Schwartz T, et al. Utility of lung biopsy for the diagnosis of idiopathic pulmonary fibrosis. *Am J Resp Crit Care Med* 2001; 164:193–196.
15. Webb WR, Stein MG, Finkbeiner WE, et al. Normal and diseased isolated lungs: high-resolution CT. *Radiology* 1988;166:81–87.
16. Kang EY, Grenier P, Laurent F, et al. Interlobular septal thickening: patterns at high-resolution computed tomography. *J Thorac Imaging* 1996;11:260–264.
17. Leung AN, Miller RR, Müller NL. Parenchymal opacification in chronic infiltrative lung diseases: CT–pathologic correlation. *Radiology* 1993;188:209–214.
18. Remy-Jardin M, Giraud F, Remy J, et al. Importance of ground glass attenuation in chronic diffuse infiltrative lung disease: pathologic–CT correlation. *Radiology* 1993;189:693–698.
19. Kondoh Y, Taniguchi H, Kawabata Y, et al. Acute exacerbation in idiopathic pulmonary fibrosis: analysis of clinical and pathologic findings in three cases. *Chest* 1993;103:1808–1812.
20. Akira M, Hamada H, Sakatani M, et al. CT findings during phase of accelerated deterioration in patients who have idiopathic pulmonary fibrosis. *Am J Roentgenol* 1997;168:79–83.
21. Akira M. Computed tomography and pathologic findings in fulminant forms of idiopathic interstitial pneumonia. *J Thorac Imaging* 1999;14:76–84.
22. Hartman TE, Primack SL, Swensen SJ, et al. Desquamative interstitial pneumonia: thin-section CT findings in 22 patients. *Radiology* 1993;187:787–790.

23. Feigin DS, Friedman PJ. Chest radiography in DIP: a review of 37 patients. *Am J Roentgenol* 1980; 134:91–99.

24. Colby TV. Bronchiolitis: pathologic considerations. *Am J Clin Pathol* 1998;109:101–109.

25. Müller NL, Miller RR. Diseases of the bronchioles: CT and histopathologic findings. *Radiology* 1995;196:3–12.

26. Myers JL, Veal CF, Shin MS, et al. Respiratory bronchiolitis causing interstitial lung disease: a clinicopathologic study of six cases. *Am Rev Respir Dis* 1987;135:880–884.

27. King TE. Respiratory bronchiolitis-associated interstitial lung disease. *Clin Chest Med* 1993;14: 693–698.

28. Remy-Jardin, Remy J, Gosselin B, et al. Lung parenchymal changes secondary to cigarette smoking: pathologic-CT correlations. *Radiology* 1993;186:643–651.

29. Gruden JF, Webb WR. CT findings in a proved case of respiratory bronchiolitis. *Am J Roentgenol* 1993;161:44–46.

30. Heyneman LE, Ward S, Lynch DA, et al. Respiratory bronchiolitis, respiratory bronchiolitis-associated interstitial pneumonia and desquamative interstitial pneumonia: different entities or part of the spectrum of the same disease process? *Am J Roentgenol* 1999;173:1617–1622.

31. Yousem SA, Colby TV, Gaensler EA. Respiratory bronchiolitis-associated interstitial lung disease and its relationship to desquamative interstitial pneumonia. *Mayo Clin Proc* 1989;64:1373–1380.

32. Park J, Tuder R, Brown KK, et al. Respiratory bronchiolitis-associated interstitial lung disease: CT–pathologic correlation. *Radiology* 1998;209:179.

33. Holt RM, Schmidt RA, Godwin JD, et al. High resolution CT in respiratory bronchiolitis-associated interstitial lung disease. *J Comput Assist Tomogr* 1993;17:46–50.

34. Epler GR, Colby TV, McLoud TC, et al. Bronchiolitis obliterans organizing pneumonia. *N Engl J Med* 1985;312:152–158.

35. Myers JL, Colby TV. Pathologic manifestations of bronchiolitis, constrictive bronchiolitis, cryptogenic organizing pneumonia and diffuse panbronchiolitis. *Clin Chest Med* 1993;14:611–623.

36. Camus P, Lombard J-N, Perrichon M, et al. Bronchiolitis obliterans-organizing pneumonia in patients taking acebutolol or amiodarone. *Thorax* 1989;44:711–715.

37. Epler GR. Bronchiolitis obliterans organizing pneumonia: definition and clinical features. *Chest* 1992;102(Suppl):2–6.

38. Colby TV, Myers JL. The clinical and histologic spectrum of bronchiolitis obliterans including bronchiolitis obliterans organizing pneumonia (BOOP). *Semin Respir Dis* 1992;13:119–133.

39. Epler GR, Colby TV, McLoud TC, et al. Idiopathic bronchiolitis obliterans with organizing pneumonia. *N Engl J Med* 1985;312:152–159.

40. Chandler PW, Shin MS, Friedman SE, et al. Radiographic manifestations of bronchiolitis obliterans with organizing pneumonia vs. usual interstitial pneumonia. *Am J Roentgenol* 1986;147:899–906.

41. Müller NL, Guerry-Force ML, Staples CA, et al. Differential diagnosis of bronchiolitis obliterans with organizing pneumonia and usual interstitial pneumonia: clinical, functional, and radiologic findings. *Radiology* 1987;162:151–156.

42. Bartter T, Irwin RS, Nash G, et al. Idiopathic bronchiolitis obliterans organizing pneumonia with peripheral infiltrates on chest roentgenogram. *Arch Intern Med* 1989;149:273–279.

43. Müller NL, Staples CA, Miller RR. Bronchiolitis obliterans organizing pneumonia: CT features in 14 patients. *Am J Roentgenol* 1990;154:983–987.

44. Bouchardy LM, Kuhlman JE, Ball WC, et al. CT findings in bronchiolitis obliterans organizing pneumonia (BOOP) with radiographic, clinical, and histologic correlation. *J Comput Assist Tomogr* 1993;17:352–357.

45. Lee KS, Kullnig P, Hartman TE, et al. Cryptogenic organizing pneumonia: CT findings in 43 patients. *Am J Roentgenol* 1994;162:543–546.

46. Gruden JF, Webb WR, Warnock M. Centrilobular opacities in the lung on high-resolution CT: diagnostic considerations and pathologic correlation. *Am J Roentgenol* 1994;162:569–574.

47. Akira M, Yamamoto S, Sakatani M. Bronchiolitis obliterans organizing pneumonia manifesting as multiple large nodules or masses. *Am J Roentgenol* 1998;170:291–295.

48. Nishimura K, Itoh H. High-resolution computed tomographic features of bronchiolitis obliterans organizing pneumonia. *Chest* 1992;102:26S–31S.

49. Katzenstein ALA, Myers JL, Mazur MT. Acute interstitial pneumonia: a clinicopathologic, ultrastructural, and cell kinetic study. *Am J Surg Pathol* 1986;10:256–267.

50. Ichikado K, Johkoh T, Ikezoe J, et al. Acute interstitial pneumonia: high-resolution CT findings correlated with pathology. *Am J Roentgenol* 1997;168:333–338.

51. Olson J, Colby TV, Elliott CG. Hamman-Rich syndrome revisited. *Mayo Clin Proc* 1990;65:1538–1548.

52. Primack SL, Hartman TE, Ikezoe J, et al. Acute interstitial pneumonia: radiographic and CT findings in nine patients. *Radiology* 1993;188:817–820.

53. Johkoh T, Müller NL, Taniguchi H, et al. Acute interstitial pneumonia: thin-section CT findings in 36 patients. *Radiology* 1999; 211:859–863.

54. Ichikado K, Johkoh T, Ikezoe J, et al. Acute interstitial pneumonia: high-resolution CT findings correlated with pathology. *Am J Roentgenol* 1997;168:333–338.

55. Katzenstein AL, Fiorelli RF. Nonspecific interstitial pneumonia/fibrosis: histologic features and clinical significance. *Am J Surg Pathol* 1994;18:136–147.

56. Park JS, Lee KS, Kim JS, et al. Nonspecific interstitial pneumonia with fibrosis: radiographic and CT findings in seven patients. *Radiology* 1995;195:645–648.

57. Nishiyama O, Kondoh Y, Taniguchi H, et al. Serial high resolution CT findings in nonspecific interstitial pneumonia/fibrosis. *J Comput Assist Tomogr* 2000;24:41–46.

58. Nagai S, Kitaichi M, Itoh H, et al. Idiopathic nonspecific interstitial pneumonia/fibrosis: comparison with idiopathic pulmonary fibrosis and BOOP. *Eur Respir J* 1998;12:1010–1019.

59. Travis WD, Matsui K, Moss J, Ferrans VJ. Idiopathic nonspecific interstitial pneumonia: prognostic significance of cellular and fibrosing patterns. *Am J Surg Pathol* 2000;24:19–33.

60. Hartman TE, Swensen SJ, Hansell DM, et al. Nonspecific interstitial pneumonia: variable appearance at high-resolution chest CT. *Radiology* 2000;217:701–705.

61. Johkoh T, Müller NL, Cartier Y, et al. Idiopathic interstitial pneumonias: diagnostic accuracy of thin-section CT in 129 patients. *Radiology* 1999;211:555–560.

62. Kim TS, Lee KS, Chung MP, et al. Nonspecific interstitial pneumonia with fibrosis: high-resolution CT and pathologic findings. *Am J Roentgenol* 1998;171:1645–1650.

9

OCCUPATIONAL LUNG DISEASE

PNEUMOCONIOSIS
Silicosis and Coal Worker's Pneumoconiosis
Acute Silicosis (Silicoproteinosis)
Asbestos-Related Disease
Miscellaneous Pneumoconioses

CHEMICAL PNEUMONITIS
Carbamates
Paraquat

Hydrogen Sulfide
Ammonia
Hydrocarbon
Mercury Inhalation

EXTRINSIC ALLERGIC ALVEOLITIS
Isocyanate-Associated Hypersensitivity Pneumonitis

Pulmonary disease associated with the workplace is caused by inhalation (or occasionally ingestion) of a wide variety of dust particles and noxious chemicals. The development of disease in an individual worker is dependent on the toxic effects of the inhaled substance, the intensity and duration of the exposure, and the susceptibility of the worker. Depending in part on the solubility and chemical nature of the inhaled substance, reactions may be acute or chronic. As might be expected, the former are associated with exudation of edema fluid and neutrophils (sometimes eosinophils) and the relatively rapid development of symptoms and radiologic abnormalities (1,2). By contrast, more indolent disease tends to be associated with a mononuclear inflammatory reaction (sometimes granulomatous) and fibrosis, and gradually progressive clinical and radiologic abnormalities. The various disorders can be grouped together under the headings *pneumoconiosis, chemical pneumonitis,* and *extrinsic allergic alveolitis.*

PNEUMOCONIOSIS

Pneumoconiosis is defined as the accumulation of dust in the lungs and the tissue reaction to its presence. Two major pathologic forms of reaction are seen. The first is characterized by fibrosis, which can be focal and nodular (as in silicosis) or diffuse (as in asbestosis). It often results in radiographic abnormalities and, if extensive enough, may lead to significant functional impairment. The second form consists of aggregates of particle-laden macrophages with minimal or no accompanying fibrosis. This is typically seen with exposure to inert dusts such as iron, tin, and barium. Although sometimes associated with chronic radiographic abnormalities, it usually leads to few or no functional or clinical manifestations (3).

Depending on their size and shape, inhaled inorganic particles may be extruded from the lung in exhaled gas or deposited on the epithelium anywhere from the nose to the alveoli. Most of those that deposit in the upper respiratory tract or bronchi are extruded in mucus via the mucociliary escalator. By contrast, many of those that land on the epithelium of the respiratory bronchioles enter the adjacent interstitium, where they accumulate in macrophages. Particles that land in the alveoli in the periphery of the lung also accumulate in macrophages in the interstitial tissue of the interlobular septa and pleura. Depending on their physical and chemical characteristics, the particles may alter macrophage function, causing a mononuclear inflammatory reaction and fibrosis. Thus, at least in their

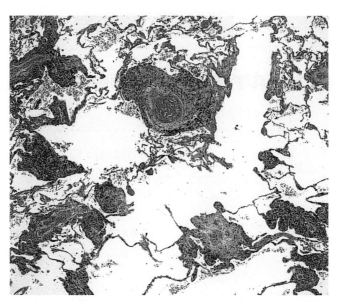

FIGURE 9.1. Mixed dust pneumoconiosis—perilymphatic distribution. A low-magnification view shows multiple, somewhat nodular foci of fibrous tissue containing abundant pigment-laden macrophages. Disease is located predominantly in the interstitial tissue adjacent to respiratory bronchioles and their accompanying arteries. The patient had worked for many years in a foundry.

early stages, most pneumoconioses are characterized histologically by thickening of the interstitial tissue in the perilymphatic regions (Fig. 9.1).

Silicosis and Coal Worker's Pneumoconiosis

Exposure to silica occurs in many occupations but is particularly important in individuals involved in mining, quarrying, and tunneling. Depending on the nature of their job and the location of the mine, coal miners may be exposed to dust that contains particles such as mica, kaolin, and silica in addition to carbon in the coal itself (4). Because of the presence of these "contaminating" particles, silicosis and coal worker's pneumoconiosis (CWP) show histologic overlap in some individuals. Despite this, the pathologic abnormalities of the two conditions are specific enough to enable diagnosis in most individuals. However, because the localization of disease is the same in silicosis and CWP, the radiographic and HRCT appearances are similar (5).

Slices of lung involved by silicosis show multiple, usually well-circumscribed nodules up to 1 cm in diameter (Fig. 9.2A). They may be black or slate gray in appearance, depending on the amount of carbon pigment they contain. Larger foci of disease (progressive massive fibrosis) tend to be more irregular in shape but are otherwise similar to the smaller nodules. The upper lobes and superior segments of the lower lobes are typically most prominently affected (Fig. 9.2B). Histologically, the nodules can be seen to be composed of relatively hypocellular fibrous tissue surrounded by a rim of particle-laden macrophages (Fig. 9.3). Needle-shaped, birefringent silicates can be identified in the macrophages by polarized light microscopy (Fig. 9.4B). Nodules located in the peribronchiolar interstitium may result in narrowing and distortion of bronchioles (6). Those present in the pleural interstitium may be associated with a "pseudoplaque" appearance on HRCT (Fig. 9.2B) (5,7).

Confluence of nodules (progressive massive fibrosis) is usually associated with an increased amount of fibrous tissue (sometimes the site of dystrophic calcification) and foci of necrosis; cavitation may be seen in larger lesions (Fig. 9.5). The latter is most often the

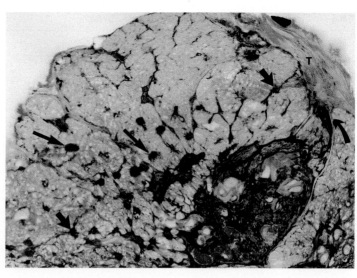

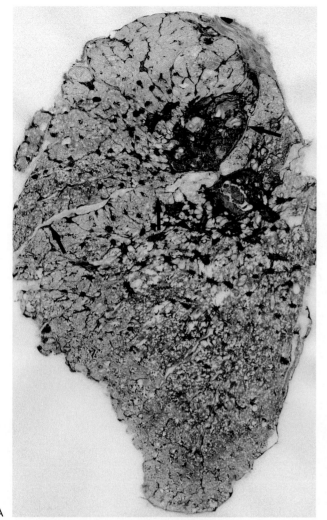

FIGURE 9.2. Silicosis—gross appearance. **A:** A paper-mounted sagittal slice of the left lung shows numerous well-circumscribed black nodules, predominantly in the upper lobe and superior segment of the lower lobe (*arrows* indicate the major fissure). Most measure 0.5 to 1.0 cm in diameter. Two foci of confluent nodules (progressive massive fibrosis) are evident, one in the posteroinferior portion of the upper lobe adjacent to the major fissure and the other in the superior segment of the lower lobe. **B:** A magnified view of the upper lobe shows some of the nodules to be located in the central portion of the lobule (*long arrows*) and others in the periphery adjacent to interlobular septa (*short arrows*). Many septa are mildly thickened and relatively easily identified because of pigmented macrophage accumulation. A focus of fibrosis adjacent to the pleura (*curved arrow*) corresponds to the pseudoplaques that are sometimes seen on HRCT (although in the case, its presence would have been masked by the fibrous tissue in adjacent pleura [T]).

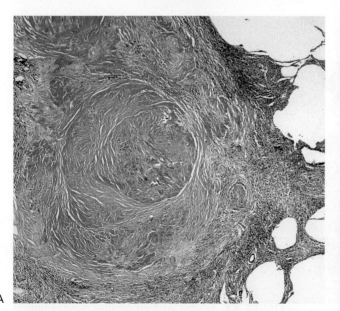

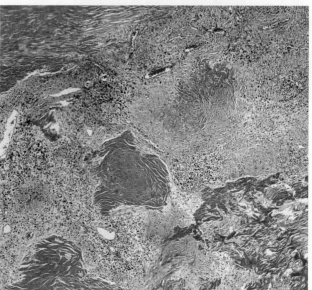

FIGURE 9.3. Silicosis—histologic appearance. **A:** A photomicrograph of a small silicotic nodule shows it to be composed of a central zone of dense collagen surrounded by a rim of macrophages that contain abundant carbon pigment. The latter is responsible for the black appearance in the gross specimen. Emphysema is evident in the adjacent lung parenchyma. **B:** A section from a focus of progressive massive fibrosis (PMF) shows multiple foci of collagen similar to that of the small nodule, suggesting that the PMF developed by expansion and confluence of individual silicotic nodules.

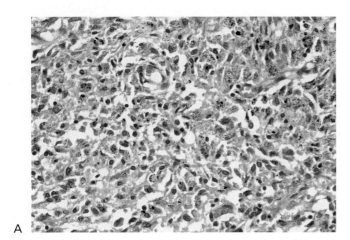 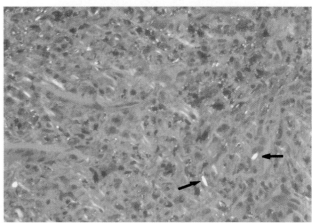

FIGURE 9.4. Silicosis—presence of carbon and silicates. Photomicrographs of macrophages in a silicotic nodule taken with routine (**A**) and polarized (**B**) light show minute black granules (carbon) and refractile silicates (*arrows*).

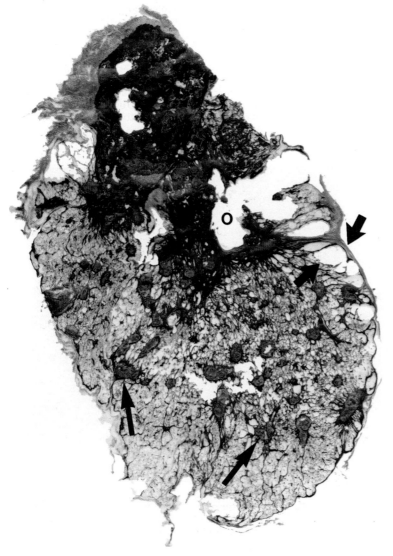

FIGURE 9.5. Silicosis with progressive massive fibrosis and cavitation. A paper-mounted sagittal slice of the left lung shows a large focus of progressive massive fibrosis containing several irregularly shaped cavities (*O*). Individual silicotic nodules (*long arrows*) and foci of emphysema (*short arrows*) are evident in the lower lobe. The patient was a coal miner who had significant silica exposure.

result of ischemia related to luminal narrowing (endarteritis obliterans) of adjacent vessels; occasionally, superimposed mycobacterial infection is the cause. The most prominent abnormality in CWP is interstitial accumulation of macrophages containing abundant carbon. Fibrosis is typically minimal, unless there is concomitant silica accumulation or extensive disease (progress massive fibrosis) (Fig. 9.5).

Radiologically, silicosis and CWP are traditionally considered to be simple or complicated in type. The former is characterized by small, well-circumscribed nodules, mainly involving the dorsal half of the upper lobes (5,7). The nodules can range from 1 to 10 mm in diameter but usually measure 2 to 5 mm (Fig. 9.6). Although there is a tendency for the nodules of silicosis to be better defined than those of CWP, this is not always the case (5). On HRCT, the nodules are seen mainly in the centrilobular regions, reflecting their peribronchiolar localization. However, because of their perilymphatic distribution, they are also seen in the subpleural regions and along the interlobular septa (6) (Fig. 9.6B). The nodules tend to involve mainly dorsal regions of the upper lobes and are most numerous in the right upper lobe (7) (Figs. 9.6C and 9.7).

Complicated silicosis or CWP is considered to be present when nodules coalesce to form opacities larger than 1 cm in diameter (progressive massive fibrosis) (Fig. 9.8). The opacities tend to develop in the periphery of the upper and middle lung zones, and often

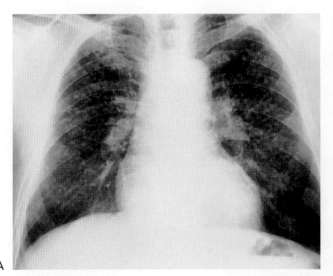

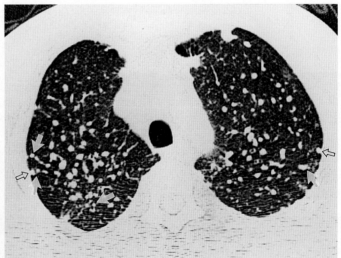

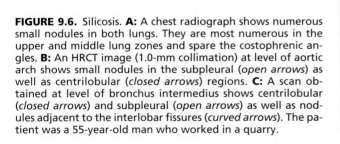

FIGURE 9.6. Silicosis. **A:** A chest radiograph shows numerous small nodules in both lungs. They are most numerous in the upper and middle lung zones and spare the costophrenic angles. **B:** An HRCT image (1.0-mm collimation) at level of aortic arch shows small nodules in the subpleural (*open arrows*) as well as centrilobular (*closed arrows*) regions. **C:** A scan obtained at level of bronchus intermedius shows centrilobular (*closed arrows*) and subpleural (*open arrows*) as well as nodules adjacent to the interlobar fissures (*curved arrows*). The patient was a 55-year-old man who worked in a quarry.

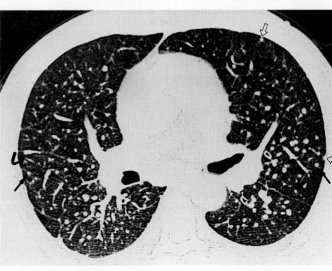

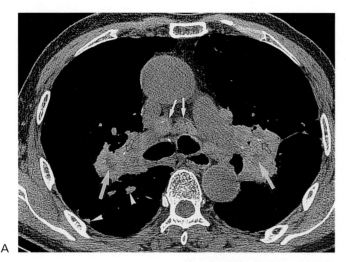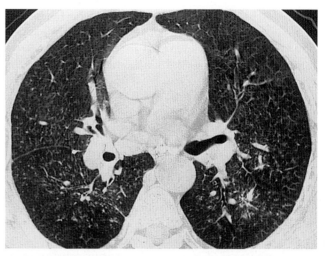

A

B

FIGURE 9.7. Coal worker's pneumoconiosis. **A:** An HRCT image (soft-tissue windows, 1.0-mm collimation) at level of main bronchi shows bilateral perihilar soft-tissue masses. Small localized areas of low attenuation (*arrows*) are present, consistent with necrosis. Foci of calcification (*open arrows*) are evident within the masses. Small pulmonary nodules (*arrowheads*) and enlarged mediastinal lymph nodes (*small arrows*) can also be seen. **B:** An image (lung windows) at level of bronchus intermedius shows small nodules most numerous in the posterior half of the lungs. The patient was a 56-year-old man.

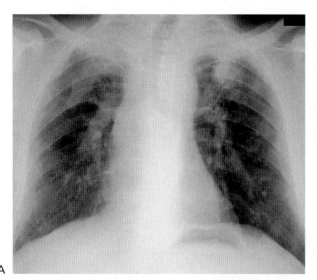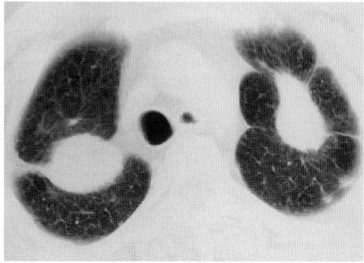

A

B

FIGURE 9.8. Silicosis with progressive massive fibrosis. **A:** A chest radiograph shows large opacities in both upper lobes and cephalad retraction of the hila. **B:** A CT image (7-mm collimation) shows bilateral conglomerate masses of fibrosis. A few centrilobular and subpleural nodules can be seen particularly in the left upper lobe. The patient was a 73-year-old man.

appear to migrate gradually toward the hila. Foci of emphysema are often present between the conglomerate mass and the pleura (8). The opacities are usually bilateral and symmetric. They are frequently calcified and often associated with egg-shell calcification of hilar and mediastinal lymph nodes (5,6). As indicated, cavitation can occur following ischemic necrosis or superimposed tuberculosis.

Acute Silicosis (Silicoproteinosis)

Acute silicosis is a rare condition that may follow heavy exposure to silica dust in enclosed spaces. Exposure times are frequently as short as 6 to 8 months. The condition is often rapidly progressive and may result in death from respiratory failure within 1 to 2 years. The pathologic and radiologic appearances are distinct from those of simple silicosis and resemble those of pulmonary alveolar proteinosis. The accumulation of granular, periodic acid-Schiff (PAS)-positive material within alveolar airspaces characterizes the process histologically (Fig. 9.9) (9,10).

The chest radiograph shows a pattern of bilateral airspace consolidation or ground-glass appearance, which can be diffuse but tends to involve mainly the perihilar regions (11). HRCT findings include ground-glass opacities (Fig. 9.10), with or without associated areas of consolidation (both as a result of the alveolar airspace filling), and poorly defined nodular opacities (12). A combination of ground-glass opacities and a linear pattern ("crazy-paving" appearance) may also occur (Fig. 9.11A). This pattern may be related to the combination of airspace filling and interlobular septal thickened by edema fluid and/or fibrous tissue.

Asbestos-Related Disease

Asbestos is the generic term for several fibrous silicate minerals that share the property of heat resistance. They are classified into two groups: the serpentines and the amphiboles. Chrysotile is the only asbestiform mineral in the serpentine group and accounts for more than 90% of the asbestos used in the United States (13). The pathologic hallmark of asbestos exposure is the asbestos body consisting of an asbestos fiber, usually 2 to 5 μm in width and 20 to 50 μm in length, surrounded by an iron-protein coat of variable thickness (Fig. 9.12). The bodies can be identified in tissue sections in interstitial fibrous tissue and intraalveolar macrophages and in bronchoalveolar lavage (BAL) fluid.

Asbestos-related disease may be manifested by fibrosis (of the pleura as focal [plaques] or diffuse thickening and of the lung as peribronchiolar or parenchymal interstitial thickening [asbestosis]) and by malignancy (pulmonary carcinoma or mesothelioma). Clinical manifestations of these abnormalities typically do not appear until 20 years or more after initial exposure (3,13). Pleural effusion may also occur, often at an earlier postexposure interval.

Benign Pleural Disease

Pleural plaques are the most common manifestation of asbestos exposure. Grossly, they are discrete foci of pearly white fibrous tissue, usually 2 to 5 mm thick (Fig. 9.13). They involve the parietal pleura almost exclusively and tend to be round on the diaphragm and linear (paralleling the ribs) on the costal pleura. Histologically, they consist of hypocellular bundles of collagen, often having an undulating "basketweave" pattern. The dense fibrous tissue has a propensity for dystrophic calcification. Foci of visceral pleural fibrosis morphologically distinct from parietal pleural plaques are also frequent, particularly on the dorsal aspects of the lower lobes. Unlike plaques, they are usually no more than 1 mm thick and are usually inapparent radiologically, unless associated with rounded atelectasis.

Radiologically, plaques are seen as discrete areas of pleural thickening. They are most numerous along the posterolateral aspects of the lower ribs and along the diaphragm. Cal-

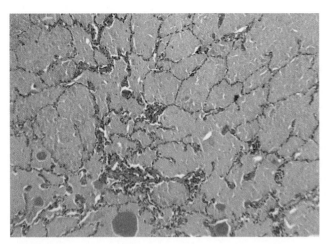

FIGURE 9.9. Acute silicoproteinosis. A photomicrograph shows filling of alveolar airspaces by finely granular eosinophilic material. Alveolar septa are normal. The patient was a 25-year-old dental technician. (Courtesy Dr. J. Majo, Barcelona, Spain.)

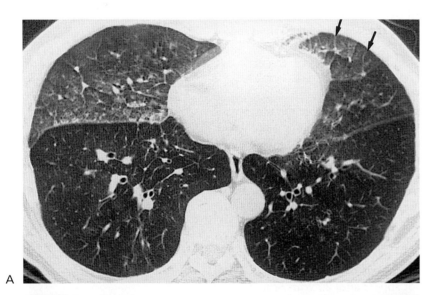

A

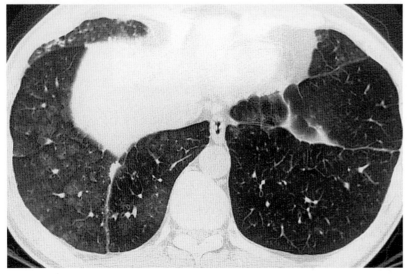

B

FIGURE 9.10. Acute silicosis. **A:** An HRCT image (1.0-mm collimation) shows ground-glass opacities in the right middle lobe and lingula. Mild interlobular septal thickening is evident (*arrows*). **B:** An image at the lung bases shows ground-glass opacities in the right middle lobe, right lower lobe, and lingula. The patient was a 52-year-old man.

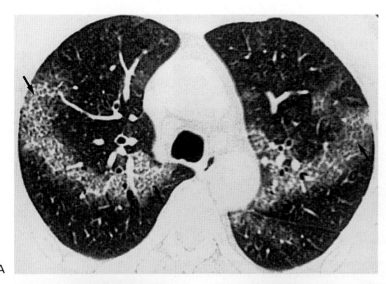

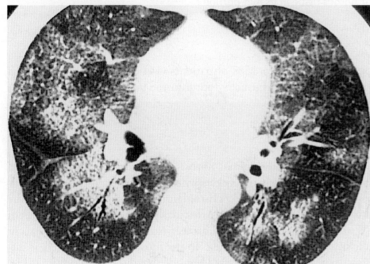

FIGURE 9.11. Acute silicosis. **A:** An HRCT image (1.5-mm collimation) at the level of the distal trachea shows patchy ground-glass opacities in both upper lobes. Also note fine intralobular linear opacities superimposed on the ground-glass opacities, resulting in an appearance known as "crazy-paving" (*arrows*). **B:** A scan obtained at the level of the right middle lobe bronchus shows more extensive abnormalities in both lungs. The patient was a 52-year-old quarry worker. (From Kim KI, Kim CW, Lee MK, et al. Imaging of occupational lung disease. *Radiographics* 2001;21: 1371–1391, with permission.)

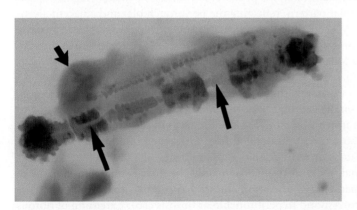

FIGURE 9.12. Asbestos body. A highly magnified photomicrograph shows an elongated macrophage (*short arrow* indicates the nucleus) that contains two asbestos bodies. Each is composed of an asbestos fiber (the translucent central portion indicated by *long arrows*) surrounded by a segmented protein-iron coat (much more prominent in the lower body).

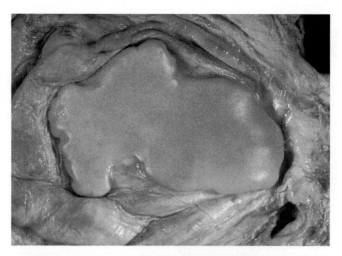

FIGURE 9.13. Diaphragmatic pleural plaque. A view of the left hemidiaphragm shows a slightly elevated, well-demarcated, and smooth-surfaced focus of fibrous tissue in its mid-portion.

cification is seen in approximately 5% to 15% of patients (14) (Fig. 9.14). Plaques that arise from the visceral pleura are rare and usually found in the lower aspects of the interlobar fissures (3).

Asbestosis

Asbestosis is defined as pulmonary parenchymal fibrosis secondary to inhalation of asbestos fibers. It develops almost exclusively in workers who have been exposed to high concentrations of the mineral, often for many years. Histologically, fibrosis is first seen in the interstitium of respiratory bronchioles (Fig. 9.15), particularly in the lower lobes adjacent to the visceral pleura. With advancing disease the fibrous tissue extends into the adjacent alveolar septa, eventually involving the entire lobule. In the most severe cases there is diffuse interstitial fibrosis associated with parenchymal remodeling and honeycombing (Fig. 9.16). Asbestos bodies are almost always identifiable microscopically in the fibrous tissue or macrophages in residual airspaces (3,13).

The initial radiographic manifestations of asbestosis consist of small, irregular opacities resulting in a fine, reticular pattern, reflecting the peribronchiolar and adjacent alveolar interstitial fibrosis (Fig. 9.17A). The fine reticulation eventually progresses to a coarse linear pattern with honeycombing. These abnormalities are usually most severe in the subpleural regions of the lower lobes (Fig. 9.17B). Pleural plaques can be identified in the vast majority of patients (13,14).

HRCT with the patient prone is the most sensitive imaging technique to detect asbestosis. It allows distinction of reversible abnormalities in the dorsal lung regions due to dependent atelectasis from irreversible fibrosis (15). Findings in early disease include subpleural dots or branching structures, intralobular lines, thickened interlobular septa, subpleural curvilinear lines, patchy areas of ground-glass attenuation, and small, cystic spaces (Fig. 9.18). These abnormalities tend to involve mainly the dorsal subpleural regions of the lower lobes. HRCT–pathology correlation studies have shown that subpleural dots and branching structures correspond to peribronchiolar fibrosis (16). Extension of fibrous tissue into the parenchyma between affected bronchioles results in pleura-based nodular irregularities (16). Thickened interlobular septa on HRCT may correspond to fibrosis of the septa themselves or to fibrosis in the periphery of the lobule. Ground-glass opacities (Fig. 9.19) are related to mild alveolar wall fibrosis (16,17).

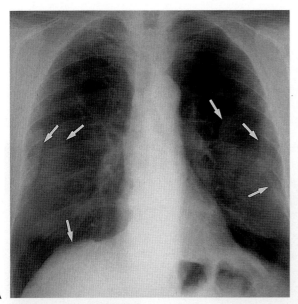

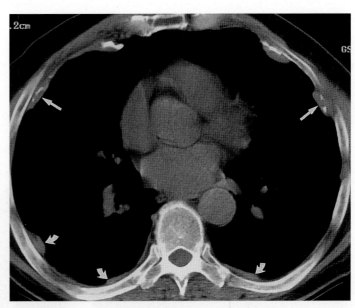

A

B

FIGURE 9.14. Pleural plaques. **A:** A chest radiograph shows multiple pleural plaques (*arrows*), seen as focal areas of increased opacity that typically have one well-defined margin (where the plaque abuts the lung) and a poorly defined margin (where the plaque abuts the chest wall). **B:** A CT image (7-mm collimation) shows bilateral calcified (*straight arrows*) and noncalcified (*curved arrows*) plaques. The patient was a 68-year-old shipyard worker.

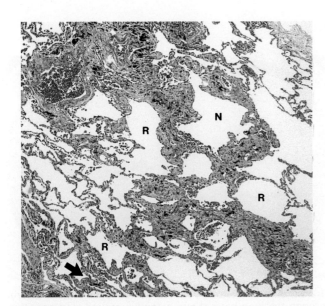

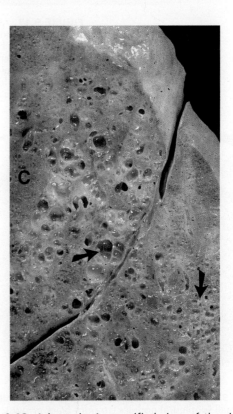

FIGURE 9.15. Asbestosis—early histologic appearance. A photomicrograph shows a moderate degree of fibrosis of the interstitial tissue of a membranous bronchiole (*N*) and several of its respiratory bronchiolar branches (*R*). Involvement of alveolar septa is also evident focally (*arrow*).

FIGURE 9.16. Asbestosis. A magnified view of the right lung shows patchy fibrosis, focally associated with a honeycomb appearance (*arrows*). The more central portion of the lobe (*C*) is less severely affected.

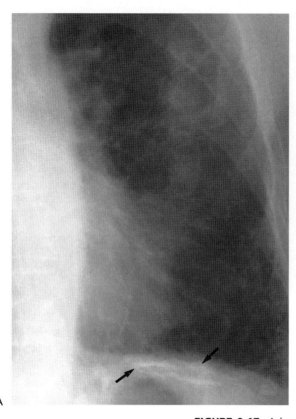
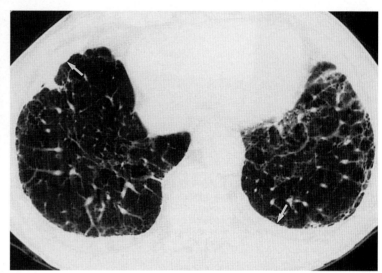

A

B

FIGURE 9.17. Asbestosis. **A:** A view of the left lower chest from a posteroanterior radiograph shows a reticular pattern most evident near the costophrenic sulcus. A calcified diaphragmatic plaque can also be seen (*arrows*). **B:** An HRCT image (1.5-mm collimation) demonstrates intralobular linear opacities and irregular septal thickening, resulting in a reticular pattern, involving mainly the subpleural lung regions. Also note bilateral pleural thickening (*arrows*). The patient was a 66-year-old man.

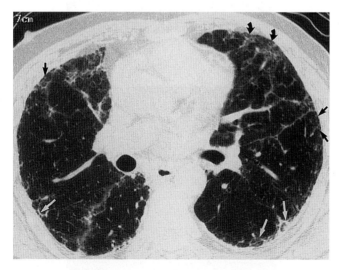

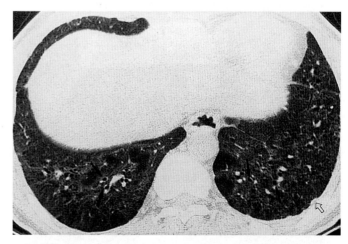

FIGURE 9.18. Asbestosis. An HRCT image (1-mm collimation) shows small subpleural nodules (*straight black arrows*), irregular linear opacities (*straight white arrows*), and patchy ground-glass opacities (*curved arrows*). The abnormalities involve mainly the subpleural lung regions. The patient was a 58-year-old man.

FIGURE 9.19. Asbestosis. An HRCT image (1.0-mm collimation) through the lung bases shows extensive ground-glass opacities and irregular linear opacities, resulting in a fine reticular pattern. Mild traction bronchiectasis (*arrows*) and pleural plaques (*open arrow*) are also evident. The patient was a 44-year-old shipyard worker.

Rounded Atelectasis

Rounded atelectasis is a form of parenchymal collapse that occurs most commonly in the peripheral lung in the dorsal regions of the lower lobes. Pathologic examination shows pleural fibrosis overlying the abnormal parenchyma as well as invaginations of fibrotic pleura into the region of collapse (Fig. 9.20). The appearance suggests that retraction of collagen in the pleura as it matures is the cause of the collapse (18).

Because of the pathogenetic association with fibrosis, the areas of atelectasis are always seen adjacent to the visceral pleura radiologically. A characteristic finding is the presence of crowding of bronchi and blood vessels that extend from the border of the mass to the hilum ("comet tail" sign) (13,19) (Fig. 9.21). In most cases, the collapsed lung has a rounded or oval shape; however, wedge-shaped and irregularly shaped masses can also occur. Volume loss of the affected lobe is uniformly present and often associated with hyperlucency of the adjacent lung. Serial examinations usually show a stable appearance (19,20).

Pulmonary Carcinoma

The association between asbestos exposure and pulmonary carcinoma is accepted as being causal. The risk of carcinoma increases with the severity of exposure and with the presence of asbestosis. It is particularly evident in workers who smoke (3,21), having been estimated to be as much as 50 to 100 times that in the nonsmoking, nonexposed population. Asbestos-related tumors frequently occur in the periphery of the lower lobes, a distribution that corresponds to the typical distribution of asbestosis (21).

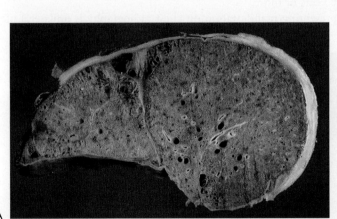

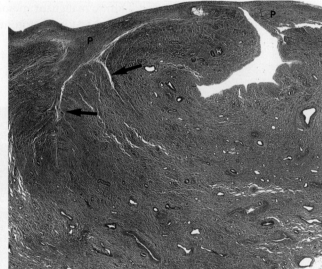

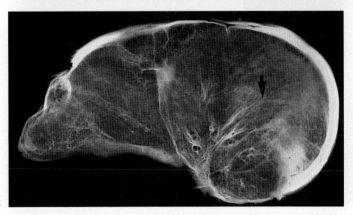

FIGURE 9.20. Rounded atelectasis. **A:** A transverse slice of the right lung shows marked pleural fibrosis, particularly over the lateral aspect of the lower lobe. The parenchyma underlying this region has a grayish appearance as a result of chronic collapse and interstitial fibrosis. **B:** A radiograph of the slice shows the focus of collapse as well as a number of vessels, some curved in appearance (*arrow*), extending into it. **C:** A low-magnification view of the edge of the lesion confirms the parenchymal collapse. (Only a few slightly expanded alveoli are evident at the bottom left of the specimen.) Fibrous tissue is present in the overlying visceral pleura (*P*) as well as in several invaginations that extend into the area of collapse (*arrows*).

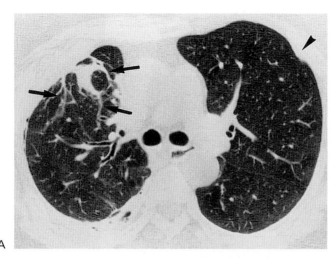 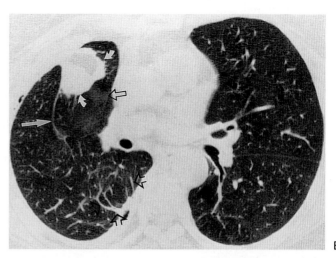

FIGURE 9.21. Rounded atelectasis. **A:** An HRCT image (1.0-mm collimation) at the level of the main bronchi shows a focal area of pleural thickening overlying a nodular opacity in the right upper lobe. Vessels can be seen sweeping toward the opacity (comet-tail sign) (*arrows*). Volume loss of the right upper lobe is evident. A pleural plaque (*arrowhead*) can be seen in left hemithorax. **B:** HRCT image at the level of the bronchus intermedius shows the inferior margin of the area of atelectasis (*curved arrows*) between right major (*straight arrow*) and minor (*open arrow*) fissures. Parenchymal bands (*open arrows* at bottom) can be seen converging to a pleural plaque in the right lower lobe. The patient was a 63-year-old woman.

Malignant Mesothelioma

Diffuse malignant mesothelioma is an uncommon neoplasm of the serosal lining of the pleural cavity or peritoneum (Fig. 9.22). The vast majority of tumors occur in association with asbestos exposure. The latency period between exposure and diagnosis is usually 20 years and often as long 40 years or more.

The most common presenting manifestation on chest radiography is unilateral pleu-

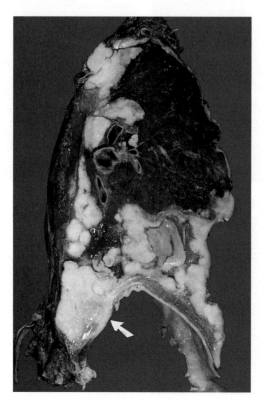

FIGURE 9.22. Malignant mesothelioma. A sagittal slice of the left lung shows marked thickening of the pleura in its inferior and posterior aspects by a somewhat nodular white tumor; mild thickening is evident anteriorly. The neoplasm has extended across the hemidiaphragm posteriorly (*arrow*).

ral effusion (22). Other manifestations include nodular and diffuse pleural thickening. Characteristic CT findings include thickening of the mediastinal pleura, nodular pleural thickening, thickening greater than 1cm, and circumferential pleural thickening (23,24) (Fig. 9.23). Since plaques rarely involve the mediastinal pleura and are usually flat and 2 to 5 mm thick, these findings have been shown to allow distinction of mesothelioma from benign pleural thickening in most cases (23). The tumor may extend into the interlobar fissures and interlobular septa or directly invade the pulmonary parenchyma. Patients with advanced disease may have invasion of the chest wall, pericardium, diaphragm, and abdomen.

Miscellaneous Pneumoconioses

Siderosis

The term *siderosis* refers to the accumulation of iron oxide in macrophages within the lung. It is seen most commonly in electric arc or oxyacetylene torch workers, who are exposed to the metal in fumes during the welding process. It is believed to be unassociated with fibrosis or functional impairment. However, when the iron is admixed with a substantial quantity of silica, the resulting silicosiderosis (mixed-dust pneumoconiosis) can be associated with appreciable pulmonary fibrosis (3). Histologically, the iron oxide particles accumulate in perivascular and peribronchiolar interstitium and the alveolar airspaces. Mild interstitial fibrosis may be present (25).

The radiographic pattern in pure siderosis consists of a diffuse, fine, reticulonodular pattern. Nodular opacities are less dense and less profuse than those of silicosis. In contrast to most cases of pneumoconiosis, these abnormalities can disappear partly or completely after cessation of dust exposure, suggesting that they are related to the presence of particle-laden macrophages that are eventually cleared rather than fibrous tissue. HRCT findings described in arc-welders include poorly defined centrilobular small nodules with or without branching linear structures (reflecting the peribronchiolar macrophage accumulation) and bilateral ground-glass attenuation without zonal predominance (reflecting the alveolar airspace macrophages) (25–27) (Fig. 9.24).

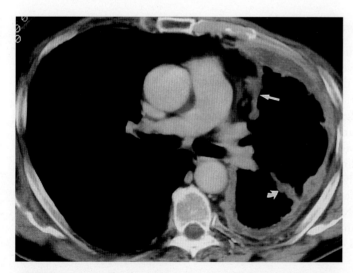

FIGURE 9.23. Malignant mesothelioma. A contrast-enhanced CT image (10-mm collimation) shows circumferential nodular thickening of the left pleura. Note involvement of the mediastinal pleura (*straight arrow*) and interlobar fissure (*curved arrow*) as well as volume loss of the ipsilateral hemithorax. The patient was a 76-year-old-man.

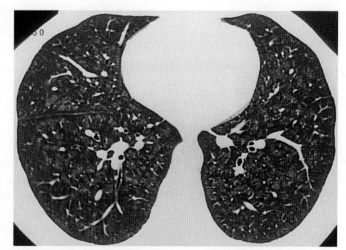

FIGURE 9.24. Siderosis. An HRCT image (1.0-mm collimation) at level of basal segmental bronchi shows bilateral ground-glass opacities and poorly defined centrilobular nodular opacities. The patient was a 57-year-old man. (From Kim KI, Kim CW, Lee MK, et al. Imaging of occupational lung disease. *Radiographics* 2001;21: 1371–1391, with permission.)

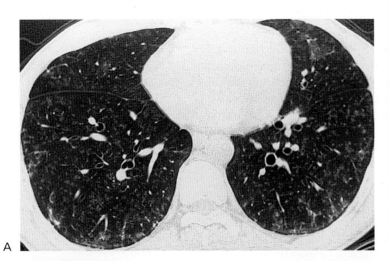

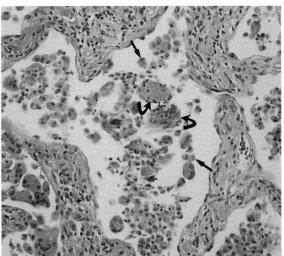

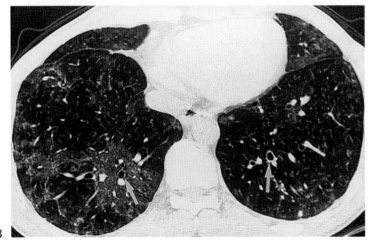

FIGURE 9.25. Giant-cell interstitial pneumonia. **A:** An HRCT image (1.0-mm collimation) at the level of the basal segmental bronchi shows patchy bilateral ground-glass opacities and irregular linear opacities. **B:** An image at a more caudad level shows slightly more severe abnormalities. Also note mild bronchial dilatation (*arrows*). **C:** A photomicrograph of a biopsy specimen shows moderate parenchymal interstitial thickening by fibrous tissue and nonspecific chronic inflammatory cell infiltrate. The adjacent airspaces contain numerous macrophages (*straight arrows*) and several multinucleated giant cells (*curved arrows*). The patient was a 47-year-old iron driller.

Hard Metal Pneumoconiosis

Hard metal is an alloy of tungsten, carbon, and cobalt. It is extremely hard and resistant to heat and is used extensively in the drilling and polishing of other metals. Exposure to hard metal dust can occur during the manufacture or use of the metal and is well recognized as a cause of interstitial pneumonitis and fibrosis (3). Although histologic findings may be those of usual or desquamative interstitial pneumonia, a pattern of giant-cell interstitial pneumonia is characteristic (28) (Fig. 9.25). With progression of the disease, parenchymal remodeling and honeycombing may be seen (25).

The radiographic findings consist of a diffuse, small, nodular and reticular pattern, sometimes associated with lymph node enlargement; the reticulation may be coarse and in advanced disease may be accompanied by small cystic spaces, reflecting the presence of honeycombing (29,30). HRCT findings consist of bilateral areas of ground-glass attenuation, areas of consolidation, and extensive reticular opacities and traction bronchiectasis indicative of fibrosis (25,31) (Fig. 9.25A).

CHEMICAL PNEUMONITIS

The inhalation of noxious chemical substances is an uncommon cause of occupational lung disease. Implicated substances include organic compounds (e.g,. carbamates and paraquat), inorganic compounds (e.g., ammonia, hydrogen sulfide, nitrogen oxide, and sulfur dioxide), and metals (e.g., mercury and nickel).

Inhalation of noxious fumes may cause disease of the tracheobronchial tree, lung parenchyma, or both. In general, more soluble gases (e.g., ammonia) result in greater irritation of the upper respiratory tract, whereas less soluble gases (e.g., nitrogen dioxide) affect mainly the distal airways and alveoli. Toxic agents also can be absorbed through the gastrointestinal tract, mucous membranes, and skin. The absorbed compound can affect the lung directly or through its metabolites. Pathologic findings include acute inflammation and (sometimes) ulceration of airway mucosa and consolidation of lung parenchyma by edema fluid (sometimes in association with a proteinaceous exudate and hyaline membranes [diffuse alveolar damage]).

Carbamates

Carbamate insecticides are commonly used as agricultural insecticides in the United States and throughout the world. They are cholinesterase inhibitors but do not effectively penetrate the central nervous system and therefore produce limited central nervous system toxicity (32). The main manifestation is noncardiogenic pulmonary edema (33).

Paraquat

Poisoning by the herbicide paraquat may be seen in an occupational setting but is often intentional for suicide. Ingestion of a large amount of the substance leads to the rapid onset of pulmonary edema. Ingestion of smaller doses results in delayed onset of pulmonary abnormalities, which may progress to respiratory failure (34). Pathologic findings are those of diffuse alveolar damage, the proliferative phase of which (pulmonary fibrosis) begins about 7 to 10 days after poisoning (Fig. 9.26C). Distortion of pulmonary architecture with dilatation of bronchioles and alveolar ducts and airspace fibrosis are late findings (35).

Radiographic manifestations include interstitial or granular opacities, or confluent bilateral opacities indicative of pulmonary edema (Fig. 9.26A). Pneumomediastinum is commonly seen. Consolidation or diffuse haziness on initial radiographs often evolves into a pattern of fibrosis (36).

The most common pattern on initial HRCT consists of diffuse bilateral areas of ground-glass attenuation, reflecting alveolar septal thickening and the early airspace exudates of diffuse alveolar damage (35,36) (Fig. 9.26B). This evolves into consolidation with reticulation and, ultimately, into architectural distortion and traction bronchiectasis.

Hydrogen Sulfide

Hydrogen sulfide is an irritant and potentially asphyxiating gas that exerts its primary toxic effects on the respiratory and neurologic systems (37). Exposure occurs in coal miners, tanners, petroleum manufacturers, and workers in geothermal power plants, aircraft factories, sewers, and rubber factories (34,38,39). When inhaled acutely in large quantities, hydrogen sulfide causes death from inhibition of the medullary respiratory center. Smaller or more prolonged exposure can lead to pulmonary edema.

Ammonia

Ammonia is a corrosive gas widely used in the production of explosives, petroleum, agricultural fertilizers, and plastics. The chemical is also used in refrigeration. Occupational exposure results from damage to storage containers and pipes. The substance is highly soluble and can cause severe mucosal damages of both upper and lower airways (34).

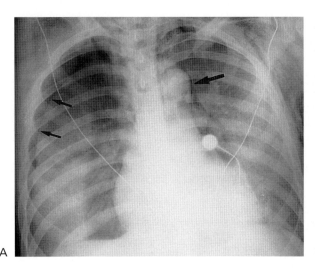

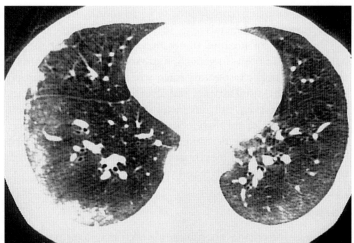

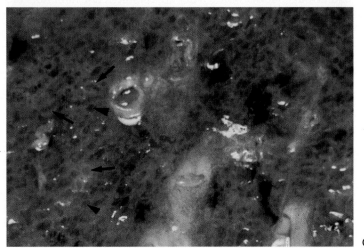

FIGURE 9.26. Paraquat poisoning. **A:** A chest radiograph shows extensive bilateral airspace consolidation. Also note the presence of pneumomediastinum (*arrow*), right pneumothorax (*small arrows*) and subcutaneous emphysema. **B:** An HRCT image (1.0-mm collimation) at the level of the basal segmental bronchi 2 days before **A** shows subpleural ground-glass opacities and airspace consolidation. The patient was an 18-year-old man. **C:** A highly magnified view of lung obtained at autopsy of another patient who ingested paraquat 10 days before death shows the lumina of transitional airways (*arrowheads*) to be particularly prominent as a result of thickening of the surrounding parenchyma (*arrows*), an appearance consistent with the proliferative phase of diffuse alveolar damage.

The radiographic appearance in ammonia inhalation varies according to the severity of the exposure. In mild exposure, the chest radiograph is normal. After larger exposures, radiographs may demonstrate airspace consolidation as a result of parenchymal edema. Patients who survive the initial insult usually recover completely; however, they may have residual bronchiectasis or bronchiolitis obliterans as a result of the airway damage (40,41) (Fig. 9.27).

Hydrocarbon

Acute pneumonitis following ingestion or aspiration of petroleum products is usually related to accidental poisonings in children. Accidental aspiration of petroleum in performers demonstrating the art of fire eating can cause a distinct type of chemical pneumonitis known as fire-eater's lung (42,43).

Histologically, the acute phase is characterized by acute inflammation of the lung parenchyma and airway walls. One to 2 weeks after the initial onset of symptoms, obliterative bronchiolitis and/or parenchymal fibrosis may be seen. Well-delimited cystic spaces 1 cm or more in diameter (pneumatoceles) may develop as a result of coalescence of several necrotic bronchioles or partial obstruction of a bronchiolar lumen with the creation

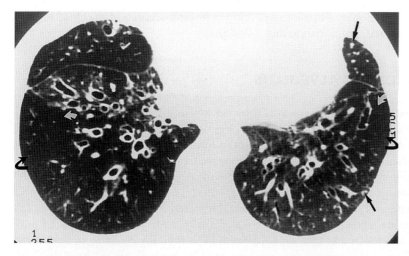

FIGURE 9.27. Ammonia inhalation—bronchiectasis and obliterative bronchiolitis. An HRCT image (1.0-mm collimation) shows extensive bilateral bronchiectasis as well as localized areas of decreased attenuation and perfusion (*curved arrows*) consistent with obliterative bronchiolitis. Centrilobular nodules and branching linear structures (*straight arrows*) consistent with mucus filled-dilated bronchioles are also evident. The patient was a 56-year-old man who had inhaled ammonia 15 years previously following a refrigerator explosion. (From Kim KI, Kim CW, Lee MK, et al. Imaging of occupational lung disease. *Radiographics* 2001;21:1371–1391, with permission.)

of a check-valve (42,43). Radiographic and HRCT findings include unilateral or bilateral airspace consolidation, and pneumatoceles (42,43) (Fig. 9.28).

Mercury Inhalation

Exposure to mercury vapor is an uncommon cause of occupational lung disease. Two primary sources of contamination are dumping of large quantities of inorganic mercury and mining. Mercury is used in electrolysis, in the manufacture of thermometers, and in the cleaning of boilers (34,44). Exposure to mercury vapor has also been described during smelting silver from dental amalgam containing mercury (45).

Exposure to more than 1 to 2 mg/m^3 of elemental mercury vapor for a few hours causes acute bronchiolitis and pneumonitis, the latter being manifested as diffuse alveolar

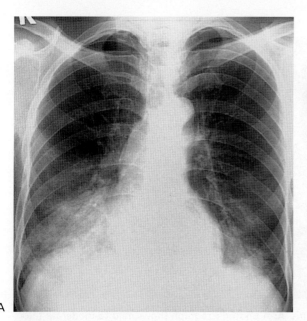

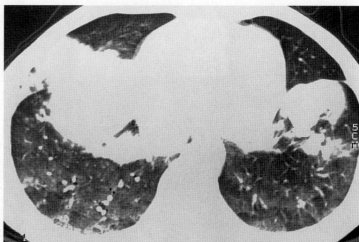

A   B

FIGURE 9.28. Hydrocarbon pneumonitis. **A:** A chest radiograph obtained 1 day after hydrocarbon ingestion shows consolidation in both lower lung zones. **B:** A CT image (10-mm collimation) shows extensive bilateral ground-glass opacities and patchy airspace consolidation. The patient was a 54-year-old man. (From Kim KI, Kim CW, Lee MK, et al. Imaging of occupational lung disease. *Radiographics* 2001;21:1371–1391, with permission.)

damage. Extensive pulmonary fibrosis can develop as healing occurs and may lead to progressive, sometimes fatal, pulmonary failure (45,46).

EXTRINSIC ALLERGIC ALVEOLITIS

Numerous organic dusts of plant or animal origin as well as some chemicals can cause extrinsic allergic alveolitis (EAA). The size of the organism or protein complex that causes EAA is small, probably no more than 1 to 2 μm in most cases. The most thoroughly investigated individuals in whom the disease develops are farmers (the causative agent being thermophilic actinomycetes) and bird fanciers or workers (the antigen being protein derived from bird serum and secreted into the gut).

The pathogenesis of the disorder is uncertain. However, it is likely that both type III and type IV immune reactions play a role. Inhaled antigens are probably deposited predominantly on bronchiolar and alveolar epithelium (47), typically resulting in both alveolitis and bronchiolitis. Histologic abnormalities tend be more severe in the vicinity of small membranous and proximal respiratory bronchioles (48). Typically, there is alveolar interstitial thickening by a mononuclear (largely lymphocytic) infiltrate (Fig. 9.29A). Poorly formed granulomas and isolated or small clusters of multinucleated giant cells are common, most often in the peribronchiolar interstitium (Fig. 9.29B). Alveolar airspaces are usually unaffected; a proteinaceous exudate and/or fibroblastic tissue are seen occasionally. The walls of small membranous and respiratory bronchioles also contain a predominantly lymphocytic infiltrate. In severe cases, bronchiolar epithelial ulceration and obliterative bronchiolitis may be seen (Fig. 9.30). Repeated or chronic exposure can result in parenchymal interstitial fibrosis.

The radiologic findings are influenced by the stage of the disease (49). Acute heavy exposure to the inciting antigen can result in diffuse airspace consolidation, which reflects the presence of pulmonary edema. More commonly, there are bilateral ground-glass opacities (Fig. 9.31) and poorly defined nodules (49,50), reflecting the presence of alveolitis and bronchiolitis, respectively (48,49). On HRCT, the nodules have a centrilobular dis-

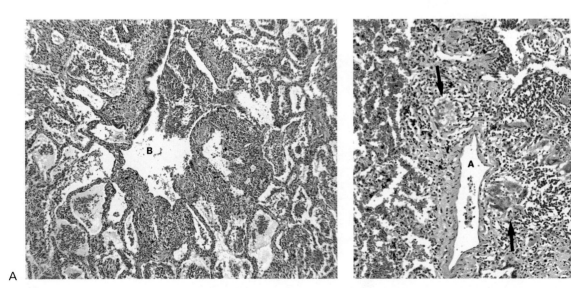

A   B

FIGURE 9.29. Extrinsic allergic alveolitis. **A:** A photomicrograph shows mild to moderate thickening of the interstitial tissue of a small membranous bronchiole (*B*) by a lymphocytic infiltrate. The adjacent alveolar septa are expanded by a similar infiltrate. Airspaces contain an increased number of macrophages. (The airspace hemorrhage was secondary to the biopsy procedure). **B:** A view elsewhere in the section shows several poorly formed granulomas (*arrows*) in the interstitial tissue adjacent to a small pulmonary artery (*A*). The patient was a 55-year-old farmer.

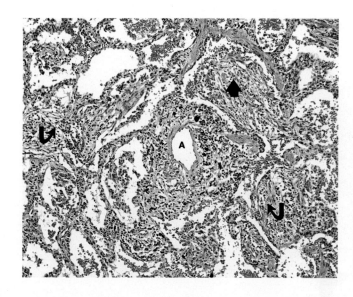

FIGURE 9.30. Extrinsic allergic alveolitis. A photomicrograph shows mild thickening of the perivascular and alveolar interstitium by a lymphocytic infiltrate (*A* = pulmonary artery). The lumina of a membranous bronchiole (*thick arrow*) and several respiratory bronchioles (*curved arrows*) are filled with fibroblastic tissue that also contains lymphocytes. The patient was 46-year-old farmer.

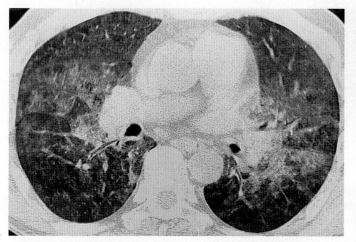

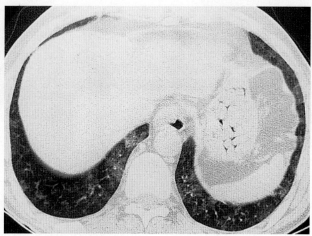

FIGURE 9.31. Acute extrinsic allergic alveolitis. **A:** An HRCT image (1-mm collimation) at the level of the bronchus intermedius shows bilateral ground-glass opacities and small areas of consolidation. **B:** Another image through lung bases shows extensive bilateral ground-glass opacities. The patient was a 54-year-old farmer.

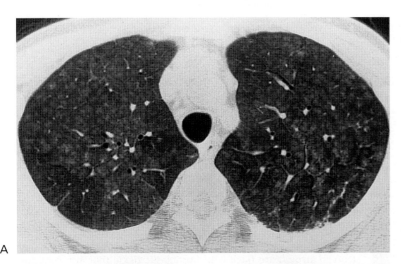

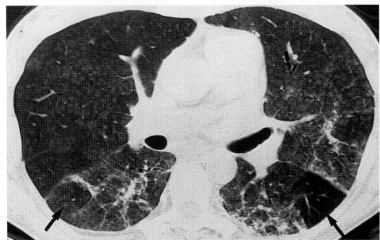

FIGURE 9.32. Subacute extrinsic allergic alveolitis. **A:** A CT image at the level of the upper lobes obtained using sliding-thin-slab (4.9 mm) maximum-intensity projection (MIP) technique shows poorly defined centrilobular nodular opacities throughout both lungs. **B:** An image at the level of the bronchus intermedius again shows nodular areas of ground-glass opacity. Focal areas of low attenuation suggesting air trapping (*arrows*) are evident in the left lower lobe. The patient was a 45-year-old woman.

tribution (Fig. 9.32A). The abnormalities can be diffuse, but tend to involve mainly the middle and lower lung zones (50). Another common finding is the presence of lobular areas of decreased vascularity and perfusion that show air trapping on expiratory HRCT (Fig. 9.32B) (51,52). These are presumably the result of bronchiolar obstruction by plugs of fibroblastic tissue.

The chronic stage of EAA is characterized by fibrosis, although evidence of active disease is often present. Radiologic findings indicative of this complication include intralobular interstitial thickening, irregular interlobular septal thickening, traction bronchiectasis, and honeycombing (Fig. 9.33). Relative sparing of the lung bases is seen in most cases, a finding that usually allows distinction of EAA from idiopathic pulmonary fibrosis (53,54).

Isocyanate-Associated Hypersensitivity Pneumonitis

Isocyanates are used for the large-scale production of polyurethane polymers, which are in turn used for manufacturing flexible and rigid foams, elastomers, adhesives, and surface coatings (55). Acute or chronic exposure to high concentrations of isocyanates can result in respiratory illness through a direct irritant effect. They can also cause occupational asthma (55,56) and, less often, extrinsic allergic alveolitis. Although these agents are not organic dusts, the hypersensitivity reaction they cause is identical radiologically and pathologically to allergic alveolitis caused by organic agents (3) (Fig. 9.34).

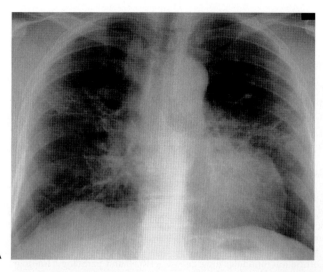

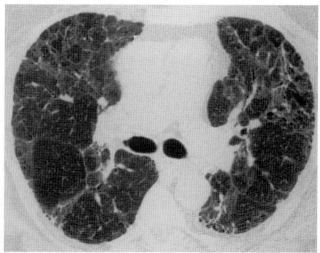

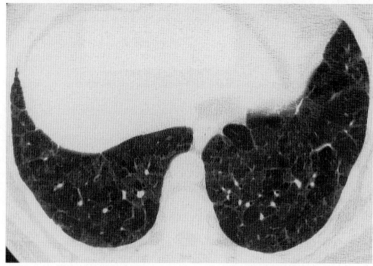

FIGURE 9.33. Chronic extrinsic allergic alveolitis. **A:** A chest radiograph shows irregular linear opacities involving the middle and lower lung zones. **B:** An HRCT image (1-mm collimation) at the level of the main bronchi shows extensive irregular linear opacities and ground-glass opacities. **C:** Another image through the lung bases shows patchy ground-glass opacities and minimal fibrosis. The patient was a 54-year-old man.

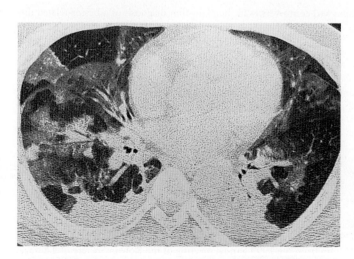

FIGURE 9.34. Isocyanate-induced acute hypersensitivity pneumonitis. An HRCT image (1-mm collimation) shows patchy ground-glass opacities and dependent airspace consolidation. The abnormalities cleared completely following treatment with corticosteroids. The patient was a 32-year-old man who had been exposed to isocyanate while painting.

REFERENCES

1. Schwartz DA, Peterson MW. Occupational lung disease. *Adv Intern Med* 1997;42:269–312.
2. Cullen M, Cherniack M, Rosenstock L. Medical progress: occupational medicine. *N Engl J Med* 1990;322:594–601.
3. Fraser RS, Müller NL, Colman N, et al. Inhalation of inorganic dust (pneumoconiosis). In: *Diagnosis of diseases of the chest,* 4th ed. Philadelphia: WB Saunders, 1999:2386–2484.
4. Stark P, Jacobson F, Shaffer K. Standard imaging in silicosis and coal worker's pneumoconiosis. *Radiol Clin North Am* 1992;30:1147–1154.
5. Webb WR, Müller NL, Naidich DP. *High-resolution CT of the lung,* 3rd ed. Philadelphia: Lippincott-Raven, 2001:259–353.
6. Fujimura N. Pathology and pathophysiology of pneumoconiosis. *Curr Opin Pulm Med* 2000;6: 140–144.
7. Remy-Jardin M, Remy J, Farre I, et al. Computed tomographic evaluation of silicosis and coal worker's pneumoconiosis. *Radiol Clin North Am* 1992;30:1155–1176.
8. Kinsella N, Müller NL, Vedal S, et al. Emphysema in silicosis: a comparison of smokers with nonsmokers using pulmonary function testing and computed tomography. *Am Rev Respir Dis* 1990;141:1497–1500.
9. Lee KS, Kim TS, Han J, et al. Diffuse micronodular lung disease: HRCT and pathologic findings. *J Comput Assist Tomogr* 1999;23:99–106.
10. Dumontet C, Biron F, Vitrey D, et al. Acute silicosis due to inhalation of a domestic product. *Am Rev Respir Dis* 1991;143:880–882.
11. Dee P, Suratt P, Winn W. The radiographic findings in acute silicosis. *Radiology* 1978;126:359–363.
12. Marchiori E, Ferreira A, Müller NL. Silicoproteinosis: high-resolution CT and histologic findings. *J Thorac Imaging* 2001;16:127–129.
13. McLoud TC. Conventional radiography in the diagnosis of asbestos-related disease. *Radiol Clin North Am* 1992;30:1177–1189.
14. Peacock C, Copley SJ, Hansell DM. Asbestos-related benign pleural disease. *Clin Radiol* 2000;55:422–432.
15. Aberle DR, Gamsu G, Ray CS, et al. Asbestos-related pleural and parenchymal fibrosis: detection with high-resolution CT. *Radiology* 1988;166:729–34.
16. Akira M, Yokoyama K, Yamamoto S, et al. Early asbestosis: evaluation with high-resolution CT. *Radiology* 1991;178:409–416.
17. Akira M, Yamamoto S, Yokoyama K, et al. Asbestosis: high-resolution CT–pathologic correlation. *Radiology* 1990;176:389–394.
18. Menzies R. Fraser R. Rounded atelectasis: pathologic and pathogenetic features. *Am J Surg Pathol* 1987;11:674–681.
19. Lynch DA, Gamsu G, Ray CS, et al. Asbestos-related focal lung masses: manifestations on conventional and high-resolution CT scans. *Radiology* 1988;169:603–607.
20. Batra P, Brown K, Hayashi K, et al. Rounded atelectasis. *J Thorac Imaging* 1996;11:187–197.
21. Sluis-Cremer GK. The relationship between asbestosis and bronchial cancer. *Chest* 1980;78: 380–381.
22. Gefter WB, Conant EF. Issues and controversies in the plain-film diagnosis of asbestos-related disorders in the chest. *J Thorac Imag* 1988;3:11–28.
23. Leung AN, Müller NL, Miller RR. CT in differential diagnosis of diffuse pleural disease. *Am J Roentgenol* 1990;154:487–492.
24. Kawashima A. Libshitz HI. Malignant pleural mesothelioma: CT manifestations in 50 cases. *Am J Roentgenol* 1990;155:965–969.
25. Akira M. Uncommon pneumoconioses: CT and pathologic findings. *Radiology* 1995;197:403–409.
26. Kim K-I, Choi SJ, Sohn HS, et al. High-resolution CT findings of welders' pneumoconiosis. *J Korean Radiol Soc* 1996;34:367–371.
27. Han D, Goo JM, Im J-G, et al. Thin-section CT findings of arc-welders' pneumoconiosis. *Korean J Radiol* 2000;1:79–83.
28. Ohori NP, Sciurba FC, Owens GR, Hodgson MJ, Yousem SA. Giant-cell interstitial pneumonia and hard-metal pneumoconiosis. A clinicopathologic study of four cases and review of the literature. *Am J Surg Pathol.* 1989;13:581–587.
29. Coates EO Jr, Watson JHL. Diffuse interstitial lung disease in tungsten carbide workers. *Ann Intern Med* 1971;75:709–716.
30. Forrest ME, Skerker LB, Nemirott MJ. Hard metal pneumoconiosis: another cause of diffuse interstitial fibrosis. *Radiology* 1978;128:609–612.
31. Lee KS, Im J-G, Kang DS. Notes from the 1999 annual meeting of the Korean Society of Thoracic Radiology. *J Thorac Imag* 2000;15:30–35.
32. Arena JM, Drew RH. *Poisoning: toxicology, symptoms, treatments,* 5th ed. Springfield, IL: Charles C Thomas, 1986:187–188.
33. Park CH, Kim K-I, Park SK, et al. Carbamate poisoning: high resolution CT and pathologic findings. *J Comput Assist Tomogr* 2000;24:52–54.

34. White CS, Templeton PA. Chemical pneumonitis. *Radiol Clin North Am* 1992;30:1231–1243.
35. Lee SH, Lee KS, Ahn JM, et al. Paraquat poisoning of the lung: thin-section CT findings. *Radiology* 1995;195:271–274.
36. Im JG, Lee KS, Han MC, et al. Paraquat poisoning: findings on chest radiography and CT in 42 patients. *Am J Roentgenol* 1991;157: 697–701.
37. Milby TH, Baselt RC. Hydrogen sulfide poisoning: clarification of some controversial issues. *Am J Ind Med* 1999;35:192–195.
38. Richardson DB. Respiratory effects of chronic hydrogen sulfide exposure. *Am J Ind Med* 1995;28:99–108.
39. Hessel PA, Herbert FA, Melenka LS, et al. Lung health in relation to hydrogen sulfide exposure in oil and gas workers in Alberta, Canada. *Am J Ind Med* 1997;31:554–557.
40. De la Hoz RE, Schlueter DP, Rom WN. Chronic lung disease secondary to ammonia inhalation injury: a report on three cases. *Am J Ind Med* 1996;29:209–214.
41. Hoeffler HB, Schweppe HI, Greenberg SD. Bronchiectasis following pulmonary ammonia burn. *Arch Pathol Lab Med* 1982;106:686–687.
42. Bankier AA, Brunner C, Lomoschitz F, et al. Pyrofluid inhalation in "fire-eaters": sequential findings on CT. *J Thorac Imag* 1999;14:303–306.
43. Franquet T, Gomez-Santos D, Gimenez A, et al. Fire eater's pneumonia: radiographic and CT findings. *J Comput Assist Tomogr* 2000;24:448–450.
44. Asano S, Eto K, Kurisaki E, et al. Review article: acute inorganic mercury vapor inhalation poisoning. *Pathol Int* 2000;50:169–174.
45. Kanluen S, Gottlieb CA. A clinical pathologic study of four adult cases of acute mercury inhalation toxicity. *Arch Pathol Lab Med* 1991;115:56–60.
46. Rowens B, Guerrero-Bentancourt D, Gottlieb CA, et al. Respiratory failure and death following acute inhalation of mercury vapor: a clinical and histologic perspective. *Chest* 1991;99:185–190.
47. Pitcher WD. Hypersensitivity pneumonitis. *Am J Med Sci* 1990;300:251–266.
48. Colby TV, Swensen SJ. Anatomic distribution and histopathologic patterns in diffuse lung disease: correlation with HRCT. *J Thorac Imag* 1996;11:1–26.
49. Silver SF, Müller NL, Miller RR, et al. Hypersensitivity pneumonitis: evaluation with CT. *Radiology* 1989;173:441–445.
50. Remy-Jardin M, Remy J, Wallaert B, et al. Subacute and chronic bird breeder hypersensitivity pneumonitis: sequential evaluation with CT and correlation with lung function tests and bronchoalveolar lavage. *Radiology* 1993;189:111–118.
51. Hansell DM, Wells AU, Padley SPG, et al. Hypersensitivity pneumonitis: correlation of individual CT patterns with functional abnormalities. *Radiology* 1996;199:123–128.
52. Small JH, Flower CDR, Traill ZC, et al. Air-trapping in extrinsic allergic alveolitis on computed tomography. *Clin Radiol* 1996;51:684–688.
53. Adler BD, Padley SPG, Müller NL, et al. Chronic hypersensitivity pneumonitis: high-resolution CT and radiographic features in 16 patients. *Radiology* 1992;185:91–95.
54. Lynch DA, Newell JD, Logan PM, et al. Can CT distinguish hypersensitivity pneumonitis from idiopathic pulmonary fibrosis? *Am J Roentgenol* 1995;165:807–811.
55. Vandenplas O, Malo JL, Saetta M, et al. Occupational asthma and extrinsic alveolitis due to isocyanates: current status and perspectives. *Br J Ind Med* 1993;50:213–228.
56. Vadern/Musk AW, Peters JM, Wegman DH. Isocyanates and respiratory disease: current status. *Am J Ind Med* 1988;13:331–349.

10

DRUG-INDUCED LUNG DISEASE

CLASSIFICATION
Interstitial pneumonitis and fibrosis
Eosinophilic pneumonia
Bronchiolitis obliterans organizing pneumonia
Diffuse alveolar damage

CHEMOTHERAPEUTIC AND IMMUNOSUPPRESSIVE DRUGS
Bleomycin
Busulfan
Cyclophosphamide

Carmustine
Methotrexate

MISCELLANEOUS DRUGS
Nitrofurantoin
Amiodarone

ILLICIT DRUGS
Narcotic and sedative drugs
Cocaine

CLASSIFICATION

Drug-induced pulmonary injury is manifested by a wide variety of histologic reaction patterns. The most common of these are interstitial pneumonitis and fibrosis (either usual interstitial pneumonia [UIP] or nonspecific interstitial pneumonia [NSIP]), eosinophilic pneumonia, bronchiolitis obliterans organizing pneumonia (BOOP), and diffuse alveolar damage (DAD) (1). Other reactions—such as granulomatous pneumonitis, vasculitis, alveolar proteinosis, obliterative bronchiolitis, and venoocclusive disease—are less common (1,2). None of these histologic patterns is specific for either drug reaction in general or the reaction to a particular drug. As a result, the diagnosis of drug-induced pulmonary disease is based on a combination of radiologic, clinical, and (sometimes) histologic findings in a patient who has received a drug known to cause the abnormalities.

Interstitial Pneumonitis and Fibrosis

One of the most common forms of drug-induced pneumonitis is nonspecific interstitial pneumonia (NSIP) (1). This is characterized histologically by more or less homogeneous alveolar wall thickening by fibrous tissue and mononuclear inflammatory cells. The reaction is seen most commonly in association with methotrexate, amiodarone, or carmustine therapy (1). The corresponding radiographic and high-resolution computed tomography (HRCT) findings usually consist of patchy or diffuse ground-glass opacities (1) (Fig. 10.1). With progression of disease there may be evidence of fibrosis, including reticulation, traction bronchiectasis, and honeycombing; these are typically predominant in the lung bases. In some patients the fibrosis is patchy in distribution and predominantly peribronchovascular; this pattern is seen most commonly in patients receiving nitrofurantoin (3).

The second most common histologic form of drug-induced interstitial pneumonitis is usual interstitial pneumonia (UIP) (1). This is characterized histologically by a heterogeneous pattern of chronic inflammation and fibrosis, the latter consisting of both dense and loose (fibroblastic) connective tissue. Progression of the interstitial disease leads to obliteration of alveolar airspaces by mature fibrous tissue associated with dilatation of residual transitional airways (honeycombing). This pattern of injury occurs most com-

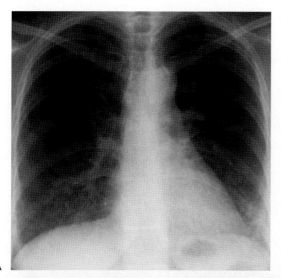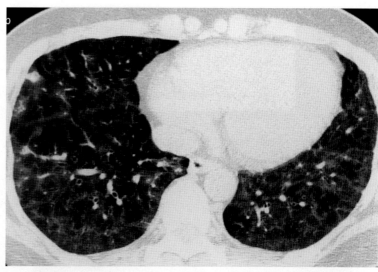

FIGURE 10.1. Nonspecific interstitial pneumonia (NSIP) secondary to cytoxan. **A:** A chest radiograph shows poorly defined ground-glass opacities involving the lower lung zones. **B:** An HRCT image (1-mm collimation) shows extensive bilateral ground-glass opacities as well as small areas of consolidation in the right middle and lower lobes and mild reticulation. The patient was a 45-year-old woman who had received cytoxan.

monly in association with cytotoxic chemotherapeutic agents, such as bleomycin, busulfan, methotrexate, doxorubicin, and carmustine (4,5). Noncytotoxic drugs, such as nitrofurantoin, amiodarone, gold, and penicillamine, also result in this reaction occasionally.

The predominant findings on the chest radiograph and HRCT are those of fibrosis with or without associated areas of consolidation (6). The fibrosis is characterized by the presence of irregular reticular opacities, honeycombing, architectural distortion, and traction bronchiectasis (Fig. 10.2). On HRCT the abnormalities are usually bilateral and symmetric, with predominant lower lung zone involvement. A peripheral and subpleural distribution of abnormalities is common (6–8).

Eosinophilic Pneumonia

Eosinophilic pneumonia is characterized histologically by the accumulation of eosinophils in the alveolar airspaces and infiltration of the adjacent interstitial space by eosinophils and variable numbers of lymphocytes and plasma cells. Peripheral eosinophilia is present in up to 40% of patients (4,9). As a drug reaction, it is seen most commonly in association with

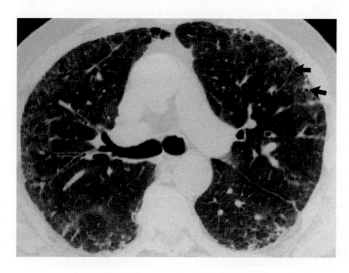

FIGURE 10.2. Usual interstitial pneumonia secondary to methotrexate. An HRCT image (1-mm collimation) shows a bilateral reticular pattern and ground-glass opacities involving the subpleural lung regions. Focal traction bronchiectasis is evident (*arrows*). The patient was a 75-year-old man.

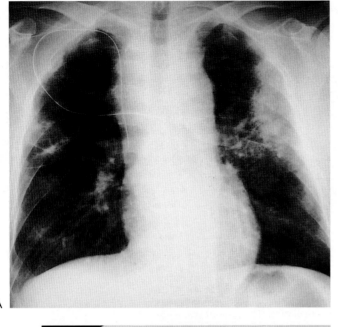

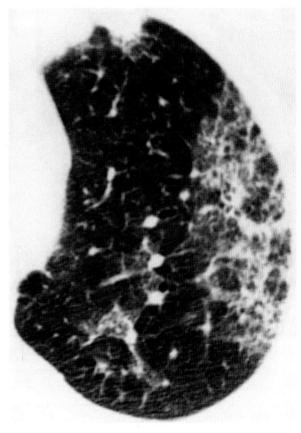

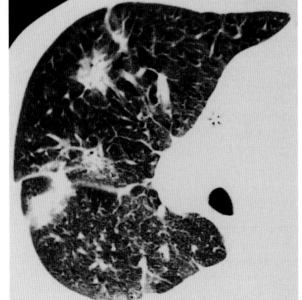

FIGURE 10.3. Eosinophilic pneumonia secondary to methotrexate. **A:** A chest radiograph shows bilateral areas of consolidation involving mainly the peripheral regions of the upper lobes. Also note evidence of mediastinal lymph node enlargement. **B:** An HRCT image (1-mm collimation) targeted to the left upper lobe shows peripheral ground-glass opacities, mild consolidation, and reticulation. **C:** A second image targeted to the right lung shows patchy peripheral and peribronchial consolidation in the right upper lobe and superior segment of right lower lobe. Patchy ground-glass opacities can be seen in the right lower lobe. The patient was a 50-year-old man.

methotrexate, sulfasalazine, para-aminosalicylic acid, nitrofurantoin, and nonsteroidal antiinflammatory drugs (1,4,10). Chest radiography and HRCT show bilateral airspace consolidation, which tends to involve mainly the peripheral lung regions and the upper lobes (1) (Fig. 10.3).

Bronchiolitis Obliterans Organizing Pneumonia

Bronchiolitis obliterans organizing pneumonia (BOOP) is characterized by parenchymal interstitial infiltration by mononuclear inflammatory cells and obliteration of the lumens of respiratory bronchioles, alveolar ducts, and (usually to a lesser extent) alveoli by fibroblastic tissue. The reaction has been reported most frequently in association with methotrexate, cyclophosphamide, gold, nitrofurantoin, amiodarone, bleomycin, and busulfan (1,11). The chest radiograph shows patchy bilateral areas of consolidation; on

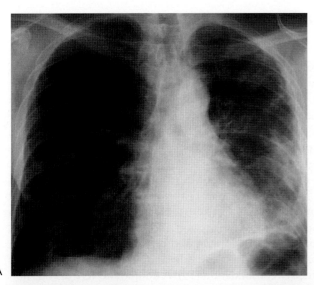 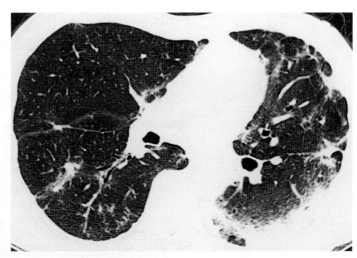

FIGURE 10.4. Bronchiolitis obliterans organizing pneumonia secondary to drug reaction. **A:** A chest radiograph shows extensive consolidation in the peripheral and basal regions of the left lung and mild consolidation in the right lung. **B:** An HRCT image (1-mm collimation) demonstrates subpleural consolidation in the left lower lobe and lingula, focal consolidation in right lower lobe and patchy ground-glass opacities. The patient was a 58-year-old man who had received cyclophosphamide and busulfan.

HRCT the areas of consolidation often have a predominantly peripheral or peribronchial distribution (1,11) (Fig. 10.4).

Diffuse Alveolar Damage

Diffuse alveolar damage (DAD) is characterized by the presence of alveolar airspace and interstitial edema, hyaline membrane formation, and proliferation of type II pneumocytes. In relation to drug-induced pulmonary disease, it occurs most commonly in association with cytotoxic agents such as bleomycin, aspirin, and narcotics (4,9). The corresponding radiologic features are those of adult respiratory distress syndrome (ARDS). The chest radiograph shows bilateral patchy or homogeneous airspace consolidation involving mainly the middle and lower lung zones (1). HRCT demonstrates extensive bilateral ground-glass opacities and dependent airspace consolidation (6,12) (Fig. 10.5).

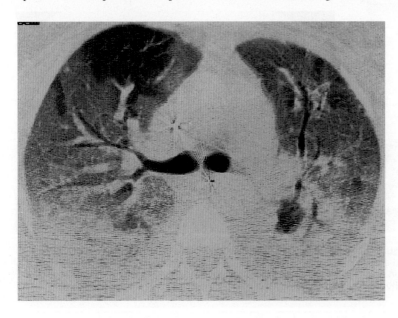

FIGURE 10.5. Diffuse alveolar damage secondary to drug reaction. An HRCT image (1-mm collimation) shows extensive bilateral ground-glass opacities and dependent airspace consolidation. The patient was a 45-year-old woman who had received several cytotoxic drugs.

CHEMOTHERAPEUTIC AND IMMUNOSUPPRESSIVE DRUGS

Bleomycin

Bleomycin is a cytotoxic drug used in the treatment of lymphomas and some carcinomas (5,13). Pulmonary toxicity is relatively common (14), with an incidence of approximately 4%. In one investigation of 100 patients receiving bleomycin, pulmonary abnormalities attributed to the drug were detected on 15% of the chest radiographs and 38% of CT scans (7). The most frequently reported histologic reactions are DAD and NSIP (1); less commonly, there is eosinophilic pneumonia (15) or BOOP (1,16).

The most common radiologic manifestations consist of bilateral bibasilar reticular, reticulonodular, or fine nodular opacities, often showing a peripheral distribution (17). These usually appear 6 weeks to 3 months after start of therapy (18). In one study of 20 patients thought to have pulmonary complications associated with combination chemotherapy regimens containing bleomycin, the region of the costophrenic angles was involved in 90%; in 33%, the opacities were confined to this region (17). With more severe disease, the abnormalities may extend into the middle and upper lung zones (17) or progress to patchy or confluent airspace consolidation (19). A unique and very uncommon manifestation of bleomycin toxicity is multiple nodules that mimic metastases; histologic correlation shows a localized BOOP reaction (16,20).

Busulfan

Busulfan is an alkylating agent used particularly in treating patients who have chronic myelogenous leukemia or who are undergoing preparation for bone marrow transplantation for hematologic and nonhematologic cancer (4,21). Clinically recognized lung toxicity occurs in approximately 5% of patients (22). It tends to occur with long-term use, ranging from 8 months to 10 years (average, 3 to 4 years) (23).

Histologic findings include NSIP, BOOP, and DAD (24), often associated with enlarged, cytologically atypical type II cells (Fig. 10.6) (24). Although similar atypical pneumocytes may be found in association with other drugs, their number is particularly great with busulfan. The atypia is likely a direct result of the drug on the type II cell nucleus.

The radiologic manifestations usually consist of a bilateral reticular or reticulonodular pattern, which may be diffuse but tends to involve mainly the lower lung zones (4). Less common radiographic and HRCT findings include patchy or widespread bilateral airspace consolidation (4,6) (Fig. 10.7).

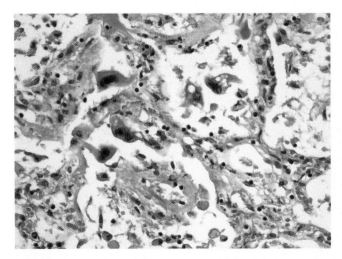

FIGURE 10.6. Interstitial pneumonitis secondary to busulfan toxicity. A magnified view of a biopsy specimen shows mild alveolar interstitial thickening as a result of capillary congestion and a lymphocytic infiltrate. Several enlarged type II cells with hyperchromatic, pleomorphic nuclei can be seen.

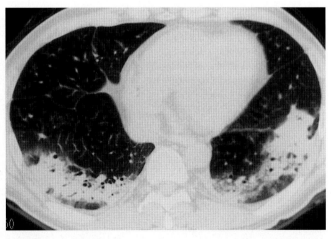

FIGURE 10.7. Nonspecific interstitial pneumonia secondary to busulfan. An HRCT image (1.5-mm collimation) shows bilateral airspace consolidation involving mainly the dorsal regions of the lower lobes. The patient was a 45-year-old man who had received busulfan.

Cyclophosphamide

Cyclophosphamide is an alkylating agent used in the treatment of a variety of malignancies and autoimmune diseases; it is commonly used in combination with other therapeutic agents (22). The incidence of pulmonary toxicity is probably less than 1% (4).

The most common histologic finding is DAD; as with busulfan, cytologically atypical type II cells are common (1,23). NSIP (1) and BOOP (12) reactions have been reported in a small number of patients. The radiological manifestations usually consist of a bilateral basilar reticular pattern, occasionally associated with focal areas of consolidation (4).

Carmustine

Carmustine (BCNU) is used mainly in the treatment of intracranial neoplasms and lymphoma (4,25). The incidence of pulmonary toxicity following its use as a single agent ranges from 1% to 20% (24). The incidence is as high as 40% to 60% of patients treated with high-dose combination chemotherapy protocols before autologous bone marrow transplantation (24).

The most common histologic reaction patterns are DAD and NSIP (1). The radiologic manifestations usually consist of a bibasilar reticular pattern (5). Less common findings include focal or patchy bilateral areas of consolidation, upper lobe reticular opacities, or pneumothorax (5). The findings on HRCT consist of bilateral areas of ground-glass attenuation involving the lower lung zones (6,26). Although the early radiographic and CT abnormalities tend to involve mainly the lower lung zones, in six patients with long-term follow-up (mean, 14 years), there was predominantly upper lobe fibrosis (27,28). The radiographic and CT findings consisted of irregular linear opacities involving mainly the subpleural lung regions and associated with elevation of the hila (28).

Methotrexate

Methotrexate is employed in the treatment of malignancy and, in lower doses, in a variety of nonmalignant diseases, including psoriasis, pemphigus, and rheumatoid arthritis (29,30). It has been estimated that drug-induced lung disease occurs in 2% to 5% of patients (31,32). In contrast to other cytotoxic agents, this is often reversible, possibly because of an underlying hypersensitivity reaction (31); however, interstitial fibrosis develops in some patients (33).

The most common histologic findings are interstitial pneumonitis and fibrosis, sometimes associated with granuloma formation and resembling extrinsic allergic alveolitis (34,35). The latter pattern is presumably the counterpart of reversible disease. DAD (36) and BOOP (37) have also been described.

The initial radiologic abnormalities consist of basal or diffuse reticular or ground-glass opacities (38,39). These progress rapidly to patchy airspace consolidation that in time reverts once again to an interstitial pattern followed by complete resolution (38,40).

MISCELLANEOUS DRUGS

Nitrofurantoin

There are two distinct clinical presentations of nitrofurantoin-induced lung disease: acute, developing hours to days after the onset of treatment; and chronic and insidious, becoming manifest after weeks to years of continuous therapy (24). The former accounts for 90% of cases (41) and presumably represents a hypersensitivity reaction (9). The radiographic manifestations consist of a diffuse reticular pattern with basilar predominance (42); septal lines may be present (6,43). The appearance suggests that the underlying abnormality is interstitial pulmonary edema, a hypothesis supported by the rapid clearing that occurs when the drug is withdrawn (43).

The most common histologic manifestation of chronic nitrofurantoin toxicity is NSIP (1). The corresponding radiographic manifestations consist of patchy bilateral areas of consolidation or reticulation that can be diffuse but tend to involve mainly the lower lung zones (1,5). HRCT may demonstrate a predominantly subpleural or peribronchovascular distribution of consolidation and fibrosis (6).

Amiodarone

Amiodarone hydrochloride is an iodinated benzofuran derivative used in the treatment of cardiac arrhythmias. It is deposited in various organs and tissues, but particularly the lungs, where the concentration is several times higher than that in other organs (44). It has been estimated that approximately 5% to 7% of patients develop pulmonary toxicity (45). Its onset is typically months after the initiation of therapy (9).

The most common histologic finding is NSIP (1); less common reactions include DAD (46,47) and BOOP (46,48). Characteristically, alveolar macrophages and type II pneumocytes have abundant, coarsely vacuolated cytoplasm (Fig. 10.8) (46,49). Ultrastructurally, the vacuoles can be seen to consist of enlarged lysosomes that contain inclusions consisting of thin lamellae surrounded by amorphous electron-dense material. Identical macrophages also can be seen in patients without evidence of disease (46), and their presence is felt to be no more than a marker of drug exposure.

The radiologic manifestations consist of bilateral reticular opacities or areas of consolidation (5,50,51). The latter may be peripheral in distribution and may involve predominantly the upper lobes, resembling chronic eosinophilic pneumonia (50,52). Less common manifestations include focal consolidation and nodular opacities (5).

Because amiodarone contains about 37% iodine by weight, it has a high attenuation value on CT; therefore CT allows confident recognition of drug deposition within pulmonary and other tissues (6,53,54) (Fig. 10.9). In one review of the CT findings in 11 patients with symptoms of amiodarone pulmonary toxicity, high-attenuation (82 to 175 HU) pulmonary lesions were present in eight (73%); increased liver or spleen attenuation, in 10 (91%); and increased myocardial attenuation, in two (18%) (53). The pattern of parenchymal abnormalities is variable and may consist of focal or confluent bilateral areas of consolidation or a reticular pattern (6,8,53). Patients who have pulmonary toxicity almost always show increased liver attenuation on CT; however, this finding is also present in patients treated with amiodarone in the absence of evidence of lung toxicity (6,8,53).

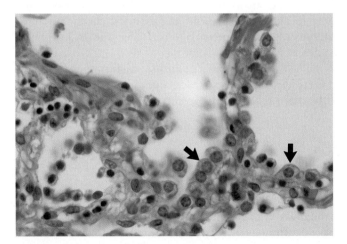

FIGURE 10.8. Interstitial pneumonitis secondary to amiodarone. A highly magnified view of a transbronchial biopsy specimen shows mild interstitial infiltration by lymphocytes. Type II cells are hyperplastic and have coarsely vacuolated cytoplasm (*arrows*). More severe interstitial inflammation was evident elsewhere in the biopsy tissue.

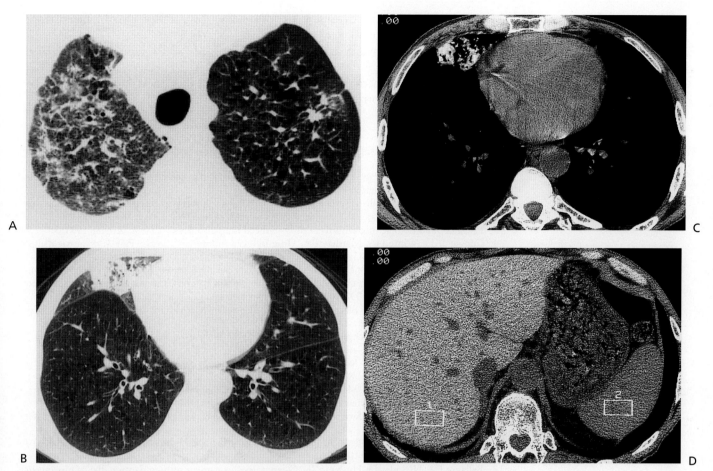

FIGURE 10.9. Amiodarone toxicity. **A:** An HRCT image (1.5-mm collimation) near the lung apices shows ground-glass opacities and mild reticulation involving mainly the right upper lobe. Two small foci of consolidation are evident in the left upper lobe. **B:** A second image at a more caudad level shows focal consolidation and ground-glass opacities in the right middle lobe. **C:** Same image as **B** photographed at soft-tissue windows demonstrates high attenuation of the area of consolidation. **D:** An image through the upper abdomen demonstrates increased attenuation of the liver. The region outlined by *rectangle 1* had a mean attenuation of 77 HU, and the spleen (*rectangle 2*) had a mean attenuation of 49 HU.

ILLICIT DRUGS

Narcotic and Sedative Drugs

Opiates are well known to cause pulmonary edema, with the incidence of the complication following heroin overdose ranging from 50% to 75% (55,56). Pulmonary edema has also been reported as a result of overdose of other narcotic and related drugs including methadone (57), propoxyphene (Darvon) (58), and naloxone (59). A high protein content of the edema fluid has been well documented in affected patients (60), indicating that the development of edema is related to increased capillary permeability. The pathologic (61) and radiographic (62,63) manifestations are indistinguishable from those of pulmonary edema from other etiologies. The findings usually consist of bilateral and symmetric airspace consolidation, often with a predominantly perihilar distribution (62). Less commonly, the edema is focal, is unilateral, or has an upper lobe distribution (62,63).

Cocaine

Cocaine, particularly in the form of the crystalline precipitate of free-base cocaine ("crack"), can result in a variety of pulmonary complications, including DAD (64), interstitial pneumonitis (64,65), eosinophilic pneumonia (66), diffuse alveolar hemorrhage (63), BOOP (67), and pulmonary edema (68).

The radiographic manifestations of edema are identical to those of opiate-related edema (69,70). Fleeting areas of consolidation resembling a Loeffler-like syndrome (65) correspond histologically to eosinophilic pneumonia and multifocal or diffuse consolidation to pulmonary hemorrhage (71) or BOOP (68,72).

REFERENCES

1. Rossi SE, Erasmus JJ, Page McAdams H, et al. Pulmonary drug toxicity: radiologic and pathologic manifestations. *Radiographics* 2000;20:1245–1259.
2. Colby TV. Anatomic distribution and histopathologic patterns in interstitial lung disease. In: Schwarz MI, King TE Jr, eds. *Interstitial lung disease.*St. Louis: Mosby–Year Book, 1993:59–77.
3. Pietra GG. Pathologic mechanisms of drug-induced lung disorders. *J Thorac Imaging* 1991;6:1–7.
4. Cooper JAD, White DA, Matthay RA. Drug induced pulmonary disease. Part 1: cytotoxic drugs. *Am Rev Respir Dis* 1986;133:321–340.
5. Aronchick JM, Gefter WB. Drug-induced pulmonary disorders. *Semin Roentgenol* 1995;30:18–34.
6. Padley SPG, Adler B, Hansell DM, et al. High-resolution computed tomography of drug-induced lung disease. *Clin Radiol* 1992;46:232–236.
7. Bellamy EA, Husband JE, Blaquiere RM, et al. Bleomycin-related lung damage: CT evidence. *Radiology* 1985;156:155–158.
8. Kuhlman JE. The role of chest computed tomography in the diagnosis of drug-related reactions. *J Thorac Imaging* 1991;6:52–61.
9. Cooper JAD, White DA, Matthay RA. Drug induced pulmonary disease: part 2. Noncytotoxic drugs. *Am Rev Respir Dis* 1986;133:488–503.
10. Searles G, McKendry RJR. Methotrexate pneumonitis in rheumatoid arthritis: potential risk factors. Four case reports and a review of the literature. *J Rheumatol* 1987;14:1164–1171.
11. Rosenow EC, Myers JL, Swensen SJ, et al. Drug-induced pulmonary disease: an update. *Chest* 1992;102:239–250.
12. Ellis SJ, Cleverley JR, Müller NL. Drug-induced lung disease: high-resolution CT findings. *Am J Roentgenol* 2000;175:1019–1024.
13. Bellamy EA, Nicholas D, Husband JE. Quantitative assessment of lung damage due to bleomycin using computed tomography. *Br J Radiol* 1987;60:1205–1209.
14. Jules-Elysee K, White DA. Bleomycin-induced pulmonary toxicity. *Clin Chest Med* 1990;11:1–20.
15. Yousem SA, Lifson JD, Colby TV. Chemotherapy-induced eosinophilic pneumonia: relation to bleomycin. *Chest* 1985;88:103–106.
16. Cohen MB, Austin JHM, Smith-Vaniz A, et al. Nodular bleomycin toxicity. *Am J Clin Pathol* 1989;92:101–104.
17. Balikian JP, Jochelson MS, Bauer KA, et al. Pulmonary complications of chemotherapy regimens containing bleomycin. *Am J Roentgenol* 1982;139:455–461.
18. Mills P, Husband J. Computed tomography of pulmonary bleomycin toxicity. *Semin Ultrasound CT MR* 1990;11:417–422.
19. Iacovino JR, Leitner J, Abbas AK, et al. Fatal pulmonary reaction from low doses of bleomycin: an idiosyncratic tissue response. *JAMA* 1976;235:1253–1255.
20. Glasier CM, Siegel MJ. Multiple pulmonary nodules: unusual manifestation of bleomycin toxicity. *Am J Roentgenol* 1981;137:155–156.
21. Crilley P, Topolsky D, Styler MJ, et al. Extramedullary toxicity of a conditioning regimen containing busulphan, cyclophosphamide and etoposide in 84 patients undergoing autologous and allogenic bone marrow transplantation. *Bone Marrow Transplant* 1995;15:361–365.
22. Rosenow EC III, Limper AH. Drug-induced pulmonary disease. *Semin Respir Infect* 1995;10:86–95.
23. Malik SW, Myers JL, De Remee RA, et al. Lung toxicity associated with cyclophosphamide use: two distinct patterns. *Am J Respir Crit Care Med* 1996;154:1851–1856.
24. Fraser RF. Müller NL, Colman N, et al. *Diagnosis of diseases of the chest.* Philadelphia: WB Saunders, 1999:2537–2583.
25. Rubio C, Hill ME, Milan S, et al. Idiopathic pneumonia syndrome after high-dose chemotherapy for relapsed Hodgkin's disease. *Br J Cancer* 1997;75:1044–1048.
26. Brown MJ, Miller RR, Müller NL. Acute lung disease in the immunocompromised host: CT and pathologic examination findings. *Radiology* 1994;190:247–454.
27. O'Driscoll BR, Hasleton PS, Taylor PM, et al. Active lung fibrosis up to 17 years after chemotherapy with carmustine (BCNU) in childhood. *N Engl J Med* 1990;323:378–382.
28. Taylor PM, O'Driscoll BR, Gattamaneni HR, et al. Chronic lung fibrosis following carmustine (BCNU) chemotherapy: radiological features. *Clin Radiol* 1991;44:299–301.
29. Carroll GC, Thomas R, Phatouros CC, et al. Incidence, prevalence and possible risk factors for

pneumonitis in patients with rheumatoid arthritis receiving methotrexate. *J Rheumatol* 1994;21:51–54.

30. Goodman TA, Polisson RP. Methotrexate: adverse reactions and major toxicities. *Rheum Dis Clin North Am* 1994;20:513–528.
31. Barrera P, Laan RF, van Riel PL, et al. Methotrexate-related pulmonary complications in rheumatoid arthritis. *Ann Rheum Dis* 1994;53:434–439.
32. Salaffi F, Manganelli P, Carotti M, et al. Methotrexate-induced pneumonitis in patients with rheumatoid arthritis and psoriatic arthritis: report of five cases and review of the literature. *Clin Rheumatol* 1997;16:296–304.
33. Bedrossian CWM, Miller WC, Luna MA. Methotrexate-induced diffuse interstitial pulmonary fibrosis. *South Med J* 1979;72:313–318.
34. Sostman HD, Matthay RA, Putman CE, et al. Methotrexate-induced pneumonitis. *Medicine* 1976;55:371–388.
35. Leduc D, De Vuyst P, Lheureux P, et al. Pneumonitis complicating low-dose methotrexate therapy for rheumatoid arthritis: discrepancies between lung biopsy and bronchoalveolar lavage findings. *Chest* 1993;104:1620–1623.
36. St. Clair E, Rice J, Snyderman R. Pneumonitis complicating low-dose methotrexate therapy in rheumatoid arthritis. *Arch Intern Med* 1985;145:2035–2038.
37. Cannon G, Ward J, Clegg D, et al. Acute lung disease associated with low-dose pulse methotrexate therapy in patients with rheumatoid arthritis. *Arthritis Rheum* 1983;26:1269–1274.
38. Clarysse AM, Cathey WJ, Cartwright GE, et al. Pulmonary disease complicating intermittent therapy with methotrexate. *JAMA* 1969;209:1861–1868.
39. Case Records of the Massachusetts General Hospital. *N Engl J Med* 1990;323:737–747.
40. Everts CS, Westcott JL, Bragg DG. Methotrexate therapy and pulmonary disease. *Radiology* 1973;107:539–543.
41. Holmberg L, Boman G, Bottiger LE, et al. Adverse reactions to nitrofurantoin: analysis of 921 reports. *Am J Med* 1980;69:733–738.
42. Nicklaus TM, Snyder AB. Nitrofurantoin pulmonary reaction: a unique syndrome. *Arch Intern Med* 1968;121:151–155.
43. Ngan H, Millard RJ, Lant AF, et al. Nitrofurantoin lung. *Br J Radiol* 1971;44:21–23.
44. Darmanata JI, van Zandwijk N, Duren DR, et al. Amiodarone pneumonitis: three further cases with a review of published reports. *Thorax* 1984;39:57–64.
45. Martin WJ II, Rosenow EC III. Amiodarone pulmonary toxicity: recognition and pathogenesis (part 1). *Chest* 1988;93:1067–1075.
46. Myers JL, Kennedy JI, Plumb VJ. Amiodarone lung: pathologic findings in clinically toxic patients. *Hum Pathol* 1987;18:349–354.
47. Dean PJ, Groshart KD, Porterfield JG, et al. Amiodarone-associated pulmonary toxicity: a clinical and pathologic study of eleven cases. *Am J Clin Pathol* 1987;87:7–13.
48. Conte SC, Pagan V, Murer B. Bronchiolitis obliterans organizing pneumonia secondary to amiodarone: clinical, radiological and histological pattern. *Monaldi Arch Chest Dis* 1997;52:24–26.
49. Kennedy JI, Myers JL, Plumb VJ, et al. Amiodarone pulmonary toxicity: clinical, radiologic, and pathologic correlations. *Arch Intern Med* 1987;147:50–55.
50. Gefter WB, Epstein DM, Pietra GG, et al. Lung disease caused by amiodarone, a new antiarrhythmia agent. *Radiology* 1983;147:339–344.
51. Olson LK, Forrest JV, Friedman PJ, et al. Pneumonitis after amiodarone therapy. *Radiology* 1984;150:327.
52. Marchlinski FE, Gansler TS, Waxman HL, et al. Amiodarone pulmonary toxicity. *Ann Intern Med* 1982;97:839–845.
53. Kuhlman JE, Teigen C, Ren H, et al. Amiodarone pulmonary toxicity: CT findings in symptomatic patients. *Radiology* 1990;177:121–125.
54. Nicholson AA, Hayward C. The value of computed tomography in the diagnosis of amiodarone-induced pulmonary toxicity. *Clin Radiol* 1989;40:564–567.
55. Duberstein JL, Kaufman DM. A clinical study of an epidemic of heroin intoxication and heroin-induced pulmonary edema. *Am J Med* 1971;51:704–714.
56. Wilen SB, Ulreich S, Rabinowitz JG. Roentgenographic manifestations of methadone-induced pulmonary edema. *Radiology* 1975;114:51–55.
57. Schaaf JT, Spivack ML, Rath GS, et al. Pulmonary edema and adult respiratory distress syndrome following methadone abuse. *Am Rev Respir Dis* 1973;107:1047–1051.
58. Bogartz LJ, Miller WC. Pulmonary edema associated with propoxyphene intoxication. *JAMA* 1971;215:259–262.
59. Taff RH. Pulmonary edema following naloxone administration in a patient without heart disease. *Anesthesiology* 1983;59:576–577.
60. Katz S, Aberman A, Frand UI, et al. Heroin pulmonary edema: evidence for increased pulmonary capillary permeability. *Am Rev Respir Dis* 1972;106:472–474.
61. Siegel H. Human pulmonary pathology associated with narcotic and other addictive drugs. *Hum Pathol* 1972;3:55–66.

62. Stern WZ, Subbarao K. Pulmonary complications of drug addiction. *Semin Roentgenol* 1983;18: 183–197.
63. Heffner JE, Harley RA, Schabel SI. Pulmonary reactions from illicit substance abuse. *Clin Chest Med* 1990;11:151–162.
64. Forrester JM, Steele AW, Waldron JA, et al. Crack lung: an acute pulmonary syndrome with a spectrum of clinical and histopathologic findings. *Am Rev Respir Dis* 1990;142:462–467.
65. Kissner DG, Lawrence WD, Selis JE, et al. Crack lung: pulmonary disease caused by cocaine abuse. *Am Rev Respir Dis* 1987;136:1250–1252.
66. Clinical Pathologic Conference. Respiratory failure and eosinophilia in a young man. *Am J Med* 1993;94:533–542.
67. Patel RC, Dutta D, Schonfeld SA. Free-base cocaine use associated with bronchiolitis obliterans organizing pneumonia. *Ann Intern Med* 1987;107:186–187.
68. Kline JN, Hirasuna JD. Pulmonary edema after freebase cocaine smoking: not due to an adulterant. *Chest* 1990;97:1009–1010.
69. Hoffman CK, Goodman PC. Pulmonary edema in cocaine smokers. *Radiology* 1989;172:463–465.
70. Eurman DW, Potash HI, Eyler WR. Chest pain and dyspnea related to "crack" cocaine smoking: value of chest radiography. *Radiology* 1989;172:459–462.
71. Murray RJ, Albin RJ, Mergner W, et al. Diffuse alveolar hemorrhage temporally related to cocaine smoking. *Chest* 1988;93:427–429.
72. Haim DY, Lippmann ML, Goldberg SK, et al. The pulmonary complications of crack cocaine: a comprehensive review. *Chest* 1995;107:233–240.

11

METABOLIC PULMONARY DISEASE

METASTATIC PULMONARY CALCIFICATION

AMYLOIDOSIS

PULMONARY ALVEOLAR PROTEINOSIS

PULMONARY ALVEOLAR MICROLITHIASIS

METASTATIC PULMONARY CALCIFICATION

Metastatic calcification is the deposition of calcium salts in otherwise normal tissue. It occurs most commonly in patients who have hypercalcemia as a result of chronic renal failure and secondary hyperparathyroidism, particularly those undergoing maintenance hemodialysis (1,2). It seldom causes any clinical symptoms.

Histologically, the calcium is seen mostly in the interstitial tissue of alveolar septa and around small vessels (Fig. 11.1). It may be focal or widespread. Although a mild to moderate degree of interstitial fibrosis also may be seen, airspaces are typically unremarkable. Given the latter observation, the histologic abnormality underlying the airspace opacities seen radiologically is unclear.

In most cases the calcification is mild and not detectable on chest radiographs. In a review of the chest radiographs and CT scans of seven patients who had biopsy-proven disease, calcification was evident on radiographs in only two cases and on CT scans in four (3).

The radiologic manifestations consist of fluffy, poorly defined nodular opacities mimicking airspace nodules (Fig. 11.2A) or, less commonly, numerous 3- to 10-mm-diameter calcified nodules (3,4). There is a predilection for the upper lung zones, possibly as a result of the relative alkalinity of this region secondary to a higher ventilation/perfusion ratio (and hence a lower regional pCO_2) (5). The calcific nature of the opacities is most readily confirmed by scanning with bone-imaging agents such as ^{99m}Tc-diphosphonate or by high-resolution computed tomography (HRCT) (3,4) (Fig. 11.2B). The latter also may demonstrate calcification of arteries in the chest wall or, less commonly, of the pulmonary arteries, superior vena cava, or myocardium (3,6). In one review of the HRCT findings in seven patients, six had evidence of calcification of the arteries in the chest wall and one had calcification of the left atrial wall (3).

PULMONARY ALVEOLAR PROTEINOSIS

Pulmonary alveolar proteinosis (PAP) is characterized by filling of the alveolar airspaces with protein- and lipid-rich material resembling surfactant (7). The disease is uncommon, with only about 330 cases reported by 1998 (8), and occurs predominantly in patients between the ages of 20 and 50 years (7,8).

It is believed that PAP results from an abnormality of surfactant production, metabolism, or clearance by type II alveolar cells and macrophages (7). Most cases are idiopathic. Some result from exposure to silica (silicoproteinosis) or occur in association with hematologic disorders, such as lymphoma or leukemia and, occasionally, HIV infection (7). Both experimental and clinical evidence suggests that some cases are related to an abnormality in granulocyte-macrophage colony stimulating factor (9,10). Patients may have no symptoms or may present with progressive shortness of breath and dry cough.

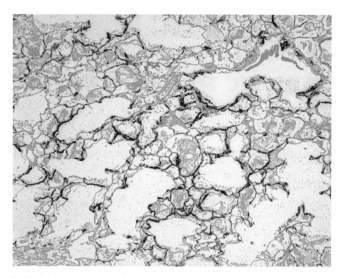

FIGURE 11.1. Metastatic pulmonary calcification. A photomicrograph of a section of lung processed by the von Kossa method shows extensive calcium phosphate (stained black) within the alveolar interstitium. The adjacent airspaces are partly filled with a proteinaceous exudate as a result of ARDS. The patient was a 62-year-old woman who had chronic renal failure.

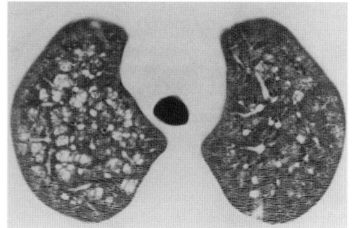

A

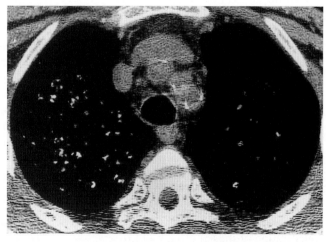

B

FIGURE 11.2. Metastatic pulmonary calcification. **A:** HRCT shows poorly defined nodular opacities and focal ground-glass opacities in both upper lobes. **B:** Soft-tissue windows demonstrate foci of calcification within the nodular opacities. The patient was a 42-year-old man with chronic renal failure.

Histologically, alveoli are filled with finely granular eosinophilic (proteinaceous) material that stains with periodic acid-Schiff (Fig. 11.3A). Scattered macrophages and small needle-shaped clefts are often present. The alveolar interstitium is usually normal but may show mild fibrosis. Ultrastructural, immunohistochemical, and biochemical investigations have shown that the intraalveolar material resembles surfactant (11,12) (Fig. 11.3B and C).

The radiographic manifestations consist of bilateral and symmetric ground-glass opacities or airspace consolidation with a vaguely nodular appearance and a predominantly perihilar or lower lobe distribution (7,8) (Fig. 11.4A). In some patients, a linear interstitial pattern can be seen superimposed on the areas of consolidation or ground-glass opacities (13,14).

The predominant finding on HRCT consists of areas of ground-glass attenuation, although areas of airspace consolidation may also be present (14–16) (Fig. 11.4B). The distribution of disease is variable; most commonly, it is random, but sometimes it is predominantly central or peripheral (14,15). The areas of ground-glass attenuation often have sharply defined straight margins, giving them a geographic appearance (15).

In most cases, a fine linear pattern forming polygonal arcades measuring 3 to 10 mm in diameter can be seen superimposed on the areas of ground-glass attenuation (15,17).

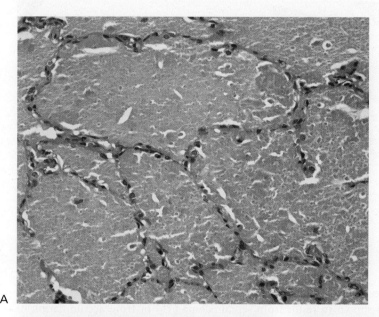

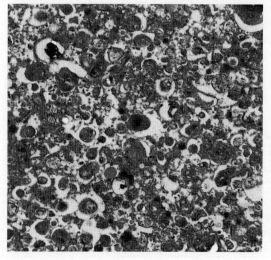

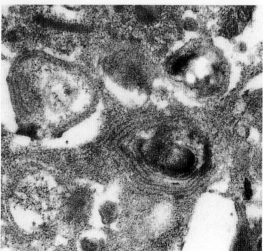

FIGURE 11.3. Pulmonary alveolar proteinosis. **A:** A high-power photomicrograph shows filling of alveolar airspaces by finely granular eosinophilic material. Alveolar septa are normal. **B, C:** Transmission electron micrographs show the material to consist of numerous minute globules, some having a lamellated appearance suggestive of surfactant.

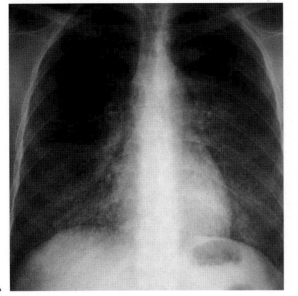

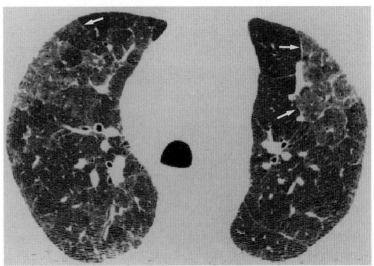

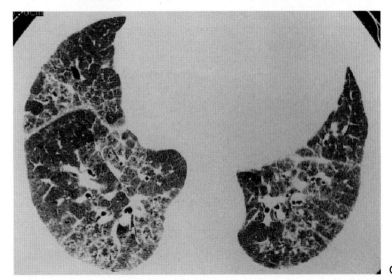

FIGURE 11.4. Pulmonary alveolar proteinosis. **A:** A chest radiograph shows bilateral ground-glass opacities with a vaguely nodular appearance involving the middle and lower lung zones. **B:** HRCT at level of upper lobes shows bilateral areas of ground-glass attenuation. In several areas, the opacities have sharply defined margins (*arrows*) corresponding to interlobular septa separating involved from uninvolved pulmonary lobules. **C:** HRCT at level of lower lobes shows a fine reticular pattern superimposed on areas of ground-glass attenuation. The patient was a 62-year-old man.

This combination gives an appearance that has been described as "crazy paving" (15,17). This pattern has been shown to result from septal edema (15) or from accumulation of lipoprotein in the airspaces adjacent to normal interlobular septa (18). The crazy-paving appearance is not specific for alveolar proteinosis; a similar abnormality has been described in some cases of bronchioloalveolar carcinoma, lipid pneumonia, pulmonary hemorrhage, hydrostatic and permeability pulmonary edema, and bacterial pneumonia (19,20).

AMYLOIDOSIS

Although originally considered to represent a single substance, amyloid is now known to consist of several proteins, each of which resembles the others morphologically but is distinctive biochemically (21). The proteins are deposited in the extracellular space, where they accumulate and cause disease by compressing the adjacent cells or tissues. The most important proteins associated with pulmonary amyloidosis are immunoglobulin (resulting in amyloid AL) and serum acute phase reactant (giving amyloid AA).

Three patterns of amyloid deposition can be seen in the lower respiratory tract: tracheobronchial, nodular parenchymal, and diffuse parenchymal (interstitial). Although there can be overlap between the three forms, particularly microscopically, most patients have only, or predominantly, one.

Tracheobronchial amyloidosis can be manifested as a localized nodule or, more commonly, as multiple discrete or confluent plaques that cause distortion of the airway wall and stenosis of its lumen (22,23). The amyloid accumulates initially in the connective tissue of the mucosa, particularly adjacent to the tracheobronchial glands, and in the walls of small bronchial vessels (Fig. 11.5). Calcification and ossification may occur (24), sometimes so extensive as to mimic tracheobronchopathia osteochondroplastica (25). The plaquelike form of disease can cause progressive dyspnea or symptoms that simulate asthma; hemoptysis and recurrent bronchitis and pneumonia are common (26,27). Discrete tracheal and endobronchial "tumors" are usually discovered incidentally at bronchoscopy; however, they can be large enough to cause airway obstruction, atelectasis, and bronchiectasis (28,29).

The radiologic manifestations of tracheobronchial amyloidosis consist of focal or diffuse thickening of the airway wall or, rarely, a localized intraluminal nodule (30,31). The involvement is generally confined to the trachea but may extend to the bronchi (Fig. 11.6). CT may demonstrate foci of calcification (31).

Nodular parenchymal amyloidosis can present as a solitary nodule or mass, or as multiple, fairly well-defined nodules, usually ranging from 0.5 to 5 cm in diameter (32,33) (Fig. 11.7). They occur most commonly in the lower lobes and typically are located peripherally (33). Calcification is seldom evident on the radiograph but is seen in 20% to 50% of nodules on CT scans (33,34). Microscopic examination shows replacement of the parenchyma by amyloid admixed with multinucleated giant cells and plasma cells (Fig. 11.8). It is presumably the last named that are the source of the light chains from which the amyloid is derived. A combination of lymphoid interstitial pneumonitis and amyloid nodules with irregular margins and cystic changes on HRCT has also been reported (35). Patients usually have no symptoms (26), with the lesion being discovered on a screening chest radiograph. Disease may progress slowly over several years, with a slight increase in size of the nodules and sometimes the development of additional nodules (36,37).

Diffuse interstitial amyloidosis is characterized by deposition of amyloid in the parenchymal interstitium and in the media of small blood vessels (Fig. 11.9). This variant is commonly manifested clinically by dyspnea and may be associated with respiratory insufficiency (26). The radiographic findings consist of a diffuse, linear interstitial pattern or, less commonly, airspace consolidation or a small nodular pattern (26,38,39) (Fig. 11.10). HRCT in one case revealed a linear interstitial pattern, small nodules, and patchy

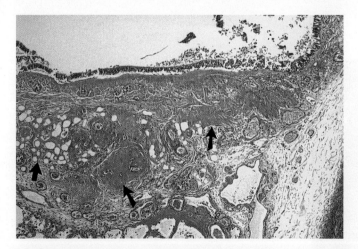

FIGURE 11.5. Tracheobronchial amyloidosis. A photomicrograph of the wall of a lobar bronchus shows diffuse thickening of the mucosa as a result of amyloid accumulation between adipocytes (*short arrow*) and adjacent interstitial tissue (*long arrows*). A small amount of amyloid is also evident in the adjacent alveolar septa.

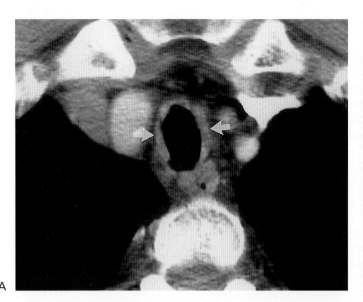

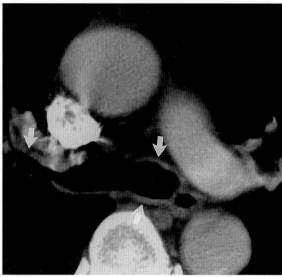

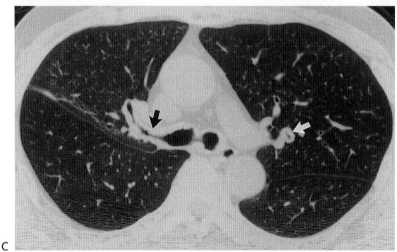

FIGURE 11.6. Tracheobronchial amyloidosis. **A, B:** CT images (3-mm collimation) at the levels of thoracic inlet (**A**) and the main and right upper lobe bronchi (**B**) show thickening of the airway wall (*arrows*) in both locations. **C:** Lung windows show wall thickening and luminal narrowing, particularly of the right upper lobe bronchus (*black arrow*), associated with partial right upper lobe atelectasis. Thickening of a segmental bronchial wall (*white arrow*) in the left upper lobe is also apparent. The patient was a 54-year-old man.

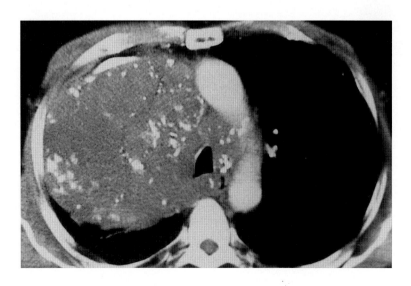

FIGURE 11.7. Nodular parenchymal amyloidosis. A contrast-enhanced CT image demonstrates a large mass in right upper lobe that extends into the adjacent mediastinum. The mass contains numerous foci of calcification. The patient was a 53-year-old man.

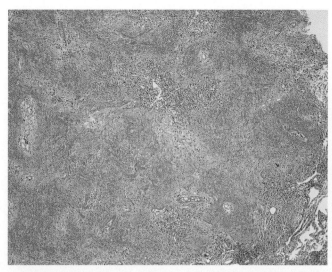

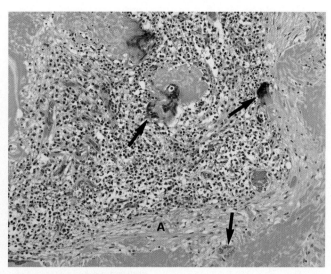

FIGURE 11.8. Nodular parenchymal amyloidosis. **A:** A photomicrograph of a well-defined parenchymal nodule shows marked accumulation of amyloid associated with loss of parenchymal architecture. **B:** A view at higher magnification shows several multinucleated giant cells (*arrows*) and numerous plasma cells. (Letter *A* designates fibrous tissue adjacent to the amyloid.)

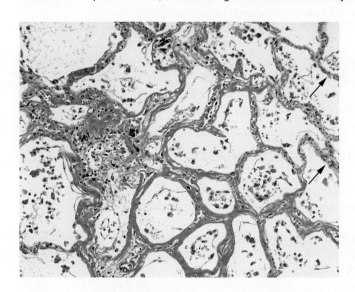

FIGURE 11.9. Diffuse interstitial amyloidosis. A photomicrograph shows extensive, mild to moderate thickening of the alveolar interstitium by amyloid. (Several normal septa are present for comparison [*arrows*]).

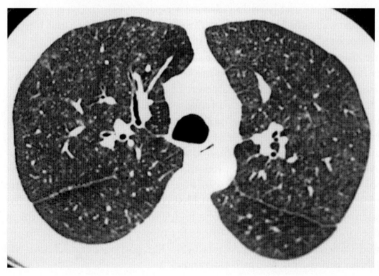

FIGURE 11.10. Diffuse interstitial amyloidosis. An HRCT image (1.5-mm collimation) shows numerous small nodules and focal areas of ground-glass attenuation. The patient was 41-year-old man.

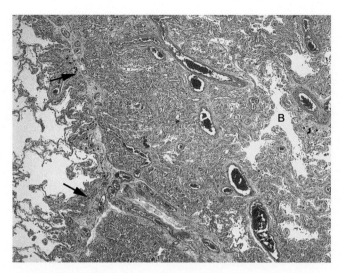

FIGURE 11.11. Marked interstitial amyloidosis resulting in apparent lobular consolidation. A photomicrograph of a region of grossly solid lung parenchyma shows marked interstitial amyloid deposition in one lobule. (*Arrows* indicate an interlobular septum that separates the abnormal lobule form a relatively normal one.) Alveolar airspaces are compressed to almost inapparent slits. The lumina of several respiratory bronchioles (*B*) are still patent.

areas of consolidation involving mainly the subpleural regions of the lower lung zones (38); several of the small nodules contained calcific foci. The areas of "consolidation" may correspond to marked interstitial deposition of amyloid associated with compression of alveolar airspaces rather than true airspace filling (Fig. 11.11).

PULMONARY ALVEOLAR MICROLITHIASIS

Pulmonary alveolar microlithiasis is a rare disease characterized by the presence of innumerable sandlike calculi ("calcispherytes") within alveolar airspaces. Although the disease can occur at any age, most of the reported cases have involved patients between the ages of 20 and 50 years (40). A familial occurrence has been noted in approximately half the reported cases (40,41). Patients may have no symptoms or may present with dyspnea on exertion or dry cough (42,43). The etiology and pathogenesis are unknown.

On histologic examination, microliths range in size from about 250 to 750 μm in diameter and are located almost invariably within alveolar airspaces (44). In the early stages of the disease, the alveolar walls are histologically normal; eventually, interstitial fibrosis develops, sometimes associated with multinucleated giant cell formation (45).

The characteristic radiologic findings consist of a very fine micronodulation diffusely involving both lungs (46,47). Individual deposits are usually identifiable as very sharply defined nodules measuring less than 1 mm in diameter. The overall density is greater over the lower than over the upper zones. In some patients, a reticular pattern or septal lines can be seen superimposed on the characteristic "sandstorm" appearance (48). The reticular pattern presumably reflects the development of interstitial fibrosis.

The HRCT manifestations consist of calcific nodules measuring 1 mm or less in diameter, sometimes confluent, and distributed predominantly along the cardiac borders and dorsal portions of the lower lung zones (46,49) (Fig. 11.12). Calcific septal lines are commonly seen (46,50) (Fig. 11.13). Correlation of HRCT and pathologic findings has shown that this apparent thickening is the result of a high concentration of microliths in the periphery of the secondary lobules (18,46). Other features seen on HRCT scans include apical bullae and thin-walled subpleural cysts (49). The pathogenetic relation between these abnormalities and the microliths is uncertain.

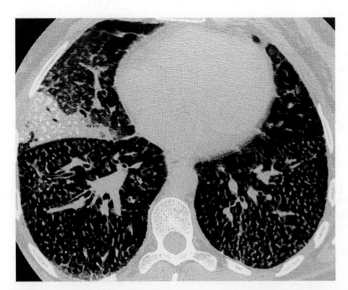

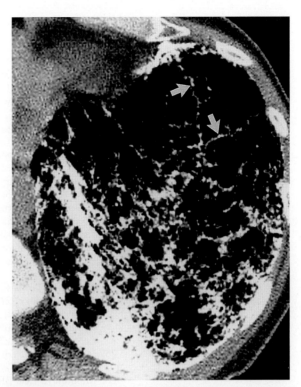

FIGURE 11.12. Pulmonary alveolar microlithiasis. An HRCT image (1-mm collimation) shows numerous well-defined small nodules. The calcific nature of the nodules is best seen within the focal area of airspace consolidation in the right middle lobe (related to an incidental bacterial pneumonia). The patient was a 38-year-old woman. (Case courtesy of Dr. Inmaculada Herráez, Department Radiology, Hospital de Leon, Leon, Spain.)

FIGURE 11.13. Pulmonary alveolar microlithiasis. An HRCT image (1-mm collimation) of left lower lobe shows numerous calcific nodules. Confluence of nodules is present particularly in the dependent lung regions. Also note calcific septal lines (*arrows*). The patient was a 60-year-old woman. (Case courtesy of Dr. Jim Barrie, University of Alberta Medical Centre, Edmonton, Alberta, Canada.)

REFERENCES

1. Faubert PF, Shapiro WB, Porush JG, et al. Pulmonary calcification in hemodialyzed patients detected by technetium-99m diphosphate scanning. *Kidney Int* 1980;18:95–102.
2. Murris-Espin M, Lacassagne L, Didier A, et al. Metastatic pulmonary calcification after renal transplantation. *Eur Respir J* 1997;10:1925–1927.
3. Hartman TE, Müller NL, Primack SL, et al. Metastatic pulmonary calcification in patients with hypercalcemia: findings on chest radiographs and CT scans. *Am J Roentgenol* 1994;162:799–802.
4. Rosenthal DI, Chandler HL, Azizi F, et al. Uptake of bone imaging agents by diffuse pulmonary metastatic calcification. *Am J Roentgenol* 1977;129:871–874.
5. West JB. *Regional differences in the lung.* New York: Academic Press, 1977:239.
6. Johkoh T, Ikezoe J, Nagareda T, et al. Case report. Metastatic pulmonary calcification: early detection by high-resolution CT. *J Comput Assist Tomogr* 1993;17:471–473.
7. Wang BM, Stern EJ, Schmidt RA, et al. Diagnosing pulmonary alveolar proteinosis: a review and an update. *Chest* 1997;111:460–466.
8. Goldstein LS, Kavuru MS, Curtis-McCarthy P, et al. Pulmonary alveolar proteinosis: clinical features and outcomes. *Chest* 1998;114:1357–1362.
9. Kavuru MS, Sullivan EJ, Piccin R, et al. Exogenous granulocyte-macrophage colony stimulating factor administration for pulmonary alveolar proteinosis. *Am J Respir Crit Care Med* 2000; 161:1143–1148.
10. Kitamura T, Tanaka N, Watanabe J, et al. Idiopathic pulmonary proteinosis as an autoimmune disease with neutralizing antibody against granulocyte-macrophage colony stimulating factor. *J Exp Med* 1999;190:875–880.
11. Gilmore LB, Talley FA, Hook GE. Classification and morphometric quantitation of insoluble materials from the lungs of patients with alveolar proteinosis. *Am J Pathol* 1988;133:252–264.
12. Mermolja M, Rott T, Debeljak A. Cytology of bronchoalveolar lavage in some rare pulmonary disorders: pulmonary alveolar proteinosis and amiodarone pulmonary toxicity. *Cytopathology* 1994;5:9–16.

13. Miller PA, Ravin CE, Smith GJW, et al. Pulmonary alveolar proteinosis with interstitial involvement. *Am J Roentgenol* 1981;137:1069–1071.

14. Godwin JD, Müller NL, Takasugi JE. Pulmonary alveolar proteinosis: CT findings. *Radiology* 1988;169:609–613.

15. Murch CR, Carr DH. Computed tomography appearances of pulmonary alveolar proteinosis. *Clin Radiol* 1989;40:240–243.

16. Zimmer WE, Chew FS. Pulmonary alveolar proteinosis. *Am J Roentgenol* 1993;161:26.

17. Lee KN, Levin DL, Webb WR, et al. Pulmonary alveolar proteinosis: high-resolution CT, chest radiographic, and functional correlations. *Chest* 1997;111:989–995.

18. Kang EY, Grenier P, Laurent F, et al. Interlobular septal thickening: patterns at high-resolution computed tomography. *J Thorac Imaging* 1996;11:260–264.

19. Tan RT, Kuzo RS. High-resolution CT findings of mucinous bronchioloalveolar carcinoma: a case of pseudopulmonary alveolar proteinosis. *Am J Roentgenol* 1997;168:99–100.

20. Franquet T, Giménez A, Bordes R, et al. The crazy-paving pattern in exogenous lipoid pneumonia: CT–pathologic correlation. *Am J Roentgenol* 1998;170:315–317.

21. Westermark P. The pathogenesis of amyloidosis: understanding general principles. *Am J Pathol* 1998;152:1125–1127.

22. Toyoda M, Ebihara Y, Kato H, et al. Tracheobronchial al amyloidosis: histologic, immunohistochemical, ultrastructural, and immunoelectron microscopic observations. *Hum Pathol* 1993;24:970–976.

23. Cordier JF, Loire R, Brune J. Amyloidosis of the lower respiratory tract: clinical and pathologic features in a series of 21 patients. *Chest* 1986;90:827–831.

24. Hui AN, Koss MN, Hochholzer L, et al. Amyloidosis presenting in the lower respiratory tract: clinicopathologic, radiologic, immunohistochemical, and histochemical studies on 48 cases. *Arch Pathol Lab Med* 1986;110:212–218.

25. Jones AW, Chatterji AN. Primary tracheobronchial amyloidosis with tracheobronchopathia osteoplastica. *Br J Dis Chest* 1977;71:268–272.

26. Rubinow A, Celli BR, Cohen AS, et al. Localized amyloidosis of the lower respiratory tract. *Am Rev Respir Dis* 1978;118:603–611.

27. Brown J. Primary amyloidosis. *Clin Radiol* 1964;15:358–367.

28. Flemming AFS, Fairfax AJ, Arnold AG, et al. Treatment of endobronchial amyloidosis by intermittent bronchoscopic resection. *Br J Dis Chest* 1980;74:183.

29. Simpson GT II, Strong MS, Skinner M, et al. Localized amyloidosis of the head and neck and upper aerodigestive and lower respiratory tracts. *Ann Otol Rhinol Laryngol* 1984;93:374–379.

30. Utz JP, Swensen SJ, Gertz MA. Pulmonary amyloidosis: the Mayo Clinic experience from 1980 to 1993. *Ann Intern Med* 1996;124:407–413.

31. Kwong JS, Müller NL, Miller RR. Diseases of the trachea and main-stem bronchi: correlation of CT with pathologic findings. *Radiographics* 1992;12:645–657.

32. Laden SA, Cohen ML, Harley RA. Nodular pulmonary amyloidosis with extrapulmonary involvement. *Hum Pathol* 1984;15:594–597.

33. Pickford HA, Swensen SJ, Utz JP. Thoracic cross-sectional imaging of amyloidosis. *Am J Roentgenol* 1997;168:351–355.

34. Urban BA, Fishman EK, Goldman SM, et al. CT evaluation of amyloidosis: spectrum of disease. *Radiographics* 1993;13:1295–1308.

35. Desai SR, Nicholson AG, Stewart S, et al. Benign pulmonary lymphocytic infiltration and amyloidosis: computed tomographic and pathological features in three cases. *J Thorac Imaging* 1997;12:215–220.

36. Gross BH, Felson B, Birnberg FA. The respiratory tract in amyloidosis and the plasma cell dyscrasias. *Semin Roentgenol* 1986;21:113–127.

37. Tamura K, Nakajima N, Makino S, et al. Primary pulmonary amyloidosis with multiple nodules. *Eur J Radiol* 1988;8:128–130.

38. Graham CM, Stern EJ, Finkbeiner WE, et al. High-resolution CT appearance of diffuse alveolar septal amyloidosis. *Am J Roentgenol* 1992;158:265–267.

39. Morgan RA, Ring NJ, Marshall AJ. Pulmonary alveolar-septal amyloidosis: an unusual radiographic presentation. *Respir Med* 1992;86:345–347.

40. Ucan ES, Keyf AI, Aydilek R, et al. Pulmonary alveolar microlithiasis: review of Turkish reports. *Thorax* 1993;48:171–173.

41. Mariotta S, Guidi L, Papale M, et al. Pulmonary alveolar microlithiasis: review of Italian reports. *Eur J Epidemiol* 1997;13:587–590.

42. Sears MR, Chang AR, Taylor AJ. Pulmonary alveolar microlithiasis. *Thorax* 1971;26:704–711.

43. Turktas I, Saribas S, Balkanci F. Pulmonary alveolar microlithiasis presenting with chronic cough. *Postgrad Med J* 1993;69:70–72.

44. Prakash UBS, Barham SS, Rosenow EC III, et al. Pulmonary alveolar microlithiasis: a review including ultrastructural and pulmonary function studies. *Mayo Clin Proc* 1983;58:290.

45. Barnard NJ, Crocker PR, Blainey AD, et al. Pulmonary alveolar microlithiasis: a new analytical approach. *Histopathology* 1987;11:639–645.

46. Cluzel P, Grenier P, Bernadac P, et al. Pulmonary alveolar microlithiasis: CT findings. *J Comput Assist Tomogr* 1991;15:938–942.

47. Helbich TH, Wojnarovsky C, Wunderbaldinger P, et al. Pulmonary alveolar microlithiasis in children: radiographic and high-resolution CT findings. *Am J Roentgenol* 1997;168:63–65.

48. Melamed JW, Sostman HD, Ravin CE. Interstitial thickening in pulmonary alveolar microlithiasis: an underappreciated finding. *J Thorac Imaging* 1994;9:126–128.

49. Korn MA, Schurawitzki H, Klepetko W, et al. Pulmonary alveolar microlithiasis: findings on high-resolution CT. *Am J Roentgenol* 1992;158:981–982.

50. Hoshino H, Koba H, Shin-Ichiroh I, et al. Pulmonary alveolar microlithiasis: high-resolution CT and MR findings. *J Comput Assist Tomogr* 1998;22:245–248.

12

RADIATION PNEUMONITIS AND FIBROSIS

PATHOLOGIC CHARACTERISTICS

BRACHYTHERAPY

RADIOLOGIC MANIFESTATIONS
Radiation Pneumonitis
Radiation Fibrosis

The development and appearance of radiation lung injury depend on a number of factors, including the volume of lung irradiated, the shape of the radiation fields, the radiation dose, the number of fractions of radiation given, the time period over which the radiation is delivered, prior irradiation, the type and dose of concomitant chemotherapy, and individual susceptibility (1–3). Generally, radiation is best tolerated if given in smaller doses, over a long period of time, and to a single lung or a small lung region. Within the therapeutic range of doses usually administered, after external beam radiotherapy, approximately 40% of patients develop radiographic abnormalities and 7% develop symptomatic radiation pneumonitis (4,5). For unilateral radiation with fractionated doses, radiographic findings of radiation pneumonitis are seldom detected with doses below 3,000 cGy, are variably present with doses between 3,000 and 4,000 cGy, and are nearly always visible at doses of 4,000 cGy or greater (3).

PATHOLOGIC CHARACTERISTICS

Radiation lung injury can be considered in early and late stages (5). The earliest abnormality is rarely seen in humans, and consists predominantly of airspace and interstitial edema (Fig. 12.1). More advanced disease is characterized grossly by poorly delimited foci of parenchymal consolidation and histologically by diffuse alveolar damage (edema and mild inflammation of alveolar septa accompanied by a proteinaceous exudate in the alveolar air spaces and hyaline membranes in alveolar ducts and respiratory bronchioles) (Fig. 12. 2) (6). Type II cells are hyperplastic and frequently have large, irregularly shaped nuclei and vacuolated cytoplasm, both characteristic features of radiation damage.

As might be expected, foci of radiation-induced fibrosis are usually not related to bronchopulmonary segments and are often clearly delimited from the adjacent unaffected lung (Fig. 12.3). A more or less linear appearance, corresponding to the direction of the x-ray beam, may be seen. Microscopic examination shows both interstitial and alveolar airspace fibrosis; an increased amount of interstitial elastic tissue is also common (Fig. 12.3). Although distorted by the adjacent fibrosis, airways can appear remarkably unaffected; however, bronchiolitis obliterans and endobronchial fibrosis may be present. Pulmonary arteries and veins often show intimal fibrosis (7).

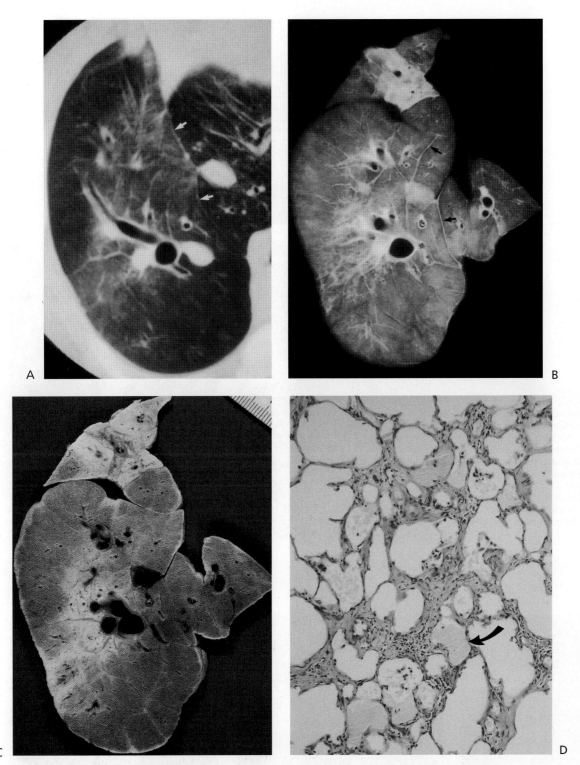

FIGURE 12.1. Radiation pneumonitis in an experimental pig model. **A:** HRCT image demonstrates ground-glass opacities and smooth thickening of interlobular septa (*arrows*). **B:** Contact radiograph of the autopsy specimen shows extensive ground-glass opacification and smooth thickening of interlobular septa (*arrows*). **C:** Corresponding lung slice shows patchy consolidation. **D:** Photomicrograph of one of the consolidated areas shows airspace edema (*arrow*) and mild interstitial fibrosis. The autopsy specimen was obtained 16 weeks after a radiation exposure of 12.5 Gy. (Courtesy of Dr. Masashi Takahashi, Department of Radiology, Shiga Medical University, Otsh, Japan.)

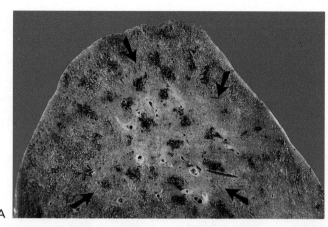

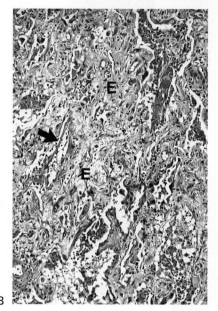

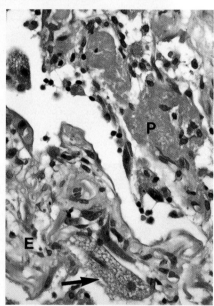

FIGURE 12.2. Radiation pneumonitis. **A:** View of the upper portion of a slice of an upper lobe shows a poorly defined area of parenchymal consolidation (*arrows*). **B, C:** Photomicrographs of tissue form this region show interstitial edema (*E*), a proteinaceous exudate (*P*) in alveolar airspaces, and a hyaline membrane (*arrow in* **B**). Note the hyperchromatic type II cell nuclei and the markedly vacuolated alveolar macrophage cytoplasm (*arrow in* **C**).

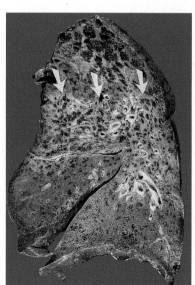

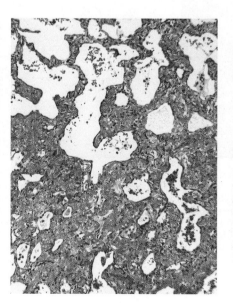

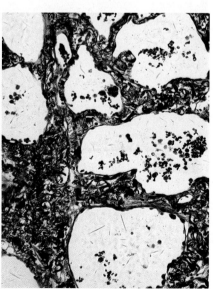

RADIOLOGIC MANIFESTATIONS

Radiation Pneumonitis

Radiographic evidence of acute radiation pneumonitis usually becomes evident about 8 weeks after completion of radiotherapy with doses of 4,000 cGy and about 1 week earlier for every additional 1,000-cGy increment (3). Abnormalities are usually most marked 3 to 4 months after completion of radiotherapy (3); they are seen rarely immediately after completion of therapy (8) and occasionally within 1 to 4 weeks (8,9).

The radiographic manifestations may be subtle, consisting of hazy ground-glass opacities with slight indistinctness of the pulmonary vessels, or more marked, consisting of patchy or homogeneous airspace consolidation (Fig. 12.4) (3,5,10). Air bronchograms are commonly present (3). The abnormalities usually have sharp boundaries corresponding to the radiation portals and therefore cross normal anatomic structures (3,11). Occasionally, mild abnormalities are seen beyond the radiation ports (5,9). Some degree of volume loss is common. This is usually the result of a surfactant deficit (10,12); however, it also may be seen following radiotherapy for an endobronchial lesion (13), in which case it may be related to radiation-induced edema of a bronchial wall that is already narrowed by the endobronchial lesion.

Evidence of acute radiation pneumonitis is seen more commonly and earlier on CT than on the chest radiograph (9,14) and is better seen on high-resolution than on conventional scans (9,15). The hallmark of radiation pneumonitis on CT is the presence of increased lung attenuation corresponding closely to the location of the radiation ports (Figs. 12.4 to 12.6) (5). Three patterns can be seen: (a) homogeneous ground-glass opacity that uniformly involves the irradiated portions of lung (see Figs. 12.5 and 12.6); (b)

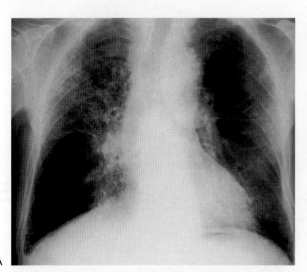
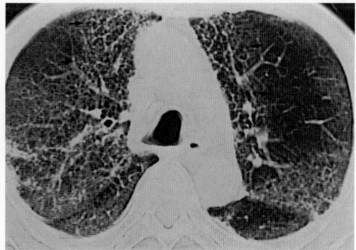

A   B

FIGURE 12.4. Radiation pneumonitis. **A:** Chest radiograph shows bilateral ground-glass opacities and a reticular pattern, most severe in right upper lobe. **B:** HRCT image at the level of the aortic arch demonstrates a reticular pattern in the paramediastinal regions of both lungs (*arrows*). Extensive ground-glass opacities are evident within and outside the radiation portals. The patient was an 85-year-old man with mediastinal lymphoma. (Courtesy of Dr. Hiroshi Moriya, Department of Radiology, Fukushima Medical University, Fukushima, Japan.)

◄───

FIGURE 12.3. Radiation fibrosis. **A:** Sagittal slice of the right lung shows a fairly well-demarcated area of fibrosis involving the superior segment of the lower lobe, the inferior portion of the upper lobe, and the superior portion of the middle lobe. The upper edge of the fibrosis is straight and extends from the anterior to the posterior pleura (*arrows*). **B, C:** Photomicrograph (**B**) shows marked interstitial thickening and airspace obliteration. Although much of this is the result of collagen deposition, as indicated in **C,** abundant elastic tissue (*wavy silver positive [black] lines*) is also present.

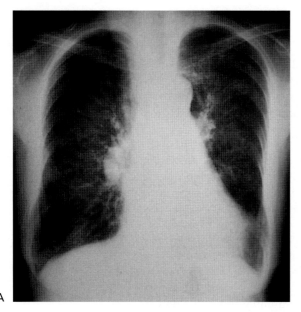
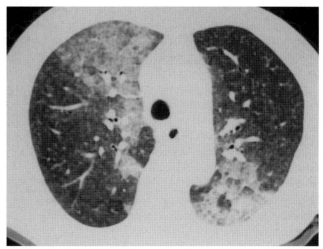

FIGURE 12.5. Radiation pneumonitis. **A:** Chest radiograph shows ground-glass opacities involving mainly the perihilar regions. **B:** HRCT image demonstrates areas of ground-glass attenuation and airspace consolidation. The patient was a 68-year-old man with esophageal carcinoma.

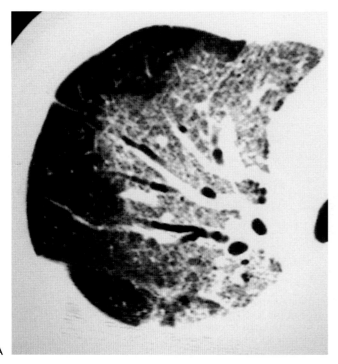
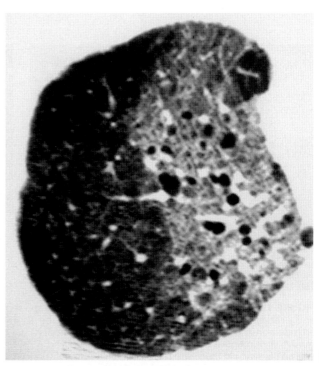

FIGURE 12.6. Radiation pneumonitis. HRCT images demonstrate areas of ground-glass attenuation and fine reticulation within the irradiated portions of lung. The patient was a 58-year-old man with mediastinal non-Hodgkin lymphoma. (Hematoxylin-eosin stain; original magnification ×10.)

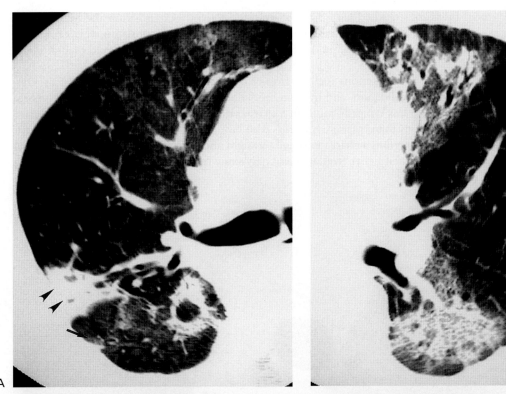

FIGURE 12.7. Radiation pneumonitis. HRCT images of the right (**A**) and left (**B**) lungs demonstrate ground-glass opacities and reticulation within the irradiated portions of lung. Patchy ground-glass opacities (*arrow*) and areas of airspace consolidation (*arrowheads*) are evident in the lung periphery, outside the radiation field. The patient was a 58-year-old man who had undergone radiation therapy for esophageal carcinoma.

patchy consolidation that is contained within the irradiated lung but does not conform to the shape of the radiation ports (Fig. 12.5); and (c) discrete consolidation that conforms to the shape of the radiation ports but does not uniformly involve the irradiated lung parenchyma (see Fig. 12.7) (9,16). The first two patterns likely represent the presence of diffuse or patchy radiation pneumonitis, whereas the third is thought to indicate the presence of early fibrosis (2,3,16). Abnormalities typically do not respect normal lung boundaries, such as interlobar fissures or segments.

Although findings of radiation pneumonitis are characteristically confined to areas of irradiated lung, abnormalities can be detected radiologically outside of the radiation portal in 10% to 20% of cases (5,9,7). These consist of subtle ground-glass opacities or patchy consolidation and are less severe than those seen within the radiation ports (16,17). Rarely, areas of consolidation initially limited to the radiation field may migrate within both lungs (18,19). This pattern has been shown to correlate histologically with a pattern of bronchiolitis obliterans organizing pneumonia (BOOP); its pathogenesis is unclear but has been hypothesized to be triggered by the irradiation (Fig. 12.7) (18,19).

Radiation Fibrosis

Radiation fibrosis develops in most patients who receive therapeutic doses of radiation and may be seen in patients who have not had radiographic evidence of acute radiation pneumonitis (3). Typically, the complication starts 3 to 4 months after completion of radiotherapy, develops gradually, and becomes stable after 9 to 12 months (3). The affected lung shows loss of volume, with obliteration of all normal architectural markings. The peripheral parenchyma is characteristically airless and opaque as a result of replacement by fibrous tissue. Dense fibrotic strands frequently extend from the hilum to the periphery. Occasionally, the radiographic findings are subtle, consisting only of mild elevation of one or both hila, mild retraction of pulmonary vessels, or mild pleural thickening (3).

The CT manifestations include streaky opacities, progressive volume loss, progressively dense consolidation, and traction bronchiectasis (Figs. 12.8 and 12.9) (2,5). Fibrosis and volume loss typically result in a sharper demarcation between normal and irradiated lung regions than is seen in patients who have radiation pneumonitis. This gives the abnormal lung regions a characteristically straight and sharply defined edge (2). The adjacent lung is frequently hyperinflated and may show bullae (5).

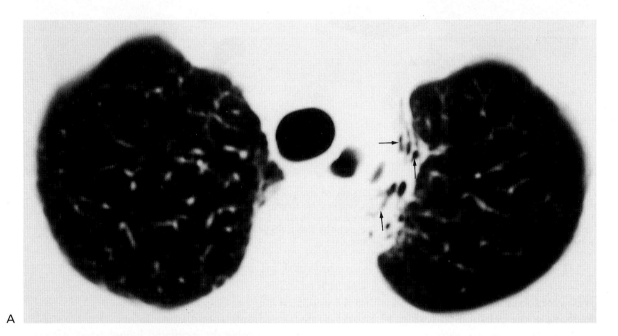

A

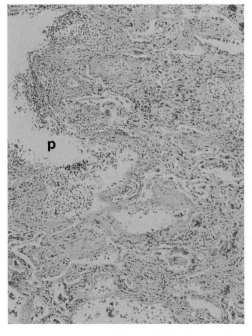

B

FIGURE 12.8. Radiation fibrosis. **A:** HRCT image demonstrates sharply marginated areas of fibrosis in the paramediastinal regions of both lungs. Traction bronchiectasis (*arrows*) can be seen within the radiated field. **B:** Photomicrograph from the left side shows marked fibrosis in the parenchyma (*p*) adjacent to a patent bronchiole. Contraction of the collagen as it matures results in dilatation of such airways and the bronchiectasis/bronchiolectasis noted on CT. The patient was a 63-year-old man with esophageal cancer.

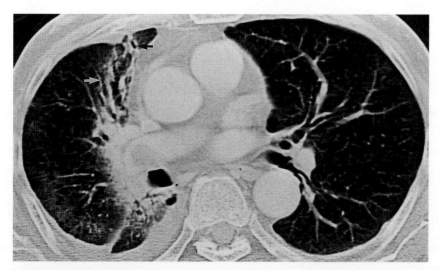

FIGURE 12.9. Radiation fibrosis. HRCT image demonstrates irregular linear opacities, consolidation, ground-glass opacities, and traction bronchiectasis (*arrows*). The radiated lung is decreased in size. Incidental note is made of small right pleural effusion. The patient was a 65-year-old man with previous radiation therapy for pulmonary carcinoma. (Courtesy of Dr. Hiroshi Moriya, Department of Radiology, Fukushima Medical University, Fukushima, Japan.)

BRACHYTHERAPY

Complications of brachytherapy include mucosal fibrosis with bronchostenosis, localized radiation pneumonitis, and bronchoesophageal fistula (20–22). In one study of 342 patients who had received brachytherapy (three fractions of 750 to 1,000 cGy at a calculated depth of 5 to 10 mm), 41 (12%) developed bronchitis and stenosis (22). At bronchoscopy, predominantly inflammatory changes were seen at a mean of about 16 weeks from the date of first brachytherapy; predominantly fibrotic changes were seen at 40 weeks. Twenty-five patients (9%) developed fatal hemoptysis. Variables associated with an increased risk of complications included large cell carcinoma, prior laser photo resection, and concurrent external-beam irradiation.

REFERENCES

1. Bush DA, Dunbar RD, Bonnet R, et al. Pulmonary injury from proton and conventional radiotherapy as revealed by CT. *Am J Roentgenol* 1999;172:735–739.
2. Davis SD, Yankelevitz DF, Henschke CI. Radiation effects on the lung: clinical features, pathology, and imaging findings. *Am J Roentgenol* 1992;159:1157–1164.
3. Libshitz HI. Radiation changes in the lung. *Semin Roentgenol* 1993;28:303–320.
4. Movsas B, Raffin TA, Epstein AH, et al. Pulmonary radiation injury. *Chest* 1997;111:1061–1076.
5. Logan PM. Thoracic manifestations of external beam radiotherapy. *Am J Roentgenol* 1998;171:569–577.
6. Fajardo LF, Berthrong M. Radiation injury in surgical pathology. *Am J Surg Pathol* 1978;2:159–199.
7. Wilkinson MJ, MacLennan KA. Vascular changes in irradiated lungs: a morphometric study. *J Pathol* 1989;158:229–232.
8. Frija J, Ferme C, Baud L, et al. Radiation-induced lung injuries: a survey by computed tomography and pulmonary function tests in 18 cases of Hodgkin's disease. *Eur J Radiol* 1988;8:18–23.
9. Ikezoe J, Takashima S, Morimoto S, et al. CT appearance of acute radiation-induced injury in the lung. *Am J Roentgenol* 1988;150:765–770.
10. Fennessy JJ. Irradiation damage to the lung. *J Thorac Imaging* 1987;1:68–79.
11. Polansky SM, Ravin CE, Prosnitz LR. Pulmonary changes after primary irradiation for early breast carcinoma. *Am J Roentgenol* 1980;134:101–105.
12. Gross NJ. The pathogenesis of radiation-induced lung damage. *Lung* 1981;159:115–125.
13. Goldman AL, Enquist R. Hyperacute radiation pneumonitis. *Chest* 1975;67:613–615.

14. Bell D, McGivern J, Bullimore J, et al. Diagnostic imaging of post-irradiation changes in the chest. *Clin Radiol* 1988;39:109–119.

15. Ikezoe J, Morimoto S, Takashima S, et al. Acute radiation-induced pulmonary injury: computed tomography evaluation. *Semin Ultrasound CT MRI* 1990;11:409–416.

16. Libshitz HI, Shuman LS. Radiation-induced pulmonary change: CT findings. *J Comput Assist Tomogr* 1984;8:15–19.

17. Mah K, Poon PY, Van DJ, et al. Assessment of acute radiation-induced pulmonary changes using computed tomography. *J Comput Assist Tomogr* 1986;10:736–743.

18. Crestani B, Kambouchner M, Soler P, et al. Migratory bronchiolitis obliterans organizing pneumonia after unilateral radiation therapy for breast carcinoma. *Eur Respir J* 1995;8:318–321.

19. Bayle JY, Nesme P, Bejui-Thivolet F, et al. Migratory organizing pneumonitis "primed" by radiation therapy. *Eur Respir J* 1995; 8:322–326.

20. Khanavkar B, Stern P, Alberti W, et al. Complications associated with brachytherapy alone or with laser in lung cancer. *Chest* 1991;99:1062–1065.

21. Gustafson G, Vicini F, Freedman L, et al. High dose rate endobronchial brachytherapy in the management of primary and recurrent bronchogenic malignancies. *Cancer* 1995;75:2345–2350.

22. Speiser BL, Spratling L. Radiation bronchitis and stenosis secondary to high dose rate endobronchial irradiation. *Int J Radiat Oncol Biol Phys* 1993;25:589–597.

13

EMPHYSEMA

CLASSIFICATION

RADIOLOGIC MANIFESTATIONS
Chest Radiograph
Computed Tomography

CENTRILOBULAR EMPHYSEMA

PANLOBULAR EMPHYSEMA

PARASEPTAL EMPHYSEMA

BULLOUS LUNG DISEASE

IRREGULAR EMPHYSEMA

Emphysema can be defined as a "condition of the lung characterized by permanent, abnormal enlargement of airspaces distal to the terminal bronchiole, accompanied by the destruction of their walls" (Fig. 13.1). The classic National Heart, Lung, and Blood Institute workshop definition includes the proviso "without obvious fibrosis" (1). Inclusion of this proviso however is controversial, because it excludes irregular (cicatricial) emphysema and some cases of paraseptal emphysema and because centrilobular emphysema is commonly associated with microscopic foci of fibrosis (2,3). Therefore, we and others (2,3) have dropped *without fibrosis* from the definition of emphysema.

The pathogenesis of emphysema is believed to be the result of an imbalance between elastolytic and anti-elastolytic processes in the lung. The former are related mostly to enzymes released from neutrophils and macrophages, either those present normally in the lung or those recruited via an inflammatory reaction. The most important antielastolytic agents are alpha$_1$-antiprotease inhibitor, normally present in circulating blood, and a bronchial mucus proteinase inhibitor, normally secreted by airway epithelial cells. The most important factors that affect the balance between these opposing processes are (a) cigarette smoke, which, in addition to other effects, can recruit neutrophils and macrophages to the vicinity of respiratory bronchioles, delay the transit of neutrophils through alveolar capillaries, and increase the synthesis and release of neutrophil enzymes; and (b) a genetically mediated deficiency of alpha$_1$-antiprotease inhibitor.

CLASSIFICATION

Emphysema can be classified into four main subtypes based on the location of the destroyed lung. Pathologically, these subtypes have been related to the distribution of abnormalities within the pulmonary acinus. (The acinus consists of all tissue distal to the terminal bronchiole, comprising three or more generations of respiratory bronchioles, followed by alveolar ducts, alveolar sacs, and their accompanying alveoli.) However, radiologically it is preferable to consider the different forms in relation to the secondary lobule. According to this, the four subtypes of emphysema are termed *centrilobular* (proximal acinar), *panlobular* (panacinar), *paraseptal* (distal acinar), and *irregular* (cicatricial) (4,5).

Centrilobular emphysema affects mainly the proximal respiratory bronchioles (proximal acinus) and therefore involves the central portion of the lobule. Panlobular emphysema involves the entire lobule. Paraseptal emphysema involves mainly the alveolar ducts and sacs (distal acinus) and therefore is characteristically situated adjacent to the interlob-

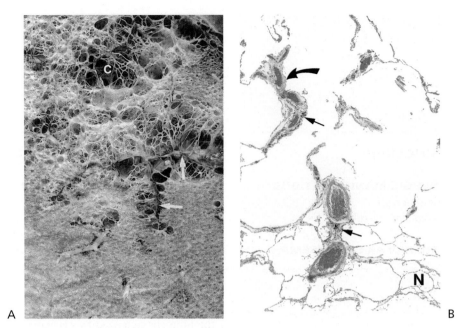

FIGURE 13.1. Emphysema: pathologic appearance. **A:** Magnified view of a slice of upper lobe shows normal parenchyma at the bottom and numerous, variably sized, cystlike spaces traversed by thin strands of residual parenchymal tissue at the top. The appearance is that of paraseptal emphysema (*arrows* indicate the pulmonary vein in an interlobular septum) combined with centrilobular emphysema (c indicates pigmented, more severely affected central portion of the lobule). **B:** Photomicrograph shows almost complete absence of alveolar septa in the central portion of a pulmonary lobule. (Compare with the normal parenchyma [*N*] at the bottom.) Note the presence of carbon pigment in the residual interstitial tissue (*straight arrows*) (responsible for the black appearance on gross specimens) and the presence of a pulmonary artery (*curved arrow*) within the emphysematous region (also see Fig. 13.4). The appearance is characteristic of centrilobular emphysema.

ular septa and visceral pleura. Emphysema that cannot be localized to a particular site within the acinus and is associated with grossly evident fibrosis is considered irregular.

Bullae can develop in association with any of the four types of emphysema but are most common with paraseptal and centrilobular emphysema. By definition, a bulla is a sharply demarcated air-containing space measuring 1 cm or larger in diameter and possessing a wall 1 mm or less in thickness (5). The space may be unilocular or separated into several compartments by thin septa. The walls may be formed by pleura, connective-tissue septa, or compressed lung parenchyma. In some patients, bullae become quite large and result in significant compromise of respiratory function, a situation that is often referred to as bullous lung disease or bullous emphysema.

Pathologically, the presence and severity of emphysema are usually assessed on gross specimens with the naked eye; such assessment can be facilitated by impregnating lung slices with barium and viewing them in water with a dissecting microscope (6) or by the use of Bouin's fixation (3,7). A number of techniques also have been proposed to characterize and quantify emphysema microscopically. These include the presence of abnormal holes (fenestrae) in the alveolar walls, the destructive index, the loss of alveolar surface area, and the loss of alveolar attachments (loss of bronchiolar traction) (8). There is, however, no universal agreement on what constitutes the most reliable method to assess "abnormal enlargement" of the airspaces distal to the terminal bronchiole and to quantify the "destruction" of their walls. It has been suggested that destruction be defined as the disorderly appearance of the acinus or the presence of holes in the alveolar walls more than 20 μm in diameter (3).

Adequate pathologic quantification of emphysema requires careful examination of a slice of inflated lung, knowledge of normal appearance, and standards to grade the emphysema as mild, moderate, or severe (8). A simple method to quantify emphysema is by comparison with a pictorial grading system in which emphysema is scored from 0 to 100 at intervals of 5 or 10 (3,8). This is referred to as the panel-grading system and has been commonly used to correlate pathologic with radiologic findings.

RADIOLOGIC MANIFESTATIONS

Chest Radiograph

The radiographic manifestations include direct signs of lung destruction and secondary alterations in the vascular pattern and increased lung volume. Direct signs of emphysema, such as bullae and irregular areas of radiolucency, can often be seen in patients with moderate or severe emphysema (9,10) (Fig. 13.2). More commonly, however, the radiographic findings reflect secondary alterations in the vascular pattern and the presence of overinflation (9,11). Vascular abnormalities related to emphysema include local avascular areas, distortion of the vessels, increased branching angles, loss of normal sinuosity of vessels, and decrease in the peripheral vascular markings (12–14) (Fig. 13.3).

The most reliable sign of overinflation is flattening of the diaphragm (9). This is considered to be present when the highest level of the diaphragmatic dome is less than 1.5 cm above a line connecting the costophrenic and vertebrophrenic junctions on the posteroanterior radiograph or a line connecting the sternophrenic and posterior costophrenic angles on the lateral view (9,15,16). In one investigation, a flattened diaphragm on the posteroanterior chest radiograph was present in 94% of patients who had severe emphysema, 76% of those who had moderate emphysema, and 21% of those who had mild emphysema; only 4% of patients without emphysema showed the abnormality (15).

Other helpful signs of overinflation include an increase in the retrosternal airspace, an increase in lung height, and a low position of the diaphragm (16). The retrosternal airspace is the space between the anterior margin of the ascending aorta and the sternum. It is con-

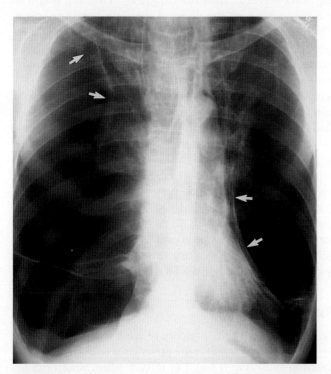

FIGURE 13.2. Emphysema: radiographic findings. A chest radiograph shows marked hyperinflation and large bullae (*arrows*) compressing the adjacent lung. The patient was a 49-year-old man.

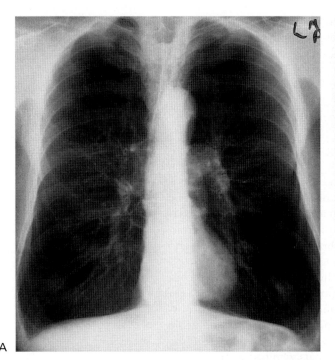
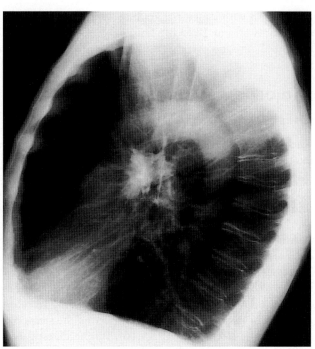

A   B

FIGURE 13.3. Emphysema: radiographic findings. **A:** Posteroanterior chest radiograph shows marked hyperinflation with flattening of the diaphragm and decrease in the peripheral vascular markings. **B:** Lateral view shows flattening of the diaphragm and an increase in the retrosternal airspace. The patient was a 53-year-old man.

sidered to be increased when the horizontal distance between the sternum and the most anterior margin of the ascending aorta is greater than 2.5 cm (9,16). The lung height is considered increased when the distance between the dome of the right hemidiaphragm and the tubercle of the first rib is 30 cm or more (16,17). The identification of the dome of the right hemidiaphragm at or below the anterior end of the seventh rib is also suggestive of hyperinflation (18); however, this finding has a low sensitivity and is less helpful in diagnosis than is a change in contour (9).

The greatest diagnostic accuracy on the radiograph is obtained by using a combination of findings. For example, in one investigation, the presence of emphysema was assessed in 60 patients (33 who had emphysema and 27 normal controls) using the following radiographic criteria: (a) depression or flattening of the diaphragm on the posteroanterior radiograph, (b) irregular radiolucency of the lungs, (c) increased retrosternal space on the lateral radiograph, and (d) flattening of the diaphragm on the lateral radiograph (15). At least two of the four criteria had to be present for a diagnosis of emphysema. Using these criteria, all 14 symptomatic and 13 of 19 (68%) asymptomatic patients who had emphysema were correctly diagnosed; no false-positive diagnoses were made. Based on these and other data (12,19), it has been estimated that the presence of two or more of the four radiographic features just listed usually requires a pathologic emphysema score (obtained by the panel grading method) of 30 out of 100 or greater (8).

Computed Tomography

The diagnosis of emphysema on CT is based on the presence of areas of abnormally low attenuation, typically without visible walls, which reflect the presence of enlarged airspaces as a result of parenchymal destruction (5,8) (Fig. 13.4). On HRCT scans, vessels can be seen within the areas of low attenuation (20). Several groups of investigators have shown that CT, particularly HRCT, findings correlate closely with the presence and severity of emphysema (7,21–23). HRCT also allows qualitative assessment of the different types of

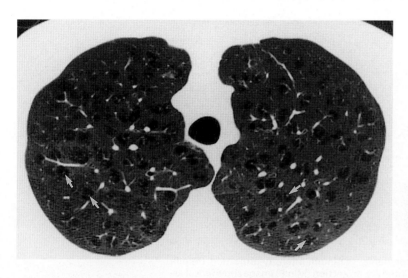

FIGURE 13.4. Emphysema: HRCT findings. An HRCT image shows focal areas of low attenuation without walls. Pulmonary vessels (*arrows*) can be seen within many of the areas of low attenuation. The findings are characteristic of centrilobular emphysema. The patient was a 49-year-old man.

emphysema (8,24). The accuracy of CT is influenced by collimation (section thickness) and by the CT window settings (7,24,25).

In one investigation, preoperative CT scans were obtained in 38 patients before lobectomy or pneumonectomy (7). Conventional 10- and 1.5-mm collimation HRCT scans were compared with the pathologic findings in the corresponding transverse slice of lung. Severity of emphysema was correlated with the severity of emphysema assessed pathologically by the panel grading method. There was good correlation between the CT and the pathologic scores for both the conventional ($r = 0.81$) and the HRCT ($r = 0.85$) scans. The areas of emphysema were more conspicuous on HRCT than on conventional CT images. However, mild emphysema was missed on CT in four patients.

Another group of investigators assessed the accuracy of 1-mm collimation HRCT and 5-mm collimation conventional CT in 42 patients who had undergone lobectomy (25). The extent of emphysema was assessed both on CT scans and in the resected lobes using a panel of standards. The severity of emphysema found pathologically was consistently underestimated on the 5-mm-collimation scans; however, there was no significant difference between the HRCT emphysema scores and the pathology scores. Subsequent studies using 1-mm-collimation HRCT scans have also shown no significant difference between the extent of emphysema as assessed on HRCT scans and in gross specimens (23,26). It should be noted, however, that mild emphysema can be missed on HRCT scans (7,8,27).

Visualization of small, subtle areas of emphysema on CT can be improved by the use of narrow window widths (800 to 1,200 HU) and low window levels (-700 to -750 HU) (8,22,24) or by the use of spiral CT with reconstruction of contiguous sections using minimum intensity projection (MinIP) (27). The latter technique consists of spiral CT performed using 1-mm collimation through a volume of lung ranging from a few millimeters to several centimeters in thickness (sliding thin-slab technique). The images can then be reconstructed individually or as a single slab. The minimum projection technique reconstructs the images based on the lowest attenuation values present within the slab and has the effect of suppressing the visualization of pulmonary vessels and optimizing visualization of low-attenuation areas (Fig. 13.5).

In one investigation of 29 patients who had no radiographic evidence of emphysema, 10 contiguous 1-mm-thick CT sections were examined before lobectomy (27). Minimum-intensity-projection images were generated including three to eight contiguous sections; slab thicknesses used were 3, 5, and 8 mm. Twenty-one of the 29 patients had emphysema; the emphysema was detected on the minimum-intensity projection images in 17 (85%), compared with 13 (62%) on standard HRCT images. The specificity of both techniques was 100%. Emphysema was easier to detect on 8-mm-thick slabs (i.e., eight contiguous 1-mm sections) than on thinner ones because of better suppression of vascular structures (27).

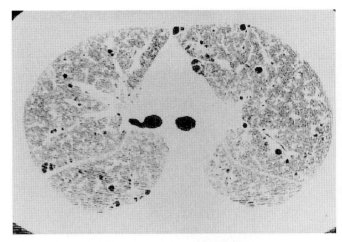

FIGURE 13.5. Emphysema: minimum-intensity-projection (MinIP) image. A minimal-intensity-projection (MinIP) image shows focal areas of low attenuation due to emphysema. The image was obtained from a sliding 1-mm collimation spiral CT study using a slab thickness of 10 mm, a technique that optimizes visualization of areas of low attenuation. The patient was a 41-year-old woman.

CENTRILOBULAR EMPHYSEMA

Centrilobular emphysema (CLE) is characterized pathologically by destruction of parenchymal tissue in the region of the proximal respiratory bronchioles. Because each secondary lobule contains several acini, early disease appears in several foci in the lobule instead of being located precisely in its center (Fig. 13.6) (28,29). The disease is found pre-

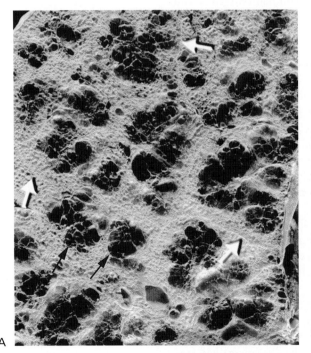

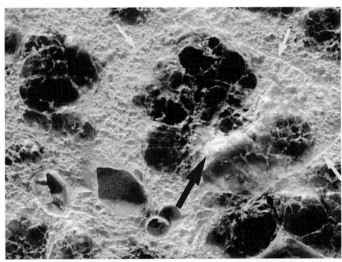

FIGURE 13.6. Centrilobular emphysema: pathologic appearance. Intermediate- (**A**) and high- (**B**) magnification views of an air-dried slice of upper lobe show multiple foci of emphysema, all of which appear black as a result of carbon accumulation. All the foci are in the central portion of the lobule (the parenchyma in the peripheral portion is normal (*white arrows* indicate interlobular septa). Several foci of emphysema are apparent in some lobules (*black arrows* in **A**), corresponding to localization of disease to the proximal respiratory bronchioles of several acini. A pulmonary artery is evident in the central portion of one focus of emphysema (*black arrow* in **B**).

dominantly in cigarette smokers, and the foci of emphysema are black as a result of carbon accumulation in the perivascular interstitial tissue. The disease is typically more severe in the apical and posterior segments of the upper lobes and the superior segment of the lower lobes (Fig. 13.7) (30,31). The reason for this upper zonal predominance is not certain and may be related to several factors, including (a) slower transit time of neutrophils in upper compared with lower lung zones because of gravity associated difference in blood flow (the increased time allowing greater opportunity for enzyme release); (b) less perfusion of upper compared with lower zones, again gravity related, leading to relative undersupply of alpha$_1$-antiprotease inhibitor; and (c) increased mechanical stress in the upper zones as a result of more negative pleural pressure and relative hyperinflation.

The earliest abnormality seen on light microscopy is dilation of respiratory bronchioles accompanied by loss of their alveolar septa. As the disease progresses, several respiratory bronchioles become confluent, creating an enlarged space supplied by a terminal bronchiole proximally and leading to relatively normal alveolar tissue distally (30). At this stage, the disease is visible grossly as relatively discrete foci of tissue loss (Fig. 13.6). With further progression, the emphysema becomes confluent, resulting in destruction of an entire lobule and, eventually, large segments of lung. At this stage, it may be difficult to distinguish centrilobular from panlobular emphysema. However, the former typically affects the parenchyma unevenly, so that areas showing early changes diagnostic of the condition can usually be found. In addition, the upper zonal predominance is usually maintained.

On HRCT, mild CLE is characterized by the presence of localized areas of low attenuation measuring a few millimeters in diameter and located in the central portion of the secondary lobule (22,32,33) (Figs. 13.4 and 13.8). As the emphysema becomes more severe, the areas of low attenuation become confluent and the centrilobular distribution becomes less apparent. In most cases, the areas of low attenuation lack visible walls; however, very thin walls may be seen, particularly when the areas of emphysema are extensive.

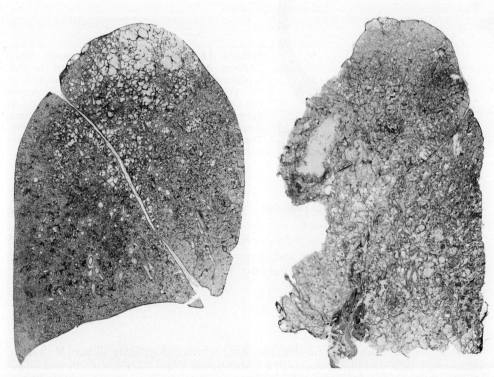

A

B

FIGURE 13.7. Emphysema: regional variation of disease. Thin paper-mounted slices of a left (**A**) and a right (**B**) lung from two patients show moderately severe centrilobular and panacinar emphysema, respectively. The disease in **A** is most prominent in the apex of the upper lobe and (to a lesser extent) the superior segment of the lower lobe. By contrast, disease in **B** is most evident in the base of the lower lobe.

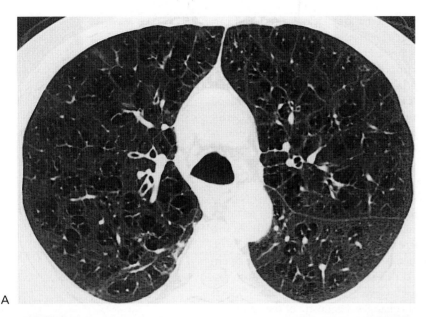

A

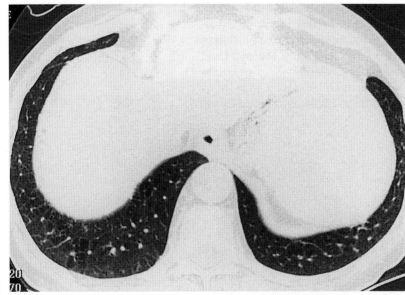

B

FIGURE 13.8. Centrilobular emphysema: HRCT findings. **A:** HRCT image at the level of the aortopulmonary window shows focal areas of low attenuation without walls. Pulmonary vessels (*arrows*) can be seen within the areas of low attenuation. **B:** Second image through lung bases shows minimal emphysema. The patient was a 66-year-old man. The findings are those of moderately severe centrilobular emphysema.

The apparent walls in such cases probably represent atelectasis or interlobular septa adjacent to the emphysematous spaces.

Several groups have shown good correlations between conventional HRCT and pathologic assessment of the extent and severity of CLE (21,22,25). However, mild CLE can be missed on both conventional and HRCT images (7,8,27).

PANLOBULAR EMPHYSEMA

Panlobular emphysema (PLE) involves the entire acinus and typically all acini within the pulmonary lobule. Mild to moderate PLE is difficult to detect macroscopically and is best seen by examination of barium-impregnated slices with a dissecting microscope. In severe disease, affected parenchyma may consist of no more than large airspaces through which strands of tissue and blood vessels pass like struts ("cotton-candy" lung). PLE tends to be more severe in the lower lung zones (Fig. 13.7) and is characteristically seen in association

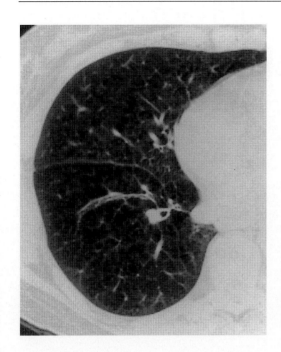

FIGURE 13.9. Panacinar emphysema: HRCT findings. HRCT image of the right lung demonstrates diffuse areas of low attenuation. The emphysema is more severe in the right lower lobe than the right middle lobe. The findings are characteristic of panacinar emphysema. The patient was a 49-year-old woman.

with alpha$_1$-antiprotease inhibitor deficiency. As with CLE, the precise factors responsible for the zonal predominance of PLE are uncertain. However, it seems likely that it is related at least partly to the increased numbers of neutrophils that transit the lower zones because of gravity-related preponderance of blood flow. For unknown reasons, PLE can also occur in association with talcosis due to intravenous drug use and in patients with Swyer-James syndrome (1,34).

The HRCT findings of PLE consist of widespread areas of abnormally low-attenuation and decreased vascularity (35,36) (Fig. 13.9). As indicated, these abnormalities are most severe in the lower lobes (Fig. 13.10). Since clinical manifestations of PLE associated with alpha$_1$-antiprotease inhibitor deficiency are often seen in cigarette smokers, focal lucencies due to centrilobular emphysema may be seen in the upper lobes. Paraseptal emphysema and bullae also can be seen but are not a major feature of the disease (35). In severe PLE, the characteristic appearance of extensive lung destruction and the associated paucity of vascular markings are easily distinguished from normal lung parenchyma on HRCT. However, mild and even moderately severe disease can be very subtle and difficult to detect (7).

The accuracy of CT in diagnosing and quantifying PLE was assessed in a study that included 10 patients who had pathologically proven disease and five normal controls (36). The correlation between the assessment of extent of PLE on CT and the pathologic grade was $r = 0.90$, $p < .01$ for conventional CT, and $r = 0.96$, $p < .01$ for HRCT. The observers missed three cases of mild disease on conventional CT and two on HRCT. In another investigation of 17 patients who had moderate to severe PLE associated with alpha$_1$-antiprotease inhibitor deficiency, all patients were found to have areas of low attenuation corresponding to parenchymal destruction and reduced vascularity (35). Bulla formation was seen in seven of 17 patients.

Panlobular emphysema secondary to alpha-1-antitrypsin deficiency can be associated with bronchiectasis (37) (Fig. 13.11). In one investigation (38), six of 14 (43%) patients who had alpha-1-antitrypsin deficiency had CT evidence of abnormality. In a second investigation (35), bronchial wall thickening, dilatation, or both were present in seven of 17 (41%) patients who had alpha-1-antitrypsin deficiency, with cystic bronchiectasis visible in one patient. Histologic findings in one patient showed destruction of elastic lamina in ectatic bronchi and bronchioles (38), suggesting that the abnormality may be the result of unopposed destructive enzymes similar to the process that occurs in the lung parenchyma.

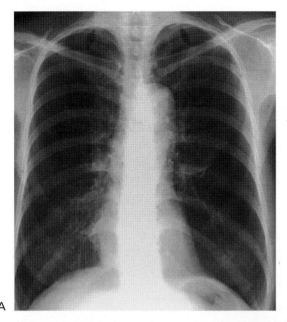

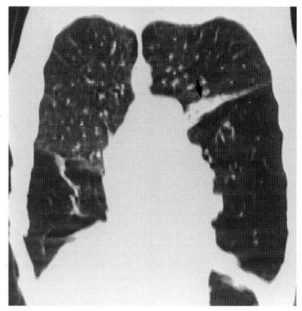

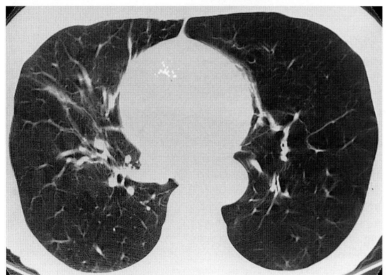

FIGURE 13.10. Panacinar emphysema. **A:** Chest radiograph shows increased lung volumes and decreased peripheral vascular markings. **B:** HRCT image shows markedly decreased attenuation and vascularity of the left lung and less severe involvement of the right lung. Note relative sparing of the right middle lobe. **C:** Coronal reconstruction from HRCT demonstrates severe emphysema throughout the lower lung zones, hyperinflation of the left lower lobe with compressive area of atelectasis of the left upper lobe (*arrow*). Only mild emphysema is evident in the upper lobes. The findings are characteristic of panacinar emphysema.

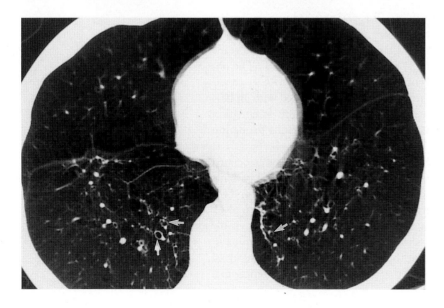

FIGURE 13.11. Panacinar emphysema and bronchiectasis. HRCT image shows diffuse areas of decreased attenuation throughout both lungs. Mild bronchiectasis (*arrows*) and localized linear areas of scarring are also evident. The patient was a 44-year-old woman with alpha$_1$-antitrypsin deficiency.

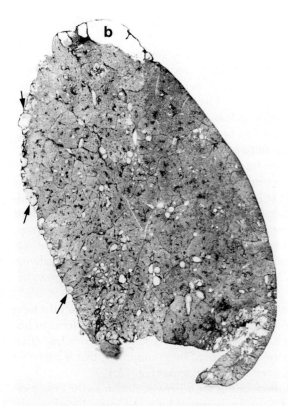

FIGURE 13.12. Paraseptal emphysema: pathologic appearance. Parasagittal paper-mounted slice of the right lung shows multiple foci of emphysema adjacent to the pleura anteriorly (*arrows*). Coalescence of such foci has led to the formation of a bulla in the apex (b).

PARASEPTAL EMPHYSEMA

Paraseptal emphysema selectively involves the pulmonary parenchyma in the peripheral portion of the acinus. Grossly, it is usually focal and consists of emphysematous spaces adjacent to the pleura or interlobular septa (Fig. 13.12). In some cases, fibrosis is associated with the emphysema, suggesting that the latter was caused by a localized inflammatory process such as infectious pneumonia. Subpleural bullae may develop from coalescence of small foci of the disease, particularly in the apex of an upper lobe. Rupture of one of these is a common cause of pneumothorax.

HRCT shows localized areas of low attenuation adjacent to interlobular septa, large bronchi and vessels, and pleura (Fig. 13.13). Because of its location adjacent to structures with soft-tissue attenuation, even mild paraseptal emphysema is easily detected on HRCT (7).

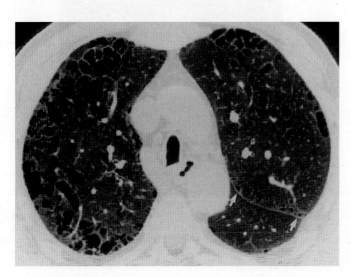

FIGURE 13.13. Paraseptal emphysema: HRCT findings. HRCT image shows focal areas of low attenuation predominantly in the subpleural region (including the pleura in the left interlobar fissure (*arrows*). The patient was a 71-year-old man.

BULLOUS LUNG DISEASE

Patients who have bullous lung disease can be divided into two groups: those who have concomitant emphysema (the vast majority of patients) and those judged to have normal pulmonary parenchyma between the bullae (39,40). A familial occurrence has been reported in patients who have the latter form (41). The incidence of bullae is increased in patients who have connective-tissue diseases such as Marfan's syndrome (42) and Ehlers-Danlos syndrome (43). The term *giant bullous emphysema* has been used to describe the presence of bullae occupying at least one-third of a hemithorax (44).

Bullae have traditionally been divided into three morphologic types (45). Type 1 lesions originate in a subpleural location or in the vicinity of parenchymal scars. They are commonly located in the apex of an upper lobe or along the costophrenic rim of the middle lobe and lingula. Each bulla characteristically has a narrow neck and usually contains only gas, without evidence of alveolar remnants or blood vessels (Fig. 13.14). When seen in an excised lung, such a bulla appears as a spherical sac projecting above the pleural surface; of necessity, it extends into the contiguous lung *in vivo,* compressing the parenchyma and causing some degree of atelectasis. Multiple bullae may be seen to extend in rows beneath the pleura.

Type 2 bullae are also superficial in location. They may occur anywhere over the lung surface but most often develop over the anterior edge of the upper and middle lobes or lingula and over the diaphragmatic surface. In contrast to type 1 lesions, this variety often contains blood vessels and strands of partially destroyed lung, indicating that it probably represents a localized exaggeration of generalized emphysema (Fig. 13.15).

Type 3 bullae lie within the lung substance but are otherwise similar to the type 2 variety and commonly contain strands of partially destroyed lung and intact blood vessels. They appear to affect both upper and lower lobes equally. Although this type usually represents an exaggerated form of generalized emphysema, it occasionally develops in its absence, in which case it probably represents the residuum of a lung abscess.

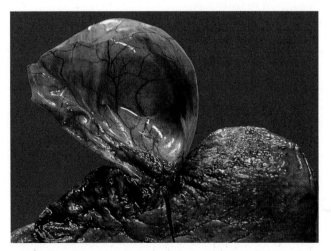

FIGURE 13.14. Bulla. A magnified view of the apex of an upper lobe shows a thin-walled bulla attached by a narrow neck to the underlying lung.

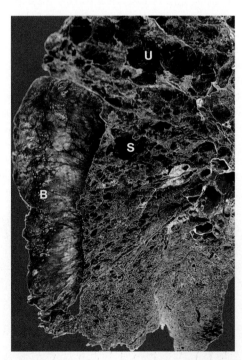

FIGURE 13.15. Emphysema with bulla formation. A magnified view of a parasagittal slice of an air-dried right lung shows severe centrilobular emphysema in the upper lobe (*U*) and superior aspect of the middle lobe (*S*). A large bulla (*B*) is evident in the anterior portion of the middle lobe.

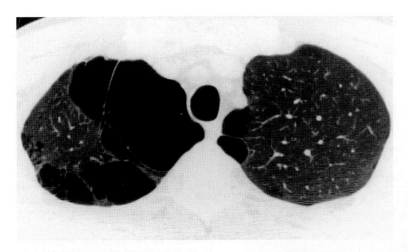

FIGURE 13.16. Bullae. An HRCT image shows bilateral subpleural areas of low attenuation with thin walls characteristic of bullae. The patient was a 37-year-old man.

Bullae are manifested on the chest radiograph and HRCT as thin-walled, sharply demarcated areas of avascularity (Fig. 13.16). They may be large enough to compress the adjacent lung parenchyma. Although such compression is usually relatively mild (44), it may result in sufficient atelectasis to appear as a masslike opacity (46) (Fig. 13.17). In one investigation of 11 patients who had such opacities, the areas of atelectasis involved mainly the upper lobes; smaller foci of atelectasis were present in the remaining lobes (46). Reexpansion of the atelectatic lung with resolution of the masslike appearance occurred in seven of the eight patients who underwent resection of bullae.

Spontaneous pneumothorax commonly occurs in association with localized areas of emphysema or bullae affecting the lung apices. In one investigation of 116 patients who had surgically treated pneumothorax, 69 had parenchymal abnormalities identified on the radiograph (47). The most common findings consisted of apical bullae (seen in 51 patients), apical scarring (in 17), and diffuse emphysema (in nine). Bullae and localized areas of emphysema can be seen on the CT scan in more than 80% of patients who have spontaneous pneumothorax (48–50). In one investigation of 35 patients who had this complication, bullae or smaller localized areas of emphysema were identified on the CT scan in 31 (89%) and on the radiograph in 11 (31%) (49). In another investigation of 27 nonsmoking patients who had spontaneous pneumothorax, 21 (81%) had localized bullae or smaller areas of emphysema visible on the CT scan (50). Focal areas of emphysema were identified at surgery in three additional patients. In none of these patients were the parenchymal abnormalities visible on the chest radiograph.

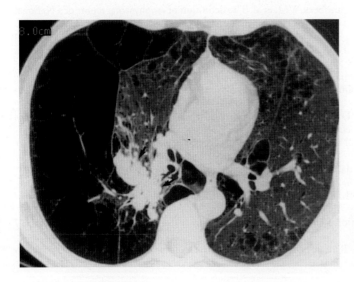

FIGURE 13.17. Emphysema with bulla formation. HRCT image shows large bullae in the right lung. Compression of the adjacent lung parenchyma has resulted in focal atelectasis (*arrows*). The right lung has an increased volume and there is a shift of mediastinum to the left. Relatively mild emphysema is present in the left lung. The patient was a 68-year-old man.

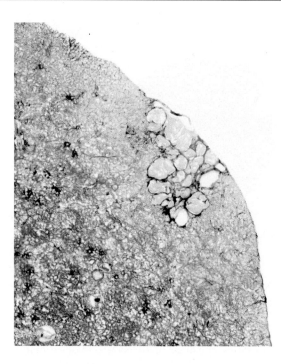

FIGURE 13.18. Irregular emphysema. Magnified view of an upper lobe shows a discrete focus of emphysema associated with mild fibrosis. Interlobular septa are inconspicuous, making interpretation somewhat difficult; however, the size and appearance of the abnormality suggest involvement of at least two lobules in an irregular fashion.

IRREGULAR EMPHYSEMA

As the name suggests, *irregular* (cicatricial) *emphysema* shows no consistent relationship to any portion of the acinus or lobule (Fig. 13.18). It is always associated with fibrosis. Most examples probably develop following an episode of pneumonia in which enzymes released from inflammatory cells cause lung destruction, leaving residual dilated airspaces and fibrous tissue. Although the abnormality is commonly seen pathologically, usually it is limited in extent and results in no functional or clinical abnormalities.

On HRCT, irregular emphysema is seen as an area of abnormally low attenuation adjacent to a scar, or in association with diffuse pulmonary fibrosis or progressive massive fibrosis (51).

REFERENCES

1. Snider GL, Kleinerman J, Thurlbeck WM, et al. The definition of emphysema: report of a National Heart, Lung, and Blood Institute, Division of Lung Diseases workshop. *Am Rev Respir Dis* 1985;132:182–185.
2. Cardoso WV, Sekhon HS, Hyde DM, et al. Collagen and elastin in human pulmonary emphysema. *Am Rev Respir Dis* 1993;48:560–565.
3. Thurlbeck WM. Emphysema then and now. *Can Respir J* 1994; 1:21–39.
4. Fraser RF, Müller NL, Colman N, et al. Diagnosis of diseases of the chest. Philadelphia: WB Saunders, 1999:2168–2263.
5. Austin JHM, Müller NL, Friedman PJ, et al. Glossary of terms for CT of the lungs: recommendations of the nomenclature committee of the Fleischner Society. *Radiology* 1996;200:327–331.
6. Heard BE. A pathological study of emphysema of the lungs with chronic bronchitis. *Thorax* 1958;13:136–149.
7. Miller RR, Müller NL, Vedal S, et al. Limitations of computed tomography in the assessment of emphysema. *Am Rev Respir Dis* 1989;139:980–983.
8. Thurlbeck WM, Müller NL. Emphysema: definition, imaging, and quantification. *Am J Roentgenol* 1994;163:1017–1025.
9. Pratt PC. Role of conventional chest radiography in diagnosis and exclusion of emphysema. *Am J Med* 1987;82:998–1006.
10. Takasugi JE, Godwin JD. Radiology of chronic obstructive pulmonary disease. *Radiol Clin North Am* 1998;36:29–55.

11. Thurlbeck WM, Henderson JA, Fraser RG, et al. Chronic obstructive lung disease: a comparison between clinical, roentgenologic, functional and morphological criteria in chronic bronchitis, emphysema, asthma and bronchiectasis. *Medicine* 1970;49:81–145.

12. Laws JW, Heard BE. Emphysema and the chest film: a retrospective radiological and pathological study. *Br J Radiol* 1962;35:750–754.

13. Thurlbeck WM, Simon G.Radiographic appearance of the chest in emphysema. *Am J Roentgenol* 1978;130:429–440.

14. Miniati M, Filippi E, Falaschi F, et al. Radiologic evaluation of emphysema in patients with chronic obstructive pulmonary disease. *Am J Respir Crit Care Med* 1995;151:1359–1367.

15. Sutinen S. Christoforidis AJ, Klugh GA, et al. Roentgenologic criteria for the recognition of nonsymptomatic pulmonary emphysema: correlation between roentgenologic findings and pulmonary pathology. *Am Rev Respir Dis* 1965;91:69–76.

16. Cleverley JR, Müller NL. Advances in radiologic assessment of chronic obstructive pulmonary disease. *Clin Chest Med* 2000;21:653–663.

17. Reich SB, Weinshelbaum A, Yee J. Correlation of radiographic measurements and pulmonary function tests in chronic obstructive pulmonary disease. *Am J Roentgenol* 1985;144:695–700.

18. Burki NL, Krumpelman JL. Correlation of pulmonary function with the chest roentgenogram in chronic airway obstruction. *Am Rev Resp Dis* 1980;121:217–223.

19. Lohela P, Sutinen S, Pääkkö P, et al. Diagnosis of emphysema on chest radiographs. *Fortschr Geb Rontgenstr Nuklearmed Erganzungsband* 1984;141:395–402.

20. Bonelli FS, Hartman TE, Swensen SJ, et al. Accuracy of high-resolution CT in diagnosing lung diseases. *Am J Roentgenol* 1998;170:1507–1512.

21. Foster WL Jr, Pratt PC, Roggli VLet al. Centrilobular emphysema: CT-pathologic correlation. *Radiology* 1986;159:27–32.

22. Hruban RH, Meziane MA, Zerhouni EA, et al. High resolution computed tomography of inflation-fixed lungs: pathologic–radiologic correlation of centrilobular emphysema. *Am Rev Respir Dis* 1987;136:935–940.

23. Gevenois PA, Koob MC, Jacobovitz D, et al. Whole lung sections for CT–pathologic correlations: modified Gough-Wentworth technique. *Invest Radiol* 1993;28:242–246.

24. Bergin CJ, Müller NL, Miller RR. CT in the qualitative assessment of emphysema. *J Thorac Imaging* 1986;1:94–103.

25. Kuwano K, Matsuba K, Ikeda T, et al. The diagnosis of mild emphysema: correlation of computed tomography and pathologic scores. *Am Rev Respir Dis* 1990;141:169–178.

26. Gevenois PA, de Maertelaer V, de Vuyst P, et al. Comparison of computed density and macroscopic morphometry in pulmonary emphysema. *Am J Respir Crit Care Med* 1995;152:653–657.

27. Remy-Jardin M, Remy J, Gosselin B, et al. Sliding thin slab, minimum intensity projection technique in the diagnosis of emphysema: histopathologic–CT correlation. *Radiology* 1996;200:665–671.

28. Thurlbeck WM. *Chronic airflow obstruction in lung disease.* Philadelphia: WB Saunders, 1976.

29. Thurlbeck WM. The pathobiology and epidemiology of human emphysema. *J Toxicol Environ Health* 1984;13:323–343.

30. Thurlbeck WM. Chronic obstructive lung disease. *Pathol Annu* 1968;3:367–398 .

31. Anderson AE Jr, Foraker AG. Centrilobular emphysema and panlobular emphysema: two different diseases. *Thorax* 1973;28:547–550.

32. Murata K, Itoh H, Todo G, et al. Centrilobular lesions of the lung: demonstration by high-resolution CT and pathologic correlation. *Radiology* 1986;161:641–645.

33. Webb WR, Stein MG, Finkbeiner WE, et al. Normal and diseased isolated lungs: high-resolution CT. *Radiology* 1988;166:81–87.

34. Stern EJ, Frank MS, Schmutz JF, et al. Panlobular pulmonary emphysema caused by i.v. injection of methylphenidate (Ritalin): findings on chest radiographs and CT scans. *Am J Roentgenol* 1994;162:555–560.

35. Guest PJ, Hansell DM. High resolution computed tomography (HRCT) in emphysema associated with alpha-1-antitrypsin deficiency. *Clin Radiol* 1992;45:260–266.

36. Spouge D, Mayo JR, Cardoso W, et al. Panacinar emphysema: CT and pathologic findings. *J Comput Assist Tomogr* 1993;17:710–713.

37. Shin MS, Ho KJ. Bronchiectasis in patients with alpha 1-antitrypsin deficiency: a rare occurrence? *Chest* 1993;104:1384–1386.

38. King MA, Stone JA, Diaz PT, et al. Alpha 1-antitrypsin deficiency: evaluation of bronchiectasis with CT. *Radiology* 1996;199:137–141.

39. Viola AR, Zuffardi EA. Physiologic and clinical aspects of pulmonary bullous disease. *Am Rev Respir Dis* 1966;94:574–580.

40. Boushy SF, Kohen R, Billig DM, et al. Bullous emphysema: clinical, roentgenologic and physiologic study of 49 patients. *Dis Chest* 1968;54:17–24.

41. Gibson GJ. Familial pneumothoraces and bullae. *Thorax* 1977;32:88–91.

42. Wood JR, Bellamy D, Child AH, et al. Pulmonary disease in patients with Marfan syndrome. *Thorax* 1984;39:780–784.

43. Ayers JG, Pope FM, Reudy JF, et al. Abnormalities of the lungs and thoracic cage in the Ehlers-Danlos syndrome. *Thorax* 1985;40:300–305.

44. Stern EJ, Webb WR, Weinacker A, et al. Idiopathic giant bullous emphysema (vanishing lung syndrome): imaging findings in nine patients. *Am J Roentgenol* 1994;162:279–282.

45. Reid L. *The pathology of emphysema.* Chicago: Year-book Medical Publishers, 1967:211–240.

46. Gierada DS, Glazer HS, Slone RM. Pseudomass due to atelectasis in patients with severe bullous emphysema. *Am J Roentgenol* 1997;168:85–92.

47. Jordan KG, Kwong JS, Flint J, Müller NL. Surgically treated pneumothorax: radiologic and pathologic findings. *Chest* 1997;111:280–285.

48. Lesur O, Delorme N, Fromaget JM, et al. Computed tomography in the etiologic assessment of idiopathic spontaneous pneumothorax. *Chest* 1990;98:341–347.

49. Mitlehner W, Friedrich M, Dissmann W. Value of computed tomography in the detection of bullae and blebs in patients with primary spontaneous pneumothorax. *Respiration* 1992;59:221–227.

50. Bense L, Lewander R, Eklund G, et al. Nonsmoking, non-alpha$_1$-antitrypsin deficiency-induced emphysema in nonsmokers with healed spontaneous pneumothorax, identified by computed tomography of the lungs. *Chest* 1993;103:433–438.

51. Kinsella N, Müller NL, Vedal S, et al. Emphysema in silicosis: a comparison of smokers with nonsmokers using pulmonary function testing and computed tomography. *Am Rev Respir Dis* 1990;141: 1497–1500.

14

PULMONARY EDEMA

HYDROSTATIC PULMONARY EDEMA
Pathogenesis
Pathologic Characteristics
Radiologic Manifestations

PERMEABILITY PULMONARY EDEMA
Pathologic Characteristics
Radiologic Manifestations

Pulmonary edema is defined as the presence of excess extravascular water in the lungs. It can result from an increase in pulmonary microvascular pressure (hydrostatic or cardiogenic pulmonary edema) or an increase in permeability of the microvascular endothelial barrier (permeability or noncardiogenic pulmonary edema). Hydrostatic pulmonary edema is usually secondary to elevated pulmonary venous pressure as a result of left ventricular failure; permeability edema usually results from microvascular endothelial injury, of which there are a variety of causes. The clinical syndrome associated with permeability edema is termed the *acute (adult) respiratory distress syndrome* (ARDS) (1). The radiologic and pathologic manifestations of ARDS are remarkably similar, regardless of cause (2,3).

HYDROSTATIC PULMONARY EDEMA

As indicated, hydrostatic pulmonary edema develops when pulmonary venous pressure is elevated secondary to disease of the left side of the heart. Increased pressure within the left atrium can be transmitted to the pulmonary veins as a result of back pressure from the left ventricle (secondary to long-standing systemic hypertension, aortic valvular disease, cardiomyopathy, and coronary artery disease with or without myocardial infarction) or can be caused by obstruction to the left atrial outflow (as a result of mitral valve stenosis or left atrial myxoma). Rarely, venous hypertension develops as a result of stenosis of the pulmonary veins themselves, such as occurs in venoocclusive disease or fibrosing mediastinitis.

Pathogenesis

Normally, a small amount of fluid escapes from the pulmonary capillaries into the adjacent interstitium. In part because of well-developed intercellular junctions, the alveolar epithelium forms an effective barrier to its flow into the airspace. In addition, the compliance of the alveolar septal interstitial tissue appears to increase as fluid accumulates, possibly because of structural and chemical changes in the connective tissue itself. As a result of these two processes, fluid does not accumulate in the alveolar interstitium and instead flows proximally into the interstitial tissue surrounding small vessels and airways. Lymphatic vessels that originate in this tissue drain the fluid to the mediastinal lymphatics and, eventually, the venous circulation (Fig. 14.1).

When the amount of fluid that leaks into the interstitium is greater than the lymphatics can handle, it accumulates in the peribronchiolar, peribronchial, and perivascular interstitial tissue. Once this tissue is "saturated," fluid accumulates in the alveolar septal interstitium and, eventually, the alveolar airspaces. The route by which the fluid gains access to the airspaces is uncertain; some evidence suggests that it comes via the airway ep-

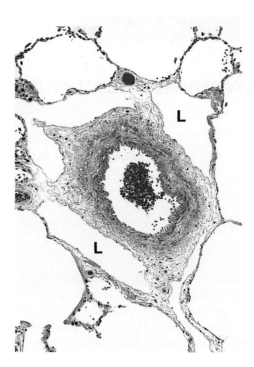

FIGURE 14.1. Perivascular lymphatic dilatation. Photomicrograph shows dilatation of several lymphatic vessels (*L*) in the interstitial tissue around a small pulmonary artery. The connective tissue itself is mildly edematous. The adjacent alveolar airspaces are free of fluid.

ithelium and spreads retrogradely, whereas other evidence indicates that it spreads directly across the alveolar epithelium.

Although the effects of gravity on the distribution of blood flow and ventilation in the normal lung have been well established, its effects on the distribution of pulmonary edema are not as clear. Gravity predisposes to dependent edema both by generating higher hydrostatic pressures toward the bases and by draining interstitial fluid toward the bases through the interstitial space. However, opposing these forces are the augmented ventilatory movements in lower zones that promote the removal of fluid through the lymphatics. The net effect of these opposing forces is difficult to predict; however, from a practical point of view, they result in maximal fluid accumulation in the lower and central lung zones.

Pathologic Characteristics

The earliest manifestation of hydrostatic pulmonary edema, both grossly and microscopically, is expansion of the connective tissue space around conducting airways, their accompanying vessels, and interlobular septa (Figs. 14.2 and 14.3). In gross specimens, this is usually best appreciated in the interlobular septa, which have a somewhat gelatinous appearance. On microscopic examination, the expansion can be seen to be a combination of dilated lymphatic vessels and edematous interstitial tissue. This fluid accumulation occurs without an appreciable increase in alveolar septal thickening and before there is airspace edema. The latter begins after the extravascular water content of the lung has increased by approximately 50% (4). At first, alveolar flooding appears to be patchy, with some alveoli filled with fluid and others immediately adjacent remaining gas filled (Fig. 14.4). However, if the process is severe enough, all alveoli within a lobule eventually become filled.

Radiologic Manifestations

Hydrostatic pulmonary edema results in two principal radiologic patterns related to whether the fluid remains localized in the interstitial space or whether it also occupies the airspaces of the lung.

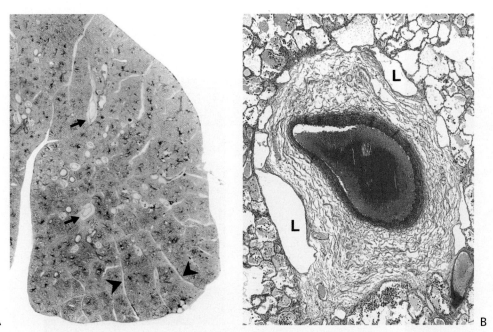

FIGURE 14.2. Interstitial and airspace edema. **A:** View of a paper-mounted slice of a lower lobe shows moderate expansion of the interstitial tissue surrounding pulmonary vessels (*arrows*) and within interlobular septa (*arrowheads*). **B:** Photomicrograph shows dilatation of lymphatic vessels (*L*) and a loose appearance of the interstitial tissue around a pulmonary vein, both caused by the accumulation of edema fluid. Airspace edema is also evident in the surrounding parenchyma.

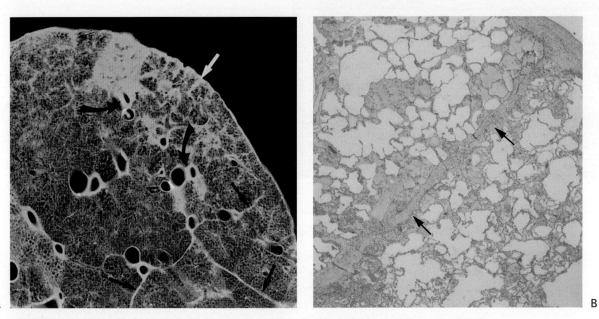

FIGURE 14.3. Interstitial and airspace edema. **A:** Contact radiograph of a portion of an upper lobe shows thickening of interlobular septa (*straight arrows*) and the interstitial tissue around several pulmonary arteries (*curved arrows*). Focal ground-glass opacities and airspace consolidation are also apparent. **B:** Photomicrograph shows thickening of an interlobular septum (*arrows*) by edema fluid and patchy foci of alveolar edema.

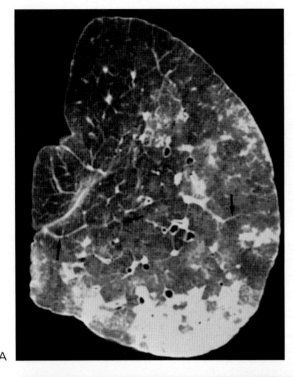

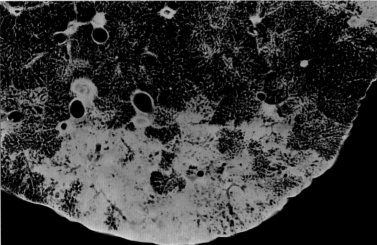

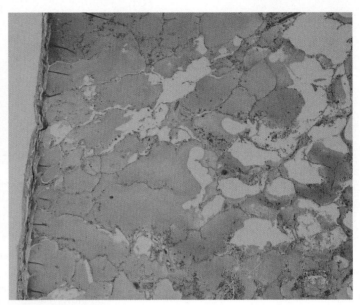

FIGURE 14.4. Airspace edema. **A:** HRCT image of a lung specimen shows smooth thickening of interlobular septa (*arrows*), ground-glass opacities, and airspace consolidation. **B:** Contact radiograph of the lower portion of the specimen demonstrates patchy airspace consolidation. **C:** Photomicrograph of the consolidated area shows extensive airspace filling by edema fluid.

Predominantly Interstitial Edema

Accumulation of fluid within the perivascular interstitial tissue results in loss of the normal sharp definition of pulmonary vascular markings (Fig. 14.5). This is initially evident radiographically at the level of the subsegmental and segmental vessels; with more severe edema, it is seen in the perihilar region (3). Edema of the peribronchial interstitial tissue results in an increase in the thickness of the walls of bronchi seen end-on, particularly in the perihilar region. These structures normally measure less than 1 mm in thickness; with edema they may be seen to measure as much as 2 mm. In addition to thickening, the airway wall loses its sharp definition. Thickening of the interlobular septa is manifested as septal lines (Kerley A and B lines). Because the pleural connective tissue is in continuity with that of the interlobular septa, accumulation of fluid in the latter site is often associated with thickening of the interlobar fissures (5). Small bilateral pleural effusions are also commonly present. When fluid accumulates in the parenchymal interstitium before the

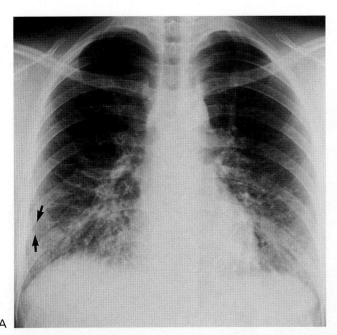
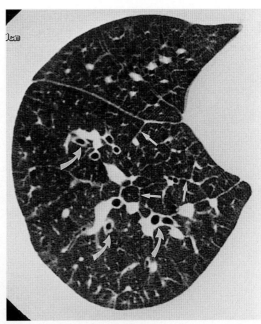

A

B

FIGURE 14.5. Interstitial pulmonary edema. **A:** Chest radiograph shows prominence of pulmonary vascular markings, a reticular pattern due to interlobular septal thickening, septal (Kerley B) lines (*arrows*), ill definition of the pulmonary vessels, and ground-glass opacities involving mainly the lower lobes. **B:** HRCT image demonstrates smooth thickening of interlobular septa (*straight arrows*) and bronchovascular bundles (*curved arrows*). The patient was a 21-year-old woman.

development of overt airspace edema, the accumulation usually is invisible or only faintly discernible radiographically as a "haze," which tends to be predominantly lower zonal or perihilar in distribution.

As on the radiograph, the findings on high-resolution computed tomography (HRCT) consist of thickening of the interlobular septa, interlobar fissures, and peribronchovascular connective tissue (peribronchial cuffing) (Fig. 14.5) (6,7). Because the fluid expands the interstitial tissue throughout, the interlobular septal thickening is generally smooth and uniform; however, focal nodularity may be seen as a result of localized dilatation of septal veins (7). Another common finding is ground-glass opacities, reflecting the presence of thickened alveolar walls. These opacities can be diffuse or patchy in distribution and usually involve mainly the dependent lung regions (6,7).

Airspace Edema

The characteristic radiographic appearance of hydrostatic airspace edema is patchy or confluent bilateral areas of consolidation that tend to be symmetric and to involve mainly the perihilar regions and the lower lung zones (Figs. 14.6 and 14.7). Air bronchograms are seen in 20% to 30% of patients (8). The consolidation sometimes extends to the subpleural zone or "cortex" of the lung; however, the cortex may be completely spared, creating a "bat's wing" or "butterfly" pattern. This pattern is seen in fewer than 10% of patients, most often those who have renal failure or rapidly developing and severe cardiac failure (3). It should be noted that the appearance of airspace edema, like that of any airspace process, may be altered when it occurs in patients with preexisting lung disease, particularly emphysema. In these patients airspace edema may simulate interstitial lung disease.

On HRCT, airspace edema results in areas of ground-glass attenuation and consolidation involving mainly the perihilar and dependent lung regions (Figs. 14.6 and 14.7) (6).

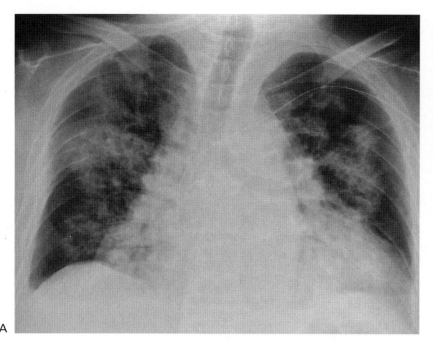
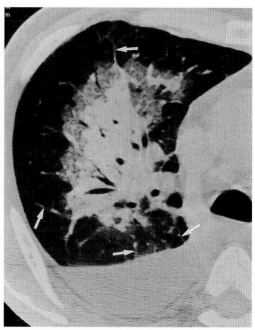

A

B

FIGURE 14.6. Airspace pulmonary edema. **A:** Chest radiograph shows bilateral airspace consolidation involving mainly the perihilar regions (butterfly pattern) and cardiomegaly. **B:** HRCT image of right lung demonstrates airspace consolidation mainly in the perihilar regions, smooth thickening of interlobular septa (*arrows*) and pleural effusion. The patient was a 52-year-old man with left heart failure.

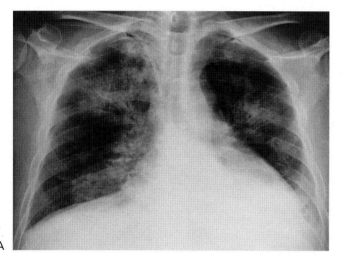
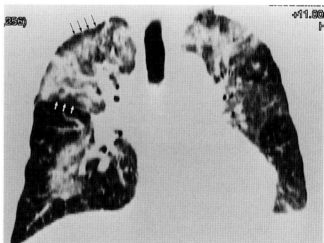

A

B

FIGURE 14.7. Airspace pulmonary edema. **A:** Chest radiograph shows bilateral airspace consolidation involving mainly the perihilar regions (butterfly pattern). **B:** Coronal multiplanar reconstruction image from HRCT shows extensive airspace consolidation with sparing of the subpleural regions (*black arrows*), including the lung adjacent to the interlobar fissure (*white arrows*). The patient was a 53-year-old man with renal failure.

PERMEABILITY PULMONARY EDEMA

Increased permeability of the pulmonary microvasculature can result from a variety of direct or indirect insults and is often associated with severe consequences. Patients typically develop progressive dyspnea. The chest radiograph reveals diffuse airspace disease, blood gas analysis demonstrates arterial oxygen desaturation that is resistant to high concentrations of inhaled oxygen, the lungs become stiff and difficult to ventilate, pulmonary vascular pressures and resistance increase, and it becomes necessary to institute prolonged ventilatory support. This combination of abnormalities is known as acute (adult) respiratory distress syndrome (1). The condition can result from a number of toxic agents or insults, including sepsis, aspiration of liquid gastric contents, trauma (including long-bone and pelvic fractures and pulmonary contusion), blood transfusions, pancreatitis, prolonged hypotension, overwhelming pneumonia, and disseminated intravascular coagulation (9,10).

Pathologic Characteristics

The pathologic changes in the lungs of patients who have ARDS are virtually the same regardless of etiology and are best described by the term *diffuse alveolar damage.* Although a continuum of histologic abnormalities exists, they can conveniently be described in three phases (11,12).

Exudative Phase

The exudative phase occurs within hours of the onset of pulmonary injury and is manifested initially by interstitial edema (affecting the perivascular, peribronchial, and interlobular interstitium as well as the alveolar wall), capillary congestion, and airspace filling by edema fluid and red blood cells. After several days, the exudate, which consists of necrotic cellular debris and fibrin as well as fluid (13,14), appears more compact and eosinophilic; similar material in alveolar ducts and respiratory bronchioles tends to become flattened against the airway wall, producing hyaline membranes (Fig. 14.8). During

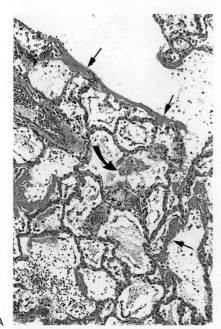
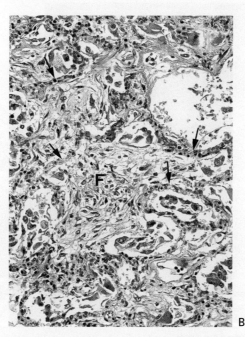

A   B

FIGURE 14.8. Diffuse alveolar damage—exudative and proliferative phases. **A:** Photomicrograph shows filling of alveolar airspaces by edema fluid, red blood cells, and a proteinaceous exudate (*curved arrow*). Similar exudate on the surface of transitional airways appears as hyaline membranes (*straight arrows*). **B:** Photomicrograph of a biopsy specimen from another patient shows filling of alveolar airspaces by loose fibroblastic tissue (*F*). Alveolar septa (*arrows*) are only mildly thickened as a result of capillary congestion.

this time, type II alveolar epithelial cells undergo proliferation, resulting in a relining of alveolar surface. Pulmonary vascular abnormalities are also common and probably result from several causes, including microvascular thrombosis associated with the initial pulmonary insult and thromboembolism (15).

Proliferative Phase

The proliferative phase begins about 7 to 14 days after the initial pulmonary insult and is characterized by organization of the airspace exudate by macrophages and fibroblasts (Fig. 14.8). It is seen predominantly within alveolar airspaces but also occurs to some extent in the parenchymal interstitium (14). The cellular proliferation is accompanied by synthesis and deposition of collagen. Transitional airways are often spared (Fig. 14.9), creating a characteristic gross appearance of multiple, evenly distributed spaces (representing the lumens of transitional airways) separated by more or less solid white-gray tissue (representing consolidated lung parenchyma).

Fibrotic Phase

In some patients, sufficient collagen is deposited to result in parenchymal fibrosis. In most, however, much of the fibroblastic proliferation resolves without functionally or histologically significant abnormality.

Radiologic Manifestations

Radiography

Good correlation has been reported between the radiographic patterns observed during life and the pathologic changes observed at autopsy (16,17).

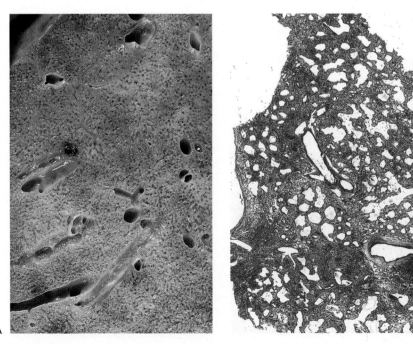

FIGURE 14.9. Diffuse alveolar damage—proliferative phase. **A:** Magnified view of a slice of lower lobe shows diffuse parenchymal consolidation. The lumens of transitional airways are easily identified as small, regularly spaced holes. **B:** Low-magnification photomicrograph confirms the presence of the patent airways, which are seen so distinctly because of extensive alveolar airspace filling by fibroblastic tissue.

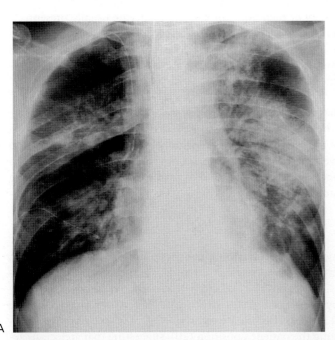
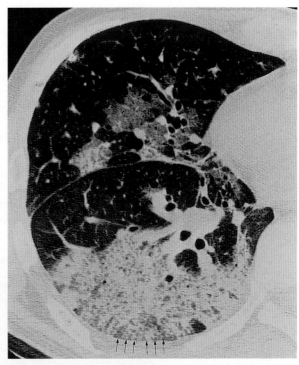

FIGURE 14.10. Acute respiratory distress syndrome. **A:** Chest radiograph shows extensive airspace consolidation and ground-glass opacities. **B:** HRCT image of the right lung demonstrates ground-glass opacities and airspace consolidation mainly in the dorsal lung regions. Also noted is a reticular pattern (*arrows*) superimposed on the ground-glass opacities ("crazy-paving" appearance). The patient was a 44-year-old man.

Exudative Phase

There is usually a delay of up to 12 hours from the clinical onset of respiratory failure to the appearance of abnormalities on the chest radiograph. The earliest findings consist of patchy, ill-defined opacities throughout both lungs (Figs. 14.10 and 14.11). Evidence of interstitial edema is variable. In one study it was documented in only five of 75 patients (17), whereas in others it has been seen more commonly (16,18).

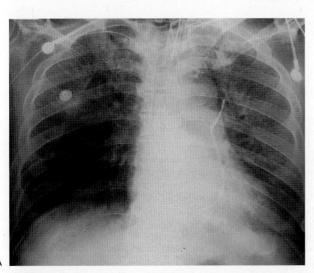
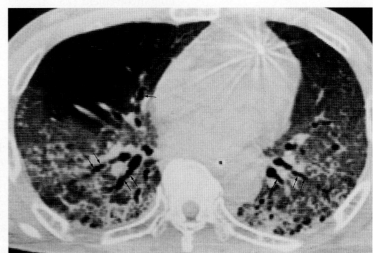

FIGURE 14.11. Acute respiratory distress syndrome. **A:** Chest radiograph shows bilateral ground-glass opacities and airspace consolidation. **B:** HRCT image demonstrates ground-glass attenuation and traction bronchiectasis (*arrows*) mainly in the dependent lung regions. The patient was 63-year-old man.

The patchy zones of consolidation rapidly coalesce to a point of massive airspace consolidation. Characteristically, involvement is diffuse, affecting all lung zones from apex to base and to the extreme periphery of each lung; air bronchograms are usually present. As distinct from hydrostatic pulmonary edema, the airspace consolidation tends to have a more peripheral distribution and septal lines are typically absent (3). Pleural effusion is usually not apparent on supine radiographs; its presence should suggest concomitant hydrostatic pulmonary edema or secondary infection.

Proliferative and Fibrotic Phases

After approximately 1 week, the pattern tends to become reticular (16,18), corresponding to the interstitial and airspace fibrosis observed pathologically (Figs. 14.10 and 14.11). In almost all patients who survive, the radiograph shows improvement within the first 10 to 14 days. Of 46 patients who were followed in one study, eight who had a relatively long survival and continuous assisted ventilation exhibited a coarse reticular pattern (16).

Computed Tomography

Early in the exudative phase of ARDS, CT commonly shows diffuse, but not uniform, ground-glass opacification or consolidation, which often does not conform to a gravity-dependent distribution (Figs. 14.10 and 14.11). Later in the exudative phase, the consolidation becomes more homogeneous and gravity dependent (19). Air bronchograms are almost always seen, and small pleural effusions are common (19). The gravitational gradient can be modified by changing the patient's position (20), suggesting that atelectasis accounts for some of the airspace consolidation (3). During the organizing phase, there is often a decrease in overall lung density and the appearance of interstitial reticulation (21). Examination at this stage often shows evidence of complications of ARDS and its treatment, such as interstitial emphysema, subpleural bullae or cysts, pneumomediastinum, and pneumothorax (5,22).

The CT appearance of ARDS secondary to pulmonary disease (e.g., pneumonia) often differs from that of ARDS resulting from extrapulmonary causes (e.g., sepsis) (23,24). Patients with the former tend to have extensive nondependent ground-glass attenuation and consolidation, a similar extent of consolidation and ground-glass attenuation, and an asymmetric distribution of abnormalities. By contrast, patients who have an extrathoracic cause of ARDS tend to have predominantly dependent ground-glass attenuation and consolidation, predominantly ground-glass opacity rather than consolidation, and symmetric lung involvement (23,24).

REFERENCES

1. Ware LB, Matthay MA. The acute respiratory distress syndrome. *N Engl J Med* 2000;342:1334–1339.
2. Greene R. Adult respiratory distress syndrome: acute alveolar damage. *Radiology* 1987;163:57–66.
3. Gluecker T, Capasso P, Schnyder P, et al. Clinical and radiologic features of pulmonary edema. *Radiographics* 1999;19:1507–1531.
4. Lai-Fook SJ. Mechanics of lung fluid balance. *Crit Rev Biomed Engin* 1986;13:171–200.
5. Ketai LH, Godwin JD. A new view of pulmonary edema and acute respiratory distress syndrome. *J Thorac Imag* 1998;13:147–171.
6. Primack SL, Müller NL, Mayo JR, et al. Pulmonary parenchymal abnormalities of vascular origin: high-resolution CT findings. *Radiographics* 1994;14:739–746.
7. Storto ML, Kee ST, Golden JA, et al. Hydrostatic pulmonary edema: high-resolution CT findings. *Am J Roentgenol* 1995;165:817–820.
8. Milne ENC, Pistolesi M, Miniati M, et al. The radiologic distinction of cardiogenic and noncardiogenic edema. *Am J Roentgenol* 1985;144:879–894.
9. Petty TL, Ashbaugh DG. The adult respiratory distress syndrome: clinical features, factors influencing prognosis and principles of management. *Chest* 1971;60:233–239.
10. Connelly KG, Repine JE. Markers for predicting the development of acute respiratory distress syndrome. *Annu Rev Med* 1997;48:429–445.

11. Hasleton PS. Adult respiratory distress syndrome: a review. *Histopathology* 1983;7:307–332.
12. Blennerhasset JB. Shock lung and diffuse alveolar damage: pathological and pathogenetic considerations. *Pathology* 1985;17:239–247.
13. Nash G, Foley FD, Langlinais PC. Pulmonary interstitial edema and hyaline membranes in adult burn patients: electron microscopic observations. *Hum Pathol* 1974;5:149–160.
14. Fukuda Y, Ishizaki M, Masuda Y, et al. The role of intraalveolar fibrosis in the process of pulmonary structural remodeling in patients with diffuse alveolar damage. *Am J Pathol* 1987;126:171–182.
15. Tomashefski JF Jr, Davies P, Boggis C, et al. The pulmonary vascular lesions of the adult respiratory distress syndrome. *Am J Pathol* 1983;112:112–126.
16. Ostendorf P, Birzle H, Vogel W, et al. Pulmonary radiographic abnormalities in shock: roentgen-clinical pathological correlation. *Radiology* 1975;115:257–263.
17. Joffe N. The adult respiratory distress syndrome. *Am J Roentgenol* 1974;122:719–732.
18. Dyck DR, Zylak CJ. Acute respiratory distress in adults. *Radiology* 1973;106:497–501.
19. Tagliabue M, Casella TC, Zincone GE, et al. CT and chest radiography in the evaluation of adult respiratory distress syndrome. *Acta Radiol* 1994;35:230–234.
20. Gattinoni L, Pelosi P, Vitale G, et al. Body position changes redistribute lung computed-tomographic density in patients with acute respiratory failure. *Anesthesiology* 1991;74:15–23.
21. Goodman LR. Congestive heart failure and adult respiratory distress syndrome: new insights using computed tomography. *Radiol Clin North Am* 1996;34:33–46.
22. Gattinoni L, Bombino M, Pelosi P, et al. Lung structure and function in different stages of severe adult respiratory distress syndrome. *JAMA* 1994;271:1772–1779.
23. Goodman LR, Fumagalli R, Tagliabue P, et al. Adult respiratory distress syndrome due to pulmonary and extrapulmonary causes: CT, clinical, and functional correlations. *Radiology* 1999;213:545–552.
24. Desai SR, Wells AU, Suntharalingam G, et al. Acute respiratory distress syndrome caused by pulmonary and extrapulmonary injury: a comparative CT study. *Radiology* 2001;218:689–693.

15

LARGE AIRWAY DISEASE

FOCAL TRACHEAL NARROWING
Tracheal Stricture
Wegener's Granulomatosis
Tuberculosis
Tracheobronchial Papillomatosis
Benign Neoplasms
Primary Malignant Neoplasms
Secondary Malignant Neoplasms

DIFFUSE TRACHEAL NARROWING
Relapsing Polychondritis
Amyloidosis

Tracheobronchopathia Osteochondroplastica
Tracheobronchitis Associated with Ulcerative Colitis
Saber-Sheath Trachea

TRACHEOBRONCHOMALACIA

TRACHEOBRONCHOMEGALY (MOUNIER-KUHN DISEASE)

BRONCHIECTASIS

BRONCHOLITHIASIS

Abnormalities of the trachea can be classified into focal and diffuse (Table 15.1). Focal disease results in decreased airway luminal diameter, whereas diffuse disease can result in decreased or increased diameter.

FOCAL TRACHEAL NARROWING

Tracheal Stricture

Strictures of the trachea are usually secondary to damage from a cuffed endotracheal or tracheostomy tube or to external neck trauma. Tube strictures are believed to occur when the cuff pressure is high enough to impede local blood circulation, with resultant ischemic necrosis of the mucosa and subsequent fibrosis (1). The most susceptible portions of the trachea are those where the mucosa overlies the cartilaginous rings.

Examination of gross specimens shows a variable degree of wall thickening and luminal narrowing. Biopsy of the affected segment early in the course of the abnormality shows granulation tissue; later on, there is dense mucosal and submucosal fibrosis that may be associated with distortion of cartilage plates.

Postintubation stenosis extends for several centimeters and typically involves the trachea above the level of the thoracic inlet. The narrowing is often concentric. Posttracheostomy stenosis typically begins 1 to 1.5 cm distal to the inferior margin of the tracheostomy stoma and involves 1.5 to 2.5 cm of tracheal wall (Fig. 15.1).

On radiographs, the stenosis may be seen as a focus of circumferential or eccentric narrowing associated with a segment of increased soft tissue or a thin membrane (web) of tissue (1). The site of narrowing is usually well seen on CT (Fig. 15.1). However, short-segment stenosis and webs may be missed because of partial volume averaging if thick sections are obtained. Spiral CT scans obtained through the stenotic area during a single breath-hold using 1- to 2-mm collimation are required for optimal assessment (2).

Wegener's Granulomatosis

Tracheal involvement in Wegener's granulomatosis is common, particularly in the subglottic region (3,4). Although most often unassociated with symptoms or a late manifes-

TABLE 15.1. DISEASE OF THE TRACHEA

Focal abnormalities
    Tracheal stricture
    Wegener's granulomatosis
    Tracheobronchial tuberculosis
    Benign neoplasms
    Primary malignant neoplasms
    Secondary malignant neoplasms

Diffuse abnormalities
    Decreased diameter
      Relapsing polychondritis
      Amyloidosis
      Tracheobronchopathia osteochondroplastica
      Tracheobronchitis associated with ulcerative colitis
      Saber-sheath trachea
      Tracheobronchomalacia
    Increased diameter
      Tracheobronchomegaly (Mounier-Kuhn disease)

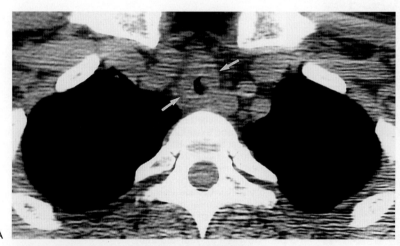

A

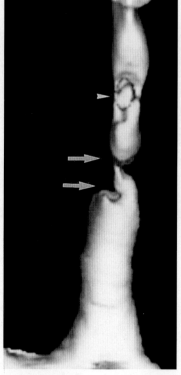

B

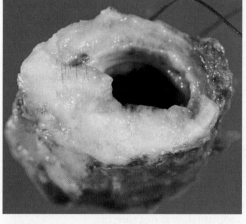

C

FIGURE 15.1. Posttracheostomy tracheal stenosis. **A:** CT image (3-mm collimation) at level of thoracic inlet shows circumferential thickening of tracheal wall (*arrows*). **B:** Three-dimensional reconstruction using shaded-surface-display technique shows focal and circumferential narrowing (*arrows*) about 2 cm distal to tracheostomy site (arrowhead). **C:** The excised specimen shows marked, somewhat eccentric thickening of the wall by fibrous tissue. The patient was a 30-year-old man.

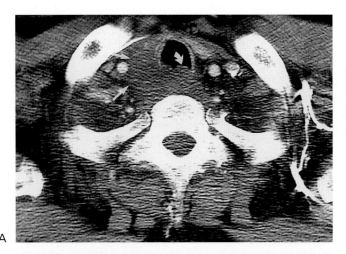

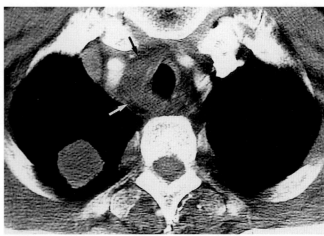

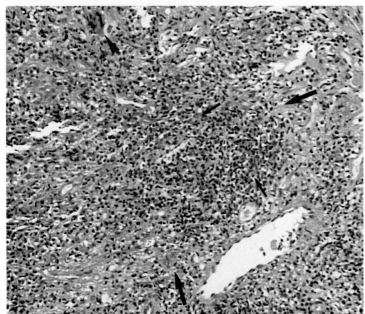

FIGURE 15.2. Wegener's granulomatosis. **A:** Intravenous contrast-enhanced conventional (7-mm collimation) CT image at level of T1 vertebral body shows both intraluminal (*curved arrow*) and extraluminal (*straight arrows*) soft-tissue lesion in cervical trachea. **B:** CT scan obtained at level of thoracic inlet shows crescentic soft tissue thickening of tracheal wall (*arrows*). A nodule is also evident in right upper lobe. **C:** Photomicrography of a biopsy specimen shows a mixed inflammatory cell infiltrate (lymphocytes, eosinophils (*small arrows*) and occasional multinucleated giant cells (*arrowhead*) characteristic of Wegener's granulomatosis. Admixed mature fibrous tissue is also evident (*large arrows*). (×100.) The patient was a 57-year-old man.

tation of well-established disease, stenosis is occasionally responsible for the initial presentation (5). Granulomatous inflammation and vasculitis typical of the disorder can be seen in the mucosa and submucosa in the early stage (Fig. 15.2). Fibrosis is seen later on. On CT, the subglottic region and proximal trachea are thickened and the lumen smoothly narrowed for a variable length (5,6). The narrowing may be symmetric or asymmetric (Fig. 15.2).

Tuberculosis

In the preantibiotic era, tracheobronchial involvement occurred in 10% to 20% of patients who had pulmonary tuberculosis (7). With improved treatment, the complication has decreased significantly in frequency. However, in areas of the world in which the disease has a high prevalence and treatment is suboptimal, it is not rare (8).

The complication probably develops most often by extension of disease from a lymph node into the adjacent airway wall or by spread of organisms from a focus of parenchymal disease within lymphatics in the airway mucosa and submucosa. The ensuing granulomatous inflammatory reaction results in swelling and, in some cases, ulceration of the mucosa (Fig. 15.3). Subsequent fibrosis may result in localized airway narrowing (8,9).

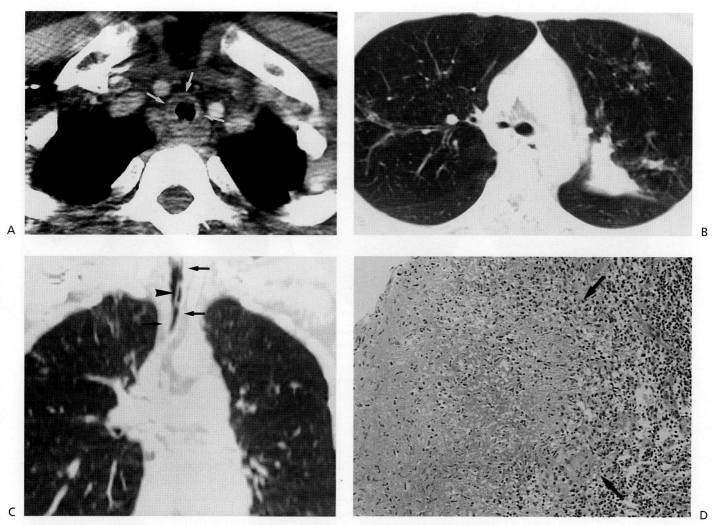

FIGURE 15.3. Active tracheal tuberculosis. **A:** Contrast-enhanced CT image (3-mm collimation) at level of thoracic inlet shows circumferential tracheal wall thickening (*arrows*). **B:** Image at the level of the azygos arch shows marked narrowing of the right main bronchus as well as parenchymal lesions consistent with tuberculosis in both upper lobes. **C:** Coronal reformation image of helical CT data shows marked narrowing of entire trachea associated with thickening of its wall (*arrows*). A pseudomembrane (*arrowhead*) is evident in the lumen. Parenchymal lesions consistent with tuberculosis are again seen in both upper lobes. **D:** Photomicrograph of a biopsy specimen from the trachea shows necrotic tissue bordered by a layer of epithelioid histiocytes (*arrows*) (necrotizing granulomatous inflammation). The epithelium has been destroyed, resulting in an intraluminal exudate (not shown) that corresponds to the pseudomembrane in the CT scan. (×100.) The patient was a 33-year-old woman.

On CT, active disease is manifested as circumferential wall thickening and irregular luminal narrowing (Fig. 15.3). When fibrosis develops, scans show areas of both smooth and irregular narrowing; wall thickening tends to be less than in patients with active disease (Fig. 15.4). Tracheal tuberculosis typically involves a long segment of the distal trachea and is almost always associated with bronchial infection (8).

Tracheobronchial Papillomatosis

Tracheobronchial papillomatosis is caused by human papillomavirus and is usually acquired at birth from an infected mother. The larynx is affected most commonly; extension into the trachea and proximal bronchi occurs occasionally. Exceptionally, the infection spreads into the lung parenchyma. The virus causes proliferation of airway

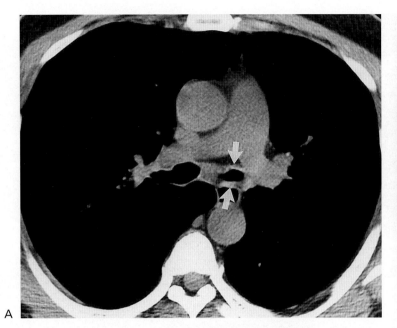
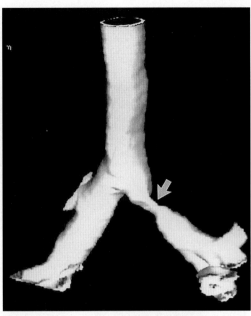

FIGURE 15.4. Bronchial narrowing due to healed tuberculosis. **A:** CT image (3-mm collimation) at the level of main bronchi shows thickening of the wall of left main bronchus (*arrows*) and narrowing of its lumen. **B:** Three-dimensional reconstruction using shaded-surface-display technique shows focal smooth narrowing of left main bronchus (*arrow*). The patient was a 47-year-old woman with previous tuberculosis.

epithelial cells, resulting in the formation of papillae that project into the airway lumen (Fig. 15.5). The resulting "tumors" may be localized and few in number or so numerous as to form a "carpet" over large areas of the mucosa. Proliferation of infected cells in the pulmonary parenchyma occurs largely within alveolar airspaces, resulting in the formation of nodules. The keratinized debris formed by the cells as they mature can accumulate in the central portion of the nodule or be expelled via the airways, resulting in a cavity. Although benign, papillomas may undergo transformation to squamous cell carcinoma (10).

The typical radiologic findings consist of multiple small nodules projecting into the airway lumen or diffuse nodular thickening of the airway wall (11,12) (Fig. 15.5). Involvement of the distal airways and parenchyma can be manifested as multiple nodules (13,14). These can measure up to several centimeters in diameter and frequently cavitate (13,14). The cavities usually have thin walls (14). Endobronchial papillomas also can result in obstructive pneumonitis and atelectasis (15).

Benign Neoplasms

Benign neoplasms constitute less than 10% of all airway neoplasms and are almost all derived from mesenchymal tissue. The most common are hamartoma, leiomyoma, neurogenic tumor (Schwannoma), and lipoma. They tend to be well demarcated, round, and less than 2 cm in diameter. Because they originate in the mucosa or submucosa, the overlying epithelium is usually intact, resulting in a smooth appearance of the tumor surface in the airway lumen (Fig. 15.6).

The radiologic appearance typically consists of a smoothly marginated intraluminal polyp (11,16). The neoplasm may appear to be limited by airway cartilage on CT (Fig. 15.6); however, some tumors, especially leiomyoma, may be seen to extend beneath the cartilage into the most peripheral portion of the airway wall. Hamartomas and lipomas may demonstrate fat attenuation on CT (16).

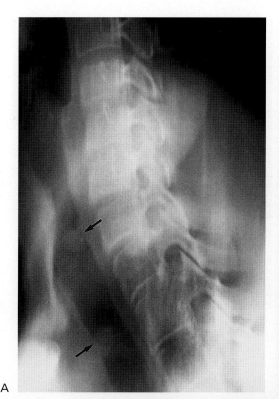

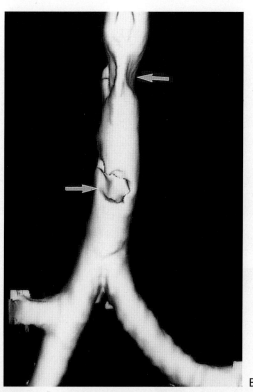

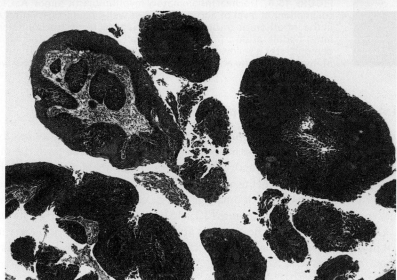

FIGURE 15.5. Tracheal papillomatosis. **A:** Sagittal image of a conventional tomogram shows multiple intraluminal nodules (*arrows*) in the tracheal air column. **B:** Three-dimensional reconstruction of the trachea from spiral CT using shaded-surface-display technique shows multifocal indentations (*arrows*) caused by the nodules. **C:** Low-magnification view of a biopsy specimen shows several papillary projections lined by squamous epithelium. The patient was a 40-year-old woman. (Courtesy of Dr. Jin Mo Goo, Department of Radiology, Seoul National University Hospital, Seoul, Korea.)

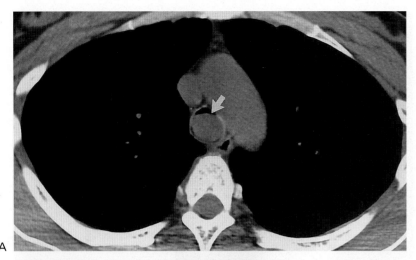

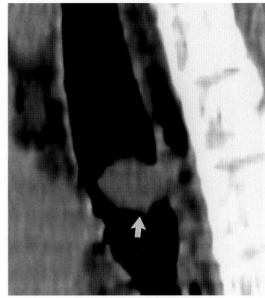

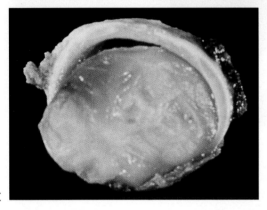

FIGURE 15.6. Tracheal inflammatory myofibroblastic tumor. **A:** CT image (3-mm collimation) at level of aortic arch shows well-circumscribed intraluminal nodule in the intrathoracic trachea (*arrow*). **B:** Sagittal reconstruction shows a pedunculated nodule arising from posterior wall of trachea. **C:** The excised specimen demonstrates a yellowish tan nodule in the tracheal lumen. There is no evidence of invasion into the adjacent wall. The patient was a 42-year-old woman.

Primary Malignant Neoplasms

Primary malignant tracheal neoplasms are uncommon, accounting for less than 1% of all thoracic malignancies. The vast majority are carcinomas derived from the surface epithelium (squamous cell carcinoma) (Fig. 15.7) or the epithelium of the tracheobronchial glands (the most common being adenoid cystic carcinoma) (Fig. 15.8). Other neoplasms, such as mucoepidermoid carcinoma (Fig. 15.9), carcinoid tumor, lymphoma, plasmacytoma, and adenocarcinoma, are rare (2,17,18).

On CT, malignant tracheal tumors appear as a mass of soft-tissue attenuation, most often in the posterior and lateral wall (2,18). They are often sessile and eccentric, result-

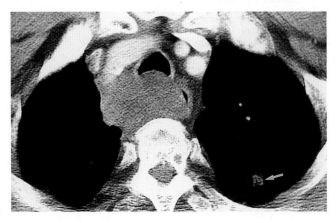

FIGURE 15.7. Tracheal squamous cell carcinoma. Conventional (7-mm collimation) CT image at level of thoracic inlet shows soft-tissue mass involving the posterior tracheal wall and infiltrating the adjacent mediastinum and right upper lobe. A small metastasis is evident in left upper lobe (*arrow*). The patient was a 77-year-old man.

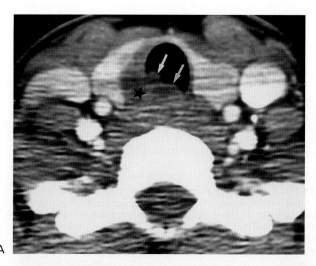

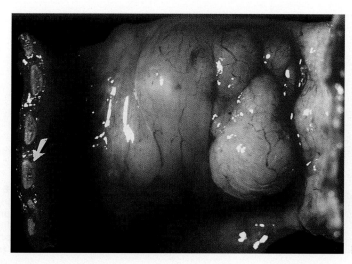

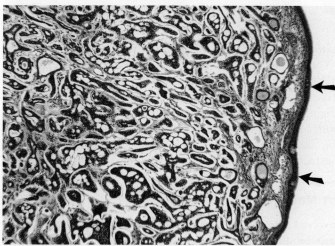

FIGURE 15.8. Tracheal adenoid cystic carcinoma. **A:** Contrast-enhanced CT image (7-mm collimation) at level of thyroid shows a heterogeneous soft-tissue lesion involving the posterolateral wall of the trachea. Both intraluminal (*arrows*) and extraluminal (star) components are evident. **B:** A surgically resected specimen from another patient shows several smooth-surfaced polypoid projections in the tracheal lumen (*arrow* indicates transected cartilage plate in the lateral wall). **C:** Low-magnification view of the tumor shows numerous irregularly shaped, smooth bordered clusters of neoplastic cells. Many of the clusters contain oval or round clear spaces (cribriform pattern), characteristic of adenoid cystic carcinoma. Note the intact tracheal epithelium (*arrows*).

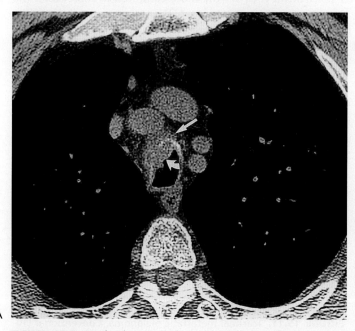

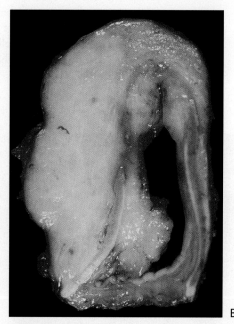

FIGURE 15.9. Tracheal mucoepidermoid carcinoma. **A:** CT image (1-mm collimation) at level of the great vessels shows an intraluminal (*curved arrow*) and extraluminal (*straight arrow*) tumor in the trachea. **B:** Sagittal section of the excised specimen also shows both intraluminal and extraluminal components. The patient was a 69-year-old man.

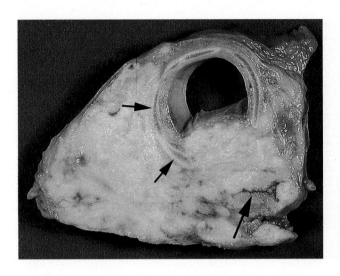

FIGURE 15.10. Esophageal carcinoma with mediastinal and tracheal invasion. A transverse section of the mediastinum shows extensive infiltration by carcinoma. The esophageal lumen has been reduced to a small slit (*long arrow*) by the primary tumor. Direct invasion of the posterior portion of the trachea is evident. *Short arrows* indicate the left lateral tracheal cartilage plates.)

ing in asymmetric luminal narrowing. About 10% are circumferential, a feature that is not seen in benign tumors (19). They can be polypoid and mostly intraluminal; however, mediastinal extension occurs in 30% to 40%. Because squamous cell carcinoma arises in the tracheal epithelium, the surface of the tumor is typically irregular (Fig. 15.7). By contrast, because of its submucosal origin, adenoid cystic carcinoma tends to be associated with an intact epithelium and a smooth contour (Fig. 15.8). Because evaluation of cephalocaudad extent of the tumors may be underestimated on cross-sectional CT images, evaluation with three-dimensional reconstructed images is recommended (20).

Secondary Malignant Neoplasms

The large airways may be involved secondarily by malignant neoplasms as a result of either hematogenous metastasis or direct invasion from the esophagus, thyroid, mediastinum, or lung. The latter mechanism is by far the more common; in most cases, the extramural source of the airway tumor is apparent on CT or gross examination (Fig. 15.10). Neoplasms that have a propensity to metastasize to the trachea and major bronchi include renal cell carcinoma and melanoma (Fig. 15.11). On CT, the resulting abnormalities are usually focal and include intraluminal soft-tissue nodules and wall thickening (2,18).

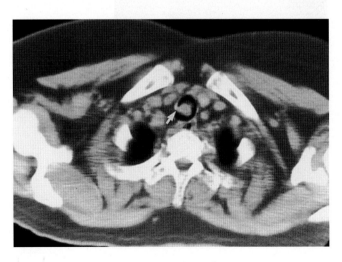

FIGURE 15.11. Tracheal metastatic melanoma. Conventional (10-mm collimation) CT image at level of thoracic inlet shows an intraluminal nodule with stalk (*arrow*). The patient was a 59-year-old woman.

DIFFUSE TRACHEAL NARROWING

Relapsing Polychondritis

Relapsing polychondritis is an unusual systemic disease that affects cartilage at various sites, including the ears, nose, joints, and tracheobronchial tree (21). The peak incidence of the disease is in the third and fourth decades; however, any age group may be affected. It is considered to have an autoimmune pathogenesis.

The larynx and subglottic trachea are often the initial sites of involvement in the lower respiratory tract. Symmetric subglottic stenosis is the most frequent manifestation. As the disease progresses, the distal trachea and bronchi may be involved (21). Histologically, the disease is characterized by an acute inflammatory infiltrate in the cartilage and perichondrial tissue. Dissolution and fragmentation of the cartilage ensue and may be followed by fibrosis.

CT scan images show smooth thickening of the airway wall associated with more or less diffuse narrowing. In the early stage, the membranous portion of the trachea (posterior wall) may be spared (Fig. 15.12). However, in advanced disease, circumferential wall

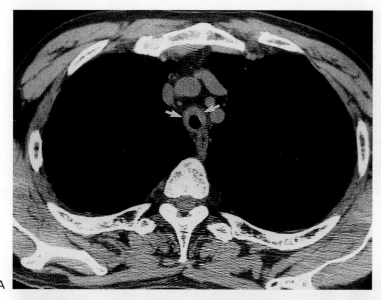

A

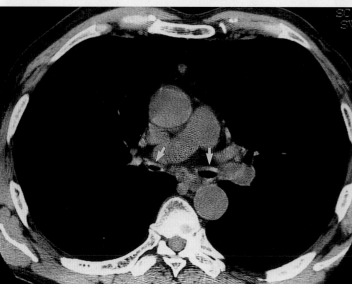

B

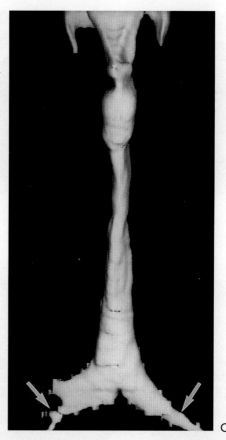

C

FIGURE 15.12. Relapsing polychondritis in a 67-year-old man. **A:** CT image (3-mm collimation) at level of the great vessels shows tracheal wall thickening. **B:** Image at the level of bronchus intermedius shows bronchial wall thickening (*arrows*) involving the anterior aspect of this bronchus and the distal left main bronchus. **C:** Three-dimensional reconstruction performed using shaded-surface-display technique shows extensive luminal narrowing of the intrathoracic trachea and some portions of left main bronchus and bronchus intermedius (*arrows*).

thickening may be seen (22,23). The trachea becomes flaccid, showing considerable collapse on expiratory images (18,22). Gross destruction of the cartilaginous rings associated with fibrosis and stenosis may occur (23).

Amyloidosis

Deposition of amyloid in the trachea and bronchi may be seen in association with systemic amyloidosis or as an isolated manifestation (17,18). The amyloid tends to be deposited initially in relation to tracheal gland acini and the walls of small blood vessels in the mucosa. As it increases in amount, the glands atrophy and the amyloid forms irregularly shaped plaques or nodules in the mucosa. These are usually multifocal; less commonly, there is a single masslike lesion. The overlying mucosa is usually intact (Fig. 15.13), resulting in a smooth appearance to the intraluminal aspect. Dystrophic calcification or ossification is frequently present histologically.

CT scan images show focal or, more commonly, diffuse thickening of the airway wall and narrowing of the lumen (18,24). Calcification may be seen (Fig. 15.13). Narrowing

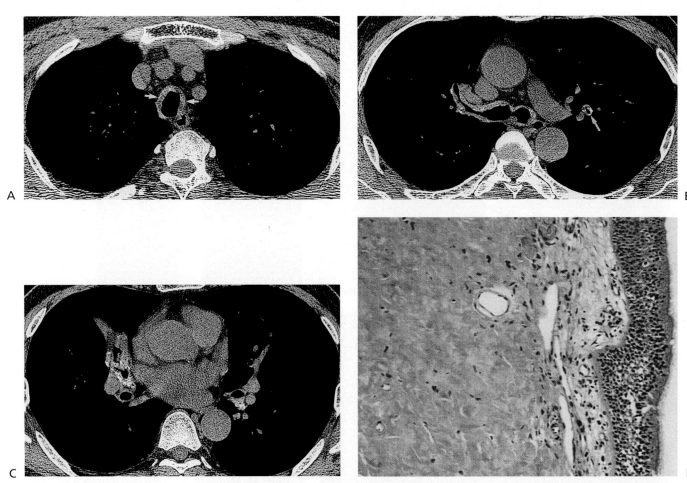

FIGURE 15.13. Tracheobronchial amyloidosis. **A:** CT image (3-mm collimation) at the level of great vessels shows circumferential tracheal wall thickening (*arrows*) with some flecks of calcification. **B:** Image at the level of main bronchi shows circumferential bronchial wall thickening with foci of calcification. Also note involvement of segmental bronchus (*arrow*) in left upper lobe. **C:** Image at the level of left atrium shows bronchial wall thickening and foci of calcification in right middle lobar bronchus and left basal trunk. Middle lobe atelectasis is also apparent. **D:** Photomicrograph of a bronchoscopic biopsy specimen shows the presence of amorphous eosinophilic material (amyloid) in the mucosa. The overlying epithelium is intact. (×40.) The patient was a 54-year-old man.

of the proximal bronchi can lead to distal atelectasis and postobstructive pneumonia (24,25).

Tracheobronchopathia Osteochondroplastica

Tracheobronchopathia osteochondroplastica is characterized by the presence of multiple osteocartilaginous nodules on the inner surface of the trachea (26). Men are more frequently involved than women and most patients are more than 50 years of age (27,28).

Histologically, the disorder is characterized by mucosal and submucosal foci of hyaline cartilage that may be calcified or contain foci of lamellar bone. The mucosal surface is intact. Connection between the osteocartilaginous nodules and the perichondrium of the tracheobronchial cartilage plates can usually be demonstrated (17). Because it contains no cartilage, the posterior wall of the trachea is spared (6,28).

The chest radiograph shows multiple sessile nodules that project into the tracheal lumen (27). Calcification may or may not be evident. The abnormalities extend over a long segment of the trachea (27). On CT, tracheal cartilages are thickened and show irregular calcification (28) (Fig. 15.14). The nodules can be seen protruding from the anterior and lateral walls into the lumen. They usually show foci of calcification.

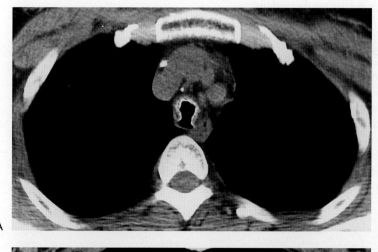

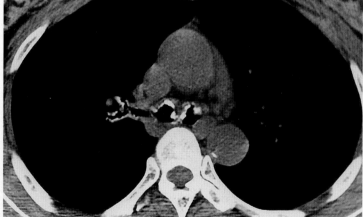

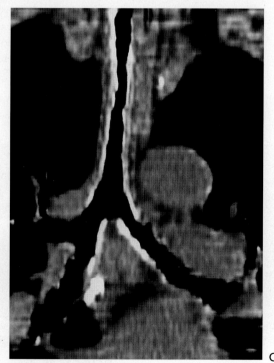

A

B

C

FIGURE 15.14. Tracheobronchopathia osteochondroplastica. **A:** Mediastinal window of CT (3-mm collimation) scan obtained at level of great vessels shows tracheal wall thickening and calcification. The posterior wall is spared. **B:** Scan obtained at level of main bronchi shows bronchial wall thickening and foci of calcification. **C:** Coronal reconstruction shows tracheal and bronchial wall thickening and foci of calcification. The patient was a 54-year-old woman.

Tracheobronchitis Associated with Ulcerative Colitis

Airway disease is relatively uncommon in ulcerative colitis but may take several forms, including ulcerative tracheitis and tracheobronchitis, bronchiectasis, and small-airway disease, most commonly obliterative bronchiolitis.

Tracheobronchitis is characterized histologically by more or less concentric mucosal and submucosal fibrosis and chronic inflammation. Ulceration and luminal narrowing may be evident. In the trachea, both the membranous and cartilaginous portions are affected (18,29). On CT, the tracheal wall is diffusely thickened and shows irregular luminal narrowing. Bronchial wall thickening also may be present (18).

Saber-Sheath Trachea

Saber-sheath trachea is defined as a trachea that has a coronal diameter equal to or less than one-half its sagittal diameter, measured at 1 cm above the top of the aortic arch (30,31). The abnormality affects only the intrathoracic trachea, with abrupt widening of the tracheal lumen above the thoracic inlet. It has been described exclusively in men (9,30). Most affected individuals have chronic obstructive pulmonary disease, and it has been suggested that mechanical forces related to hyperinflated lungs cause the coronal diameter of the intrathoracic trachea to narrow and the sagittal diameter to elongate. The trachea usually shows a smooth inner margin but occasionally has a nodular contour (32). Calcification of the tracheal cartilage is frequently evident.

Tracheobronchomalacia

The term *tracheobronchomalacia* refers to a weakening of the tracheal and proximal bronchial walls that is manifested by collapse during forced expiration. The condition has been associated with intubation, chronic obstructive pulmonary disease, trauma, recurrent infections, and polychondritis. The underlying feature of most of these conditions is necrosis of cartilage and its replacement by relatively flaccid fibrous tissue.

On CT, tracheobronchomalacia is diagnosed when the airways show narrowing of their luminal diameter by more than 50% on expiration, compared with that on inspiration (18) (Fig. 15.15).

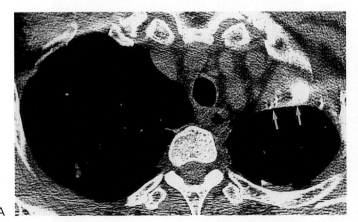
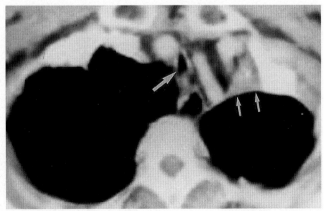

A   B

FIGURE 15.15. Tracheomalacia. **A:** Inspiratory HRCT image (1-mm collimation) at the level of the thoracic inlet shows a normal tracheal diameter. Note left upper lobe atelectasis (*arrows*). The foci of calcification within left upper lobe are presumably related to previous granulomatous infection. **B:** Expiratory CT (10-mm collimation) image at a similar level as **A** shows marked narrowing (*large arrow*) of the tracheal lumen. The atelectatic left upper lobe is also evident (*small arrows*). The patient was a 61-year-old woman.

TRACHEOBRONCHOMEGALY (MOUNIER-KUHN DISEASE)

Tracheobronchomegaly is considered to be present when the coronal and sagittal diameters of the trachea are greater than 3 cm. It is an uncommon condition that is seen predominantly in men in the fourth and fifth decades.

The abnormality has been documented in association with connective-tissue disorders such as Ehlers-Danlos syndrome and in some congenital syndromes affecting the skeleton, suggesting an intrinsic abnormality in airway structure. In fact, histologic examination of the airways in some patients has shown thinning of muscle, cartilage, and/or elastic tissue (33). In some cases, the cartilaginous rings of the tracheal wall dilate and the intercartilaginous portions bulge outward, forming diverticula-like protrusions that may have an irregularly corrugated or scalloped appearance on CT (34,35). The entire trachea and the carina are involved. Bronchiectasis of the first to fourth order bronchi is commonly present (18, 36) (Fig. 15.16).

The diagnosis is made on the radiograph and on CT when the diameter of tracheal lumen is more than 3 cm and those of the right and left mainstem bronchi are more than 2.4 and 2.3 cm, respectively (18) (Fig. 15.16).

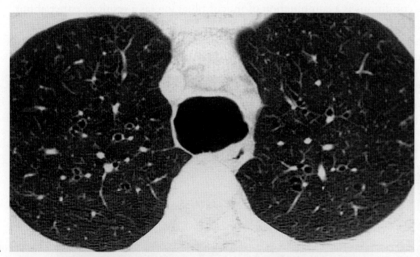

A

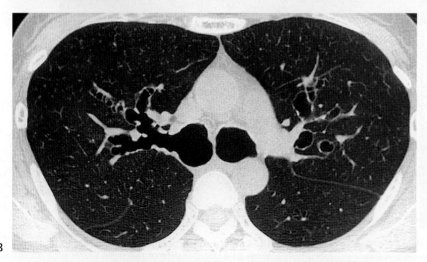

B

FIGURE 15.16. Tracheobronchomegaly (Mounier-Kuhn disease). **A:** HRCT image (1-mm collimation) at the level of the great vessels shows a markedly enlarged trachea as well as mild dilatation of segmental and subsegmental upper lobe bronchi. **B:** Image at the level of the main bronchi shows markedly enlarged luminal diameter of main, lobar and segmental airways. The patient was a 50-year-old woman.

BRONCHIECTASIS

Bronchiectasis is defined as chronic irreversible dilatation of bronchi. Although there are many specific underlying causes, from a pathogenetic point of view there are three mechanisms by which the dilatation can develop: bronchial obstruction, bronchial wall damage, and parenchymal fibrosis (traction bronchiectasis). Bronchial obstruction is caused most often by an intraluminal lesion, the most frequent of which is a carcinoma (Fig. 15.17); rarely, a benign process such as a fibrous stricture (e.g., after tuberculosis) or broncholithiasis is the cause. Occasionally, the airway obstruction is the result of extrinsic compression by enlarged lymph nodes or a neoplasm within the parenchyma. Whether the cause of the obstruction is intrinsic or extrinsic, there is usually enough atelectasis and obstructive pneumonitis in the associated lung parenchyma as well as mucus plugging of the ectatic airways that the bronchiectasis is not apparent radiographically. However, its presence can be detected in some cases on CT by the presence linear, sometimes branching bands of decreased attenuation (corresponding to intraluminal mucus) in the area of obstructive pneumonitis.

Bronchial wall injury is the underlying mechanism behind a variety of causes of bronchiectasis, including cystic fibrosis, childhood viral and bacterial infection (Fig. 15.18), immunodeficiency disorders, dyskinetic cilia syndrome, allergic bronchopulmonary aspergillosis, and lung and bone marrow transplantation. The common factor in many of these conditions is a combination of mucus plugging (as a result of either abnormal mucus or a deficiency in its clearance by the bronchial mucociliary escalator) and bacterial colonization. The latter is likely to be particularly important, as the cytokines and enzymes released by inflammatory cells attracted to the bronchus as well as toxins derived from the bacteria themselves result in a cycle of increasing airway wall damage, mucus retention, and bacterial proliferation.

Parenchymal fibrosis from a variety of causes, including tuberculosis, sarcoidosis, and idiopathic pulmonary fibrosis, can also cause bronchiectasis. As might be anticipated, the

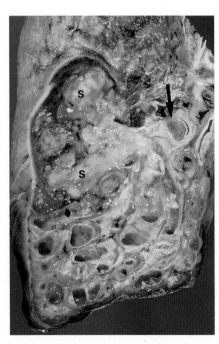

FIGURE 15.17. Postobstructive bronchiectasis. A sagittal slice of a resected right lung shows marked varicose bronchiectasis of the basal segmental airways. (The mucus with which they were filled was washed away to demonstrate the lumina.) Squamous cell carcinoma can be seen obstructing the lower lobe bronchus (*arrow*) and distending the subsegmental bronchi of the superior segment (*s*).

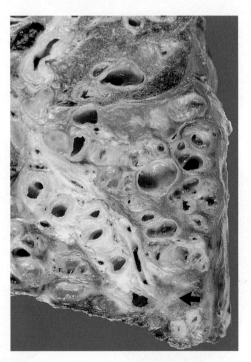

FIGURE 15.18. Lower lobe bronchiectasis following childhood pneumonia. View of a sagittal slice of the right lower lobe shows extensive bronchiectasis (varicose and cylindrical patterns). Patchy foci of parenchymal fibrosis and organizing pneumonia (*arrow*) are evident between the ectatic airways. The patient was a 39-year-old woman who had a history of pneumonia (presumed viral) as a child.

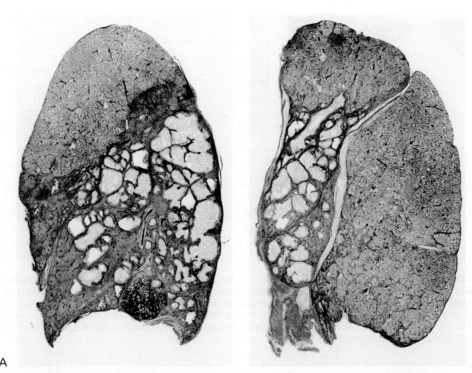

A   B

FIGURE 15.19. Bronchiectasis—gross appearance. Whole-mount slices of the right (**A**) and left (**B**) lungs show patchy bronchiectasis in the lower and middle lobes on the right and the lingula on the left. On the right side, the disease can be classified as cystic in the superior segment of the lower lobe, varicose in the middle lobe, and cylindrical in the posterior basal portion of the lower lobe.

dilatation is caused by maturation and retraction of fibrous tissue located in the parenchyma adjacent to an airway (hence the term *traction bronchiectasis*) (37,38). Such bronchiectasis is usually localized; identification of the specific region affected may give a clue to the underlying cause (e.g., bronchiectasis localized to or most severe in the apicoposterior segment of an upper lobe is suggestive of tuberculosis).

Grossly, bronchiectasis has been traditionally classified into three subtypes, reflecting increasing severity of disease (Fig. 15.19): (a) cylindrical, characterized by relatively uniform airway dilatation; (b) varicose, characterized by nonuniform, somewhat serpiginous dilatation; and (c) cystic. As the extent and degree of airway dilatation increases, the lung parenchyma distal to the affected airways shows increasing collapse or fibrosis. Thus the ends of the dilated airway segments appear closer to the pleura than normal airways of the same diameter.

Histologically, the bronchial wall is usually thickened as a result of an infiltrate of mononuclear inflammatory cells and an increase in fibrous tissue (Fig. 15.20). Neutrophils also may be seen, both within the airway wall and in its lumen (39,40); they are particularly abundant in the latter location in cystic fibrosis. With progression of disease, mucosal elastic tissue and muscle is lost and there may be destruction of cartilage. Bronchiolitis, often associated with fibrosis and luminal distortion, is common (41).

Bronchiectasis may manifest on the chest radiograph as thickened bronchial walls visible as parallel lines (so-called tram lines). When seen end-on, bronchiectatic airways appear as poorly defined ring shadows. Dilated bronchi filled with mucus and pus result in tubular or ovoid opacities. Cystic bronchiectasis manifests as multiple thin-walled ring shadows often containing air–fluid levels.

HRCT findings include lack of tapering of bronchial lumina, internal diameter of bronchi greater than that of the adjacent pulmonary artery, visualization of bronchi within 1 cm of the costal pleura or abutting the mediastinal pleura, and mucus-filled dilated bronchi (41,42) (Figs. 15.20 to 15.22). Associated CT findings of bronchiolitis—areas of

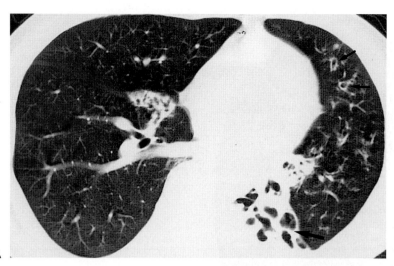

A

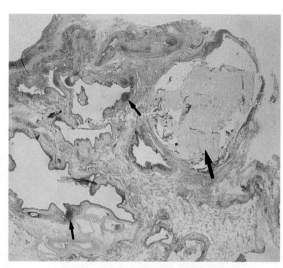

B

FIGURE 15.20. Bronchiectasis. **A:** CT image (2.5-mm collimation) at the level of the right inferior pulmonary vein shows cystic (*large arrow*) and cylindrical (*small arrows*) bronchiectasis. **B:** A low-magnification photomicrograph shows several dilated bronchi, the walls of which are thickened by fibrous tissue and an inflammatory cell infiltrate (focally with lymphoid follicles [*small arrows*]). Abundant mucus is present in one airway (*large arrow*) (×2.). The patient was a 53-year-old man who had previous tuberculosis.

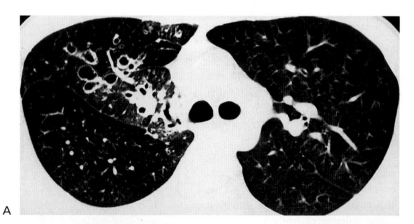

A

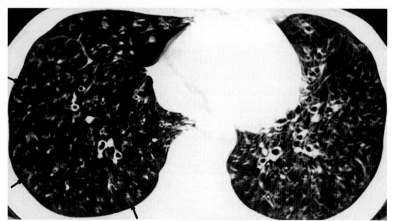

B

FIGURE 15.21. Bronchiectasis. **A:** HRCT image (1-mm collimation) at the level of the main bronchi shows ectatic right upper lobe bronchi. Some areas of ground-glass opacity are also evident, presumably representing aspirated blood (the patient presented with hemoptysis). **B:** HRCT image at the level of the basal segments shows bronchiectasis and centrilobular nodules and branching linear structures (*arrows*) reflecting bronchiolitis and/or filling of ectatic bronchioles with mucus. The patient was a 28-year-old man with ciliary dyskinesia.

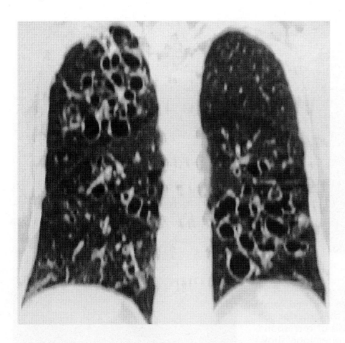

FIGURE 15.22. Cystic bronchiectasis. A coronal (1.5-mm collimation) reformation image shows clusters of cysts in both lungs. The distribution of the bronchiectasis suggests that it was a complication of previous viral infection. The patient was a 34-year-old man.

decreased attenuation and vascularity, bronchiolectasis, and centrilobular nodules or branching structures (tree-in-bud appearance)—are seen in about 75% of patients (41–43) (Fig. 15.21).

BRONCHOLITHIASIS

Broncholithiasis is defined as the presence of calcified material within the bronchial lumen. Most broncholiths are composed of fragments of calcified material that were originally located in a peribronchial lymph node. The underlying abnormality is usually granulomatous lymphadenitis caused by *Mycobacterium tuberculosis* or fungi such as *Histoplasma capsulatum*. The process begins when foci of necrotic tissue associated with the inflammation undergo dystrophic calcification. Over time, rubbing of the overlying bronchial wall against the node results in erosion of the calcified focus into the lumen. Identification of calcified material within an acute inflammatory exudate or granulation tissue should suggest the diagnosis on bronchoscopic biopsy specimens (Fig. 15.23).

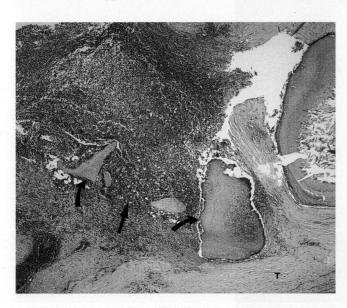

FIGURE 15.23. Broncholithiasis. A photomicrograph of bronchial wall shows fibrous tissue (*T*) and granulation tissue (*straight arrow*) containing irregularly shaped fragments of calcified necrotic material (*curved arrows*). The last named were shown to contain fungal organisms consistent with *Histoplasma capsulatum*. Similar material was found in a lymph node adjacent to the airway wall.

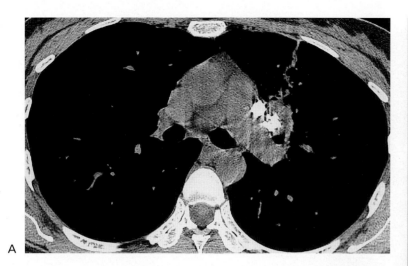

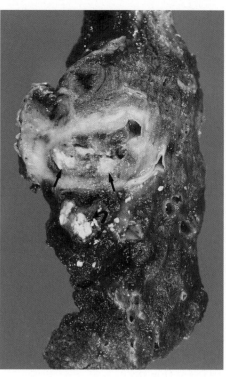

FIGURE 15.24. Broncholithiasis in a 44-year-old woman. **A:** CT image (1-mm collimation) at the level of the main bronchi shows calcified lymph nodes in the aortopulmonary window. Obstruction of the anterior segmental bronchus of left upper lobe and partial atelectasis of corresponding segment are also evident. **B:** The resected left upper lobe shows bronchial wall fibrosis and luminal obstruction by an inflammatory exudate and granulation tissue. Calcified debris is evident in the airway lumen (*straight arrows*) and peribronchial lymph node (*curved arrow*).

Bronchial wall fibrosis (Fig. 15.24) and obstructive pneumonitis (Fig. 15.25) may be apparent in gross specimens.

Radiographic findings are nonspecific and include lymph node calcification, and lobar or segmental atelectasis. In the majority of cases, the diagnosis can be made on CT by identifying a focus of calcified material within a bronchial lumen; peribronchial lymph node calcification is common (44,45) (see Fig. 15.24). When broncholithiasis is suspected, 2- to 3-mm collimation CT should be obtained to minimize the effect of partial volume averaging and to allow better localization of the calcified lymph node.

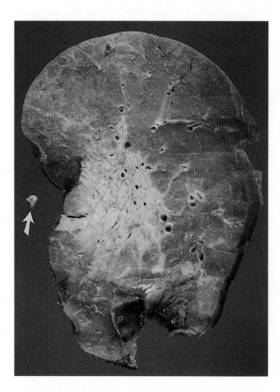

FIGURE 15.25. Broncholithiasis in a 50-year-old man. A sagittal slice of a left upper lobe shows a fairly well-circumscribed focus of parenchymal consolidation and interlobular septal fibrosis in the region of the superior lingular segment. Microscopic examination showed obstructive pneumonitis. An irregularly shaped broncholith (*arrow*) was found in the subtending bronchus.

REFERENCES

1. James AE, MacMillan AS, Eaton SB, et al. Roentgenology of tracheal stenosis resulting form cuffed tracheostomy tube. *Am J Roentgenol* 1970;109:455–458.
2. Marom EM, Goodman PC, McAdams HP. Focal abnormalities of the trachea and main bronchi. *Am J Roentgenol* 2001;176:707–711.
3. McDonald TJ, Neel HB, DeRemee RA. Wegener's granulomatosis of the subglottis and the upper portion of the trachea. *Ann Otol Rhinol Laryngol*1982;91:588–592.
4. Langford CA, Sneller MC, Hallahan CW, et al. Clinical features and therapeutic management of subglottic stenosis in patients with Wegener's granulomatosis. *Arthritis Rheum*1996;39:1754–1760.
5. Stein MG, Gamsu G, Webb WR. et al. Computed tomography of diffuse tracheal stenosis in Wegener granulomatosis. *J Comput Assist Tomogr* 1986;10:868–870.
6. Shepherd JO, McLoud TC. Imaging the airways: computed tomography and magnetic resonance imaging. *Clin Chest Med* 1991;12:151–168.
7. Lukomsky GI, Tetarchenko VE. *Bronchology.* St. Louis: Mosby, 1979:287–305.
8. Kim Y, Lee KS, Yoon JH, et al. Tuberculosis of the trachea and main bronchi: CT findings in 17 patients. *Am J Roentgenol* 1997;168:1051–1056.
9. Kim YH, Kim HT, Lee KS, et al. Serial fiberoptic bronchoscopic observations of endobronchial tuberculosis before and early after antituberculous chemotherapy. *Chest* 1993;103:673–677.
10. Guillou L, Sahli R, Chaubert P, et al. Squamous cell carcinoma of the lung in a non-smoking, non-irradiated patient with juvenile papillomatosis: evidence of human papillomavirus-11 DNA in both carcinoma and papillomas. *Am J Surg Pathol* 1991;15:891–898.
11. McCarthy MJ, Rosado-de-Christenson ML. Tumors of the trachea. *J Thorac Imaging* 1995;10:180–198.
12. Takasugi JE, Godwin JD. The airway. *Semin Roentgenol*1991;26:175–190.
13. Gruden JF, Webb R, Sides DM. Adult-onset disseminated tracheobronchial papillomatosis: CT features. *J Comput Assist Tomogr* 1994;18:640–642.
14. Kotylak TB, Barrie JR, Raymond GS. Tracheobronchial papillomatosis with spread to pulmonary parenchyma and the development of squamous cell carcinoma. *Can Assoc Radiol J* 2001;52:126–128.
15. Kramer SS, Wehunt WD, Stocker JT, et al. Pulmonary manifestations of juvenile laryngotracheal papillomatosis. *Am J Roentgenol* 1985;144:687–694.
16. Reittner P, Müller NL. Tracheal hamartoma: CT findings in two patients. *J Comput Assist Tomogr* 1999;23:957–958.
17. Choplin RH, Wehunt WD, Theros EG. Diffuse lesions of the trachea. *Semin Roentgenol* 1983;18:38–50.
18. Kwong JS, Müller NL, Miller RR. Diseases of the trachea and main-stem bronchi: correlation of CT with pathologic findings. *Radiographics* 1992;12:645–657.
19. Houston HE, Payne WS, Harrison EG, et al. Primary cancers of the trachea. *Arch Surg* 1969;99:132–140.
20. Lee KS, Yoon JH, Kim TK, et al. Evaluation of tracheobronchial disease with helical CT with multiplanar and three-dimensional reconstruction: correlation with bronchoscopy. *Radiographics* 1997;17:555–567.
21. Kilman WJ. Narrowing of the airway in relapsing polychondritis. *Radiology* 1978;126:373–376.
22. Müller NL, Miller NL, Ostrow DN, et al. Clinico-radiologic-pathologic conference: diffuse thickening of the tracheal wall. *Can Assoc Radiol J* 1989;40:213–215.
23. Im J-G, Chung JW, Han SK, et al. CT manifestations of tracheobronchial involvement in relapsing polychondritis. *J Comput Assist Tomogr* 1988;12:792–793.
24. Pickford HA, Swensen SJ, Utz JP. Thoracic cross-sectional imaging of amyloidosis. *Am J Roentgenol* 1997;168:351–355.
25. Kim HY, Im JG, Song KS, et al. Localized amyloidosis of the respiratory system: CT features. *J Comput Assist Tomogr* 1999;23:627–631.
26. Lundgren R, Stjernberg NL. Tracheobronchopathia osteochondroplastica: a clinical bronchoscopic and spirometric study. *Chest* 1981;80:706–709.
27. Young RH, Sandstrom RE, Mark GJ. Tracheopathia osteoplastica: clinical, radiologic, and pathological correlations. *J Thorac Cardiovasc Surg* 1980;79:537–541.
28. Onitsuka H, Hirose N, Watanabe K, et al. Computed tomography of tracheopathia osteoplastica. *Am J Roentgenol* 1983;140:268–270.
29. Wilcox P, Miller R, Miller G, et al. Airway involvement in ulcerative colitis. *Chest* 1987;92:18–22.
30. Greene R. "Saber-sheath" trachea: relation to chronic obstructive pulmonary disease. *Am J Roentgenol* 1978;130:441–445.
31. Trigaux JP, Hermes G, Dubois P, et al. CT of saber-sheath trachea: correlation with clinical, chest radiographic and functional findings. *Acta Radiol* 1994;35:247–250.
32. Rubenstein J, Weisbrod G, Steinhardt MI. Atypical appearances of "saber-sheath" trachea. *Radiology* 1978;127:41–42.
33. Al-mallah Z, Quantock OP. Tracheobronchomegaly. *Thorax* 1968;23:230–232.

34. Shin MS, Jackson RM, Ho KJ. Tracheobronchomegaly (Mounier-Kuhn syndrome): CT diagnosis. *Am J Roentgenol* 1988;150:770–779.
35. Dunne MG, Reiner B. CT features of tracheobronchomegaly. *J Comput Assist Tomogr* 1988;12:388–391.
36. Bateson EM, Woo-Ming M. Tracheobronchomegaly. *Clin Radiol* 1973;24:354–358.
37. Westcott JL, Cole SR. Traction bronchiectasis in end-stage pulmonary fibrosis. *Radiology* 1986;161:665–669.
38. Austin JHM, Müller NL, Friedman PJ, et al. Glossary of terms for CT of the lungs: recommendations of the nomenclature committee of the Fleischner Society. *Radiology* 1996;200:327–331.
39. Hansell DM. Bronchiectasis. *Radiol Clin North Am* 1998;36:107–128.
40. Lapa E, Silva JR, Jones JAH, et al. The immunologic component of the cellular inflammatory infiltrate in bronchiectasis. *Thorax* 1989;44:668–673.
41. Kang EY, Miller RR, Müller NL. Bronchiectasis: comparison of preoperative thin-section CT and pathologic findings in resected specimens. *Radiology* 1995;195:649–654.
42. Kim JS, Müller NL, Park CS, et al. Cylindrical bronchiectasis: diagnostic findings on thin-section CT. *Am J Roentgenol* 1997;168:751–754.
43. Hartman TE, Primack SL, Lee KS, et al. CT of bronchial and bronchiolar disease. *Radiographics* 1994;14:991–1003.
44. Shin MS, Ho K-J. Broncholithiasis: its detection by computed tomography in patients with recurrent hemoptysis of unknown etiology. *J Comput Tomogr* 1993;7:189–193.
45. Conces DJ, Tarver RD, Vix VA. Broncholithiasis: CT features in 15 patients. *Am J Roentgenol* 1991;157:249–253.

16

BRONCHIOLITIS

PATHOLOGIC CLASSIFICATION

RADIOLOGIC MANIFESTATIONS

SPECIFIC FORMS OF BRONCHIOLITIS
Infectious Bronchiolitis
Chronic Bronchiolitis
Obliterative Bronchiolitis
Bronchiolitis Obliterans Organizing Pneumonia

Bronchioles are, by definition, airways that do not contain cartilage. They are classified into membranous bronchioles, which are purely conductive, and respiratory bronchioles, which contain alveoli in their walls. The lobular bronchiole and pulmonary artery are located in the center of the secondary lobule. The lobular bronchiole divides into terminal bronchioles, which is the last generation of purely conductive airways. The terminal bronchioles themselves divide into two or three generations of respiratory bronchioles. The latter, along with alveolar ducts and sacs, comprise the gas-exchanging portion of the lung.

PATHOLOGIC CLASSIFICATION

Abnormalities that involve the bronchioles may originate in the bronchioles themselves or result by extension of disease that affects the bronchi, such as bronchiectasis; the adjacent lung parenchyma (such as in bronchopneumonia) may or may not be affected. Inflammation of the bronchioles (bronchiolitis) can be classified histologically based on a consideration of two pathologic processes: inflammation and fibrosis (Table 16.1). Although both processes are present in most examples of bronchiolitis, one or the other often predominates. The inflammatory component may be acute or chronic. As might be expected, the former (acute bronchiolitis) is usually associated with processes that cause bronchiolar injury over a short period of time, such as viral or mycoplasma infection (Fig. 16.1) or the inhalation of toxic gases. Chronic cellular bronchiolitis is associated with more prolonged injury and can itself have a variety of pathologic forms. Some of these are histologically distinctive and have been described by specific terms, such as *respiratory bronchiolitis, follicular bronchiolitis,* and *diffuse panbronchiolitis.*

Chronic bronchiolitis in which fibrosis is a prominent feature (sometimes referred to as *bronchiolitis obliterans*) is manifested by two major histologic patterns. The first, which we prefer to call *obliterative bronchiolitis* but which has also been termed *constrictive bronchiolitis,* is characterized by proliferation of fibrous tissue between the epithelium and the muscularis mucosa (Fig. 16.2). The proliferation results in more or less concentric narrowing of the airway lumen, which, in its most extreme form, can lead to complete obliteration. The epithelium overlying the abnormal fibrous tissue may be flattened or metaplastic but is usually intact (i.e., without evidence of ulceration).

By contrast, the epithelium in the second form of bronchiolitis obliterans is invariably absent, at least focally (Fig. 16.3). Granulation tissue and, eventually, fibroblastic tissue extend from the site of epithelial damage into the airway lumen, resulting in partial or complete obstruction. Although this histologic pattern may be the only abnormality seen in the lung, in most cases it is associated with similar epithelial injury and fibroblastic reaction in the adjacent alveolar airspaces (Fig. 16.3); that is, there is a combination of bron-

TABLE 16.1. BRONCHIOLITIS: HISTOLOGIC CLASSIFICATION

Predominantly inflammatory (cellular)
  Acute bronchiolitis
    Infection (viruses, *Mycoplasma pneumoniae,* some bacteria, and fungi)
    Toxic fumes and gases
  Chronic bronchiolitis
    Lymphoid hyperplasia (follicular bronchiolitis)
    Cigarette smoke (respiratory bronchiolitis)
    Inhaled allergens (extrinsic allergic alveolitis)
    Panbronchiolitis

Predominantly fibrotic
  Obliterative bronchiolitis
    Posttransplant (lung, bone marrow)
    Postinfectious (e.g., Swyer-James syndrome)
    Rheumatoid disease
  Bronchiolitis obliterans organizing pneumonia
    Infection
    Aspiration
    Drugs
    Connective-tissue disease
    Idiopathic (cryptogenic organizing pneumonia)

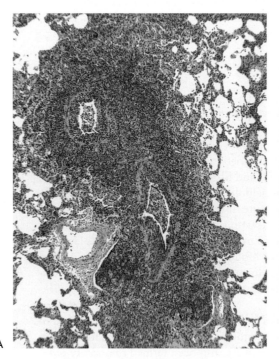
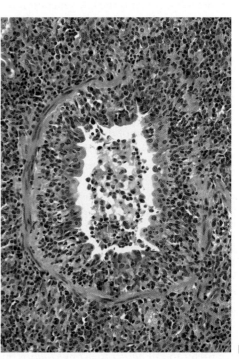

A

B

FIGURE 16.1. Acute bronchiolitis—*Mycoplasma pneumoniae.* **A:** Low-magnification photomicrograph shows marked inflammation of the wall of a membranous bronchiole; the adjacent parenchyma is relatively unaffected. **B:** Higher magnification shows a mixed cellular infiltrate (predominantly lymphocytes with scattered neutrophils) in the airway mucosa and epithelium. An exudate is evident in the airway lumen.

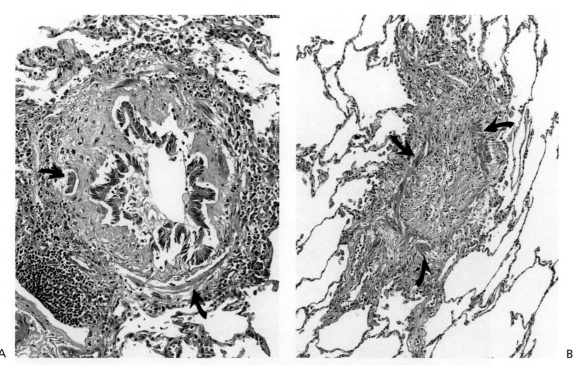

A

B

FIGURE 16.2. Chronic (obliterative) bronchiolitis. **A:** Photomicrograph of a membranous bronchiole shows a mild increase in the thickness of the lamina propria (tissue between the muscularis mucosa (*arrows*) and the epithelium) as a result of fibrous tissue. A moderately severe mononuclear inflammatory cell infiltrate is present in the peribronchiolar interstitial tissue; relatively few inflammatory cells are evident in the lamina propria itself. The airway epithelium is intact (its separation from the airway wall represents postmortem artifact). The patient was a 47-year-old man with rheumatoid disease. **B:** Photomicrograph of a more severely affected airway shows complete obliteration of the lumen by fibrous tissue (*arrows* indicate muscularis mucosa). The surrounding lung parenchyma is normal. The patient was a 39-year-old woman who had undergone bone marrow transplantation.

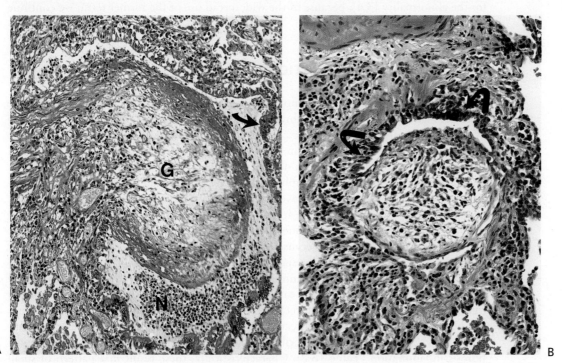

A

B

FIGURE 16.3. Chronic bronchiolitis with organizing pneumonia (BOOP). **A:** Photomicrograph shows focal ulceration of a membranous bronchiole with the presence of a polyp of granulation tissue (G) in the adjacent lumen. Residual epithelium is apparent opposite the area of ulceration (*arrow*) and an infiltrate of neutrophils (*N*) is present in the lumen. Incidental finding of uncertain (presumably infectious) etiology at autopsy. **B:** Second photomicrograph from a patient who had a clinical diagnosis of idiopathic BOOP shows a plug of fibroblastic tissue in the lumen of a membranous bronchiole. The epithelium is again intact focally (*arrows*). This appearance represents an advanced (healing) stage of the abnormality seen in **A.** (*Figure continues*)

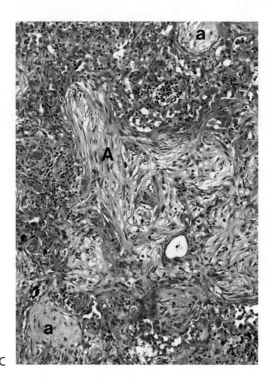

C

FIGURE 16.3. *(continued)* **C:** Third photomicrograph of the parenchyma adjacent to the bronchiole illustrated in **B** shows fibroblastic tissue completely occluding the lumen of a transitional airway (*A*) and several alveoli (*a*).

chiolitis and pneumonitis. As a result, the term *bronchiolitis obliterans organizing pneumonia* (BOOP) is frequently used to describe this form of disease (1,2). (Although we and others believe the term *cryptogenic organizing pneumonia* is a more appropriate designation for the abnormality [3,4], because of the widespread use of the former term, we continue to use it in this text.)

RADIOLOGIC MANIFESTATIONS

The radiographic features of bronchiolitis are related to a number of factors, including the extent of airway involvement, the chronicity of the disorder, and the presence or absence of underlying parenchymal disease. The manifestations are limited to three patterns: nodular or reticulonodular pattern in cellular bronchiolitis, hyperinflation and peripheral attenuation of vascular markings in obliterative bronchiolitis, and airspace consolidation in BOOP (2,5). The chest radiograph is also frequently normal in the presence of extensive bronchiolar abnormalities. However, because the radiographic findings are usually nonspecific, it plays a limited role in the differential diagnosis. Several radiologic and pathologic correlative studies have shown that HRCT reflects the predominant histologic pattern of bronchiolitis (2,5). Because of this ability, HRCT is the imaging method of choice for investigating a patient suspected of having this abnormality.

Normal bronchioles that have luminal diameters of approximately 0.6 mm and a wall thickness of approximately 0.1 mm cannot be identified on HRCT. However, the various forms of bronchiolitis often result in characteristic findings on HRCT (2,5). The findings can be classified as direct and indirect (2,6). Direct signs result from the presence of intraluminal exudate or tissue, peribronchiolar inflammation, or bronchiolar wall fibrosis/inflammation (Table 16.2). Characteristically, these result in a pattern of small centrilobular nodules and branching lines giving an appearance that resembles a tree in bud (7) (Fig. 16.4). A less common finding is the presence of centrilobular lucencies with well-defined walls, which represent bronchiolectasis (8,9) (Fig. 16.5). Indirect signs result from reflex vasoconstriction secondary to airway obstruction. The most important are areas of decreased attenuation and perfusion on inspiratory scans and air trapping on scans obtained at end expiration (10,11) (Fig. 16.6).

A tree-in-bud pattern is characteristic of acute infectious bronchiolitis, such as that caused by viruses and *M. pneumoniae* and by endobronchial spread of tuberculosis or non-tuberculous mycobacteria (12,13) (Fig. 16.4). It also may be seen in diffuse panbronchiolitis (14,15) (Fig. 16.5). Small centrilobular nodules reflecting bronchiolar inflammation and wall thickening can be seen sometimes in patients who have diseases that affect the larger airways, such as asthma, chronic obstructive pulmonary disease, and bronchiectasis (9). The centrilobular nodules in infectious bronchiolitis and panbronchiolitis usually have well-defined, sharp margins (2,9) (Fig. 16.4), whereas those seen in patients who have respiratory bronchiolitis typically have poorly defined margins (2,16) (Fig. 16.7).

Narrowing of the bronchiolar lumen, as is seen in obliterative (constrictive) bronchiolitis, results in decreased ventilation and reflex vasoconstriction (i.e., areas of decreased attenuation and vascularity). Redistribution of blood flow to uninvolved lung results in a heterogeneous pattern of attenuation known as mosaic attenuation (17,18) (Fig. 16.6). The variation in attenuation of individual lobules is accentuated on HRCT scans after maximal expiration (19,20).

Small, focal areas of low attenuation as well as small areas of air trapping can also be seen in healthy individuals (21,22). Although these can affect one or several lobules at various sites, they are most commonly seen in the superior segments of the lower lobes and near the tip of the lingula. Usually they involve less than 25% of the cross-sectional area of one lung at one scan level (21). Mosaic attenuation and air trapping can be considered abnormal when they affect a volume of lung equal to or greater than a pulmonary segment and are not limited to the superior segment of the lower lobe or the lingula tip (22,23). Mosaic attenuation and air trapping are seen on HRCT in patients who have obliterative bronchiolitis regardless of etiology (2,10), extrinsic allergic alveolitis (24), asthma (22,25), and bronchiectasis.

Unilateral or bilateral areas of consolidation are characteristic of BOOP. The consolidation is often patchy. Although it may have a random distribution, in about 60% of cases it affects mainly the peribronchial or subpleural lung regions (26,27). The consolidation

TABLE 16.2. BRONCHIOLITIS: DIFFERENTIAL DIAGNOSIS ON HRCT

Tree-in-bud pattern
  Infection
    Endobronchial spread of tuberculosis
    Mycobacterium-avium complex
    Viral, mycoplasmal, bacterial and fungal infections
  Panbronchiolitis
  Follicular bronchiolitis

Poorly defined centrilobular nodules
  Extrinsic allergic alveolitis
  Respiratory bronchiolitis
  RB-ILD

Decreased attenuation and airtrapping
  Obliterative (constrictive) bronchiolitis
    Lung, heart–lung, bone-marrow transplantation
    Postinfectious (Swyer-James syndrome)
    Toxic fume inhalation
    Collagen vascular disease
  Extrinsic allergic alveolitis

Airspace consolidation
  BOOP reaction associated with infection
  BOOP reaction due to drug reaction
  BOOP reaction associated with collagen vascular disease
  Idiopathic BOOP (cryptogenic organizing pneumonia)

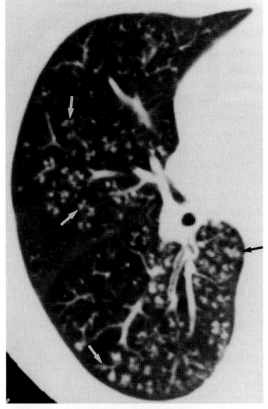

FIGURE 16.4. Tree-in-bud pattern—HRCT appearance and pathologic correlate. **A:** HRCT image of the right lung shows centrilobular nodules and branching lines (*arrows*) that have an appearance resembling a tree in bud. This pattern is typically seen in patients with infectious bronchiolitis or endobronchial spread of tuberculosis. The patient was a 68-year-old woman who had the latter abnormality. **B:** Magnified view of a slice of lung from another patient shows numerous foci of whitish consolidation, some of which have a branching appearance similar to that in the CT image. The patient also had endobronchial spread of tuberculosis. **C:** Photomicrograph of an open biopsy specimen from a third patient shows a longitudinal section of a bronchiole and two of its branches (*arrows* indicate the accompanying pulmonary artery). The histologic correlate of the tree-in-bud pattern is clearly evident. The bronchiolar lumens are obliterated by fibrous tissue and a chronic inflammatory infiltrate, indicating a healing stage of bronchiolitis. The cause was not identified but was presumed to be a virus. (HRCT courtesy of Dr. Jim Barrie, University of Alberta Medical School, Edmonton, Alberta, Canada.)

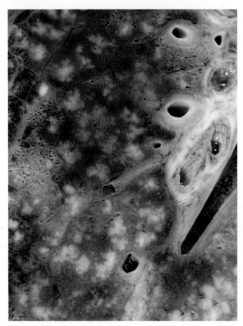

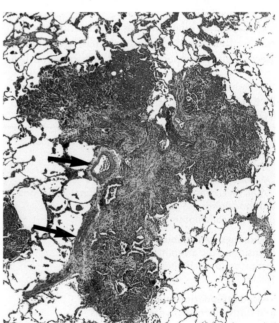

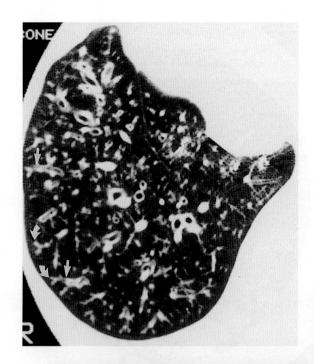

FIGURE 16.5. Bronchiolectasis. HRCT image of the right lower lobe shows thick-walled and dilated bronchioles (*straight arrows*), bronchial wall thickening, and centrilobular branching linear and nodular opacities (tree-in-bud appearance [*curved arrows*]). The patient was a 32-year-old man with panbronchiolitis and recurrent respiratory infections.

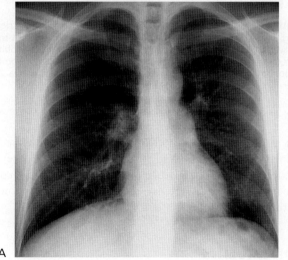

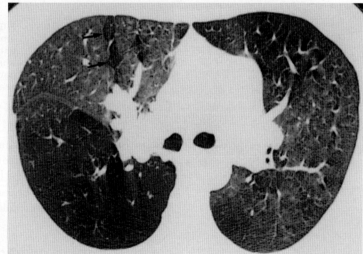

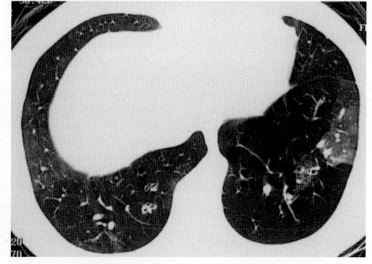

FIGURE 16.6. Obliterative bronchiolitis. **A:** Chest radiograph shows subtle areas of decreased vascularity. **B:** HRCT image at the level of the tracheal carina demonstrates markedly decreased attenuation in most of the right lower lobe, lobular areas of decreased attenuation in the right upper lobe (*arrows*) and patchy areas of decreased attenuation in the left lower lobe. Note areas with increased attenuation and vascularity in the right upper and left upper lobes secondary to blood flow redistribution. **C:** HRCT image through the lung bases shows extensive areas of low attenuation. The patient was a 36-year-old man with obliterative bronchiolitis presumed to be secondary to childhood viral infection.

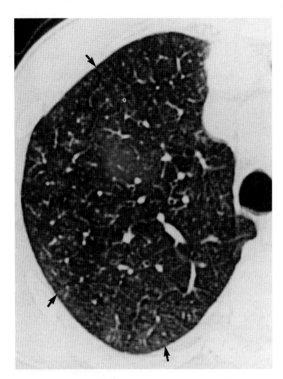

FIGURE 16.7. Respiratory bronchiolitis. HRCT image of the right upper lobe shows numerous poorly defined centrilobular nodules (*arrows*). The patient was a 49-year-old man. (Case courtesy of Dr. Martine Remy-Jardin, Hôpital Calmette, Lille, France.)

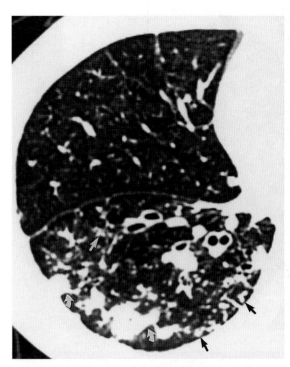

FIGURE 16.8. *Mycoplasma pneumonia.* HRCT image of the right lung shows branching linear and nodular opacities (tree-in-bud pattern; *straight arrows*) and lobular areas of airspace consolidation (*curved arrows*). The findings are characteristic of a combination of bronchiolitis and pneumonia. The patient was a 24-year-old woman with *Mycoplasma pneumonia.*

reflects the presence of organizing pneumonia. Centrilobular nodular opacities may be related to expansion of the bronchiolar lumen by fibroblastic tissue or (more commonly) to a combination of fibrosis in the lumen and adjacent alveolar airspaces. Focal areas of consolidation can also be seen in association with centrilobular nodular and branching linear opacities in infectious bronchiolitis and bronchopneumonia (13,28) (Fig. 16.8).

SPECIFIC FORMS OF BRONCHIOLITIS

Infectious Bronchiolitis

Infectious bronchiolitis is most often caused by viruses, *Mycoplasma pneumoniae*, *Haemophilus influenzae*, and *Chlamydia* species (1). It occurs most frequently in infants and children. However, it can occur in adults (28), particularly those who are immunocompromised (13,29).

The radiographic findings usually consist of a nodular or reticulonodular pattern. The characteristic finding on HRCT consists of a tree-in-bud pattern (Fig. 16.8). This pattern correlates pathologically with the presence of an intraluminal exudate and an inflammatory cell infiltrate within the walls of terminal and respiratory bronchioles (Fig. 16.4) (12). The abnormalities are characteristically centrilobular in distribution and are most easily identified in the lung periphery. Ill-defined nodules associated with branching airways also reflect the presence of bronchiolar and peribronchiolar granulomatous inflammation in patients who have endobronchial spread of tuberculosis (9,12) and chronic infection by *Mycobacterium avium-intracellulare* (30) (Fig. 16.4).

In some cases extension of infection from the airways into the adjacent lung parenchyma results in pneumonia. This is manifested as focal areas of ground-glass attenuation or consolidation, usually superimposed on the tree-in-bud pattern (13,28). These areas of parenchymal opacification frequently have a lobular distribution (Fig. 16.8).

Chronic Bronchiolitis

Chronic cellular bronchiolitis is commonly seen in association with extrinsic allergic alveolitis. The characteristic HRCT manifestations of EAA consist of diffuse, poorly defined centrilobular nodular opacities (31), reflecting the presence of an inflammatory cellular infiltrate in the bronchiolar wall and the peribronchiolar parenchyma (Fig. 16.9). More extensive alveolitis results in diffuse ground-glass attenuation. Most patients have lobular areas of air trapping caused by partial obstruction of the small airways (24).

Specific forms of chronic bronchiolitis include *respiratory bronchiolitis, follicular bronchiolitis,* and *diffuse panbronchiolitis.*

Respiratory Bronchiolitis

Respiratory bronchiolitis (RB) is characterized histologically by fibrosis and chronic inflammation (usually mild) of the walls of respiratory bronchioles accompanied by the accumulation of pigmented macrophages in their lumen and the lumen of adjacent alveoli (Fig. 16.10) (32). It has been hypothesized to be part of a spectrum of smoking-related diseases that includes respiratory bronchiolitis–interstitial lung disease (RB-ILD) and desquamative interstitial pneumonitis (DIP) (33,34). RB is typically identified as an incidental finding in asymptomatic smokers. Occasionally, smokers present with cough and dyspnea, and a combined restrictive and obstructive pattern on lung function testing (RB-ILD). Histologically, these patients appear to have an exaggerated form of RB, in which inflammation and fibrosis extends into the peribronchiolar parenchyma (Fig. 16.11). Patients

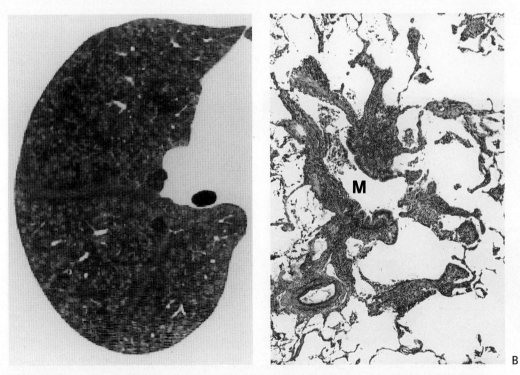

A   B

FIGURE 16.9. Extrinsic allergic alveolitis. **A:** HRCT image of the right lung shows poorly defined centrilobular nodular opacities throughout all lobes. **B:** Photomicrograph shows moderately severe chronic inflammation of the wall of a membranous bronchiole (*M*) and proximal respiratory bronchioles. The adjacent lung parenchyma shows mild interstitial inflammation. The patient was a 35-year-old woman.

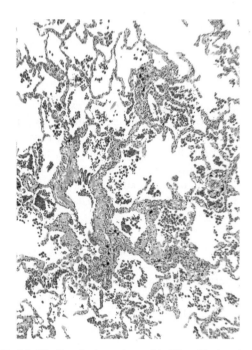

FIGURE 16.10. Respiratory bronchiolitis. Photomicrograph shows mild thickening of the walls of several respiratory bronchioles by mature fibrous tissue and an infiltrate of lymphocytes. Numerous tan macrophages are present in the airway lumen and the adjacent alveolar airspaces.

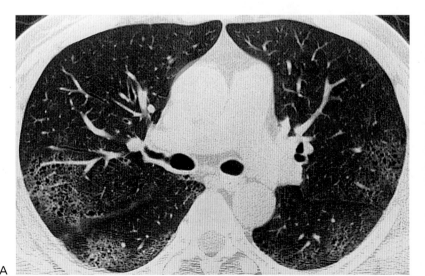

A

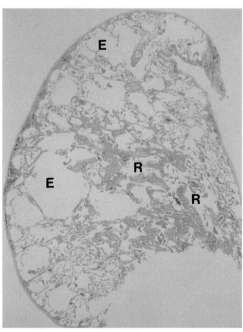

B

FIGURE 16.11. Respiratory bronchiolitis–interstitial lung disease. **A:** HRCT image demonstrates patchy bilateral ground-glass opacities in a predominantly peripheral distribution. Also note mild emphysema. **B:** Biopsy specimen shows a moderate degree of fibrosis in the walls of several respiratory bronchioles (*R*). Focal emphysema (*E*) is evident.

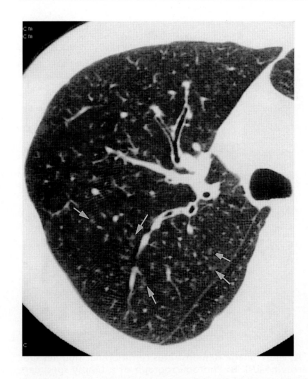

FIGURE 16.12. Respiratory bronchiolitis–interstitial lung disease. HRCT image of the right lung shows poorly defined centrilobular nodules (*arrows*). The patient was a 60-year-old smoker.

who have DIP have more diffuse involvement with a greater likelihood of developing parenchymal fibrosis and progressive lung disease.

Most patients with RB have normal radiographs and HRCT scans. In a small number, HRCT shows poorly defined centrilobular nodules or ground-glass opacities (16,35) (Fig. 16.7). These may be diffuse but often involve predominantly or exclusively the upper lobes. Most patients with RB-ILD have abnormalities evident on the radiograph and HRCT. The radiographic findings consist of ground-glass opacities with or without associated fine reticular or reticulonodular interstitial opacities (2,34). On HRCT, the abnormalities consist of diffuse or patchy areas of ground-glass attenuation (Fig. 16.11) or poorly defined nodular opacities (Fig. 16.12) often superimposed on a background of centrilobular emphysema (16,36). Occasionally a fine reticular pattern due to fibrosis may also be seen.

One group of investigators compared the HRCT findings in 16 patients who had pathologically proven respiratory bronchiolitis, eight who had respiratory bronchiolitis-associated interstitial lung disease (RB-ILD), and 16 who had DIP (16). The predominant abnormalities in respiratory bronchiolitis were centrilobular nodules seen in 12 (75%) patients and ground-glass attenuation occurred in six (38%). No single abnormality predominated in the respiratory bronchiolitis-associated interstitial lung disease group; findings included ground-glass attenuation (four [50%] patients), centrilobular nodules (three [38%], and mild fibrosis (two [25%] patients). All patients who had DIP had ground-glass attenuation, and 10 of the 16 (63%) showed evidence of fibrosis.

Follicular Bronchiolitis

The term *follicular bronchiolitis* refers to a form of bronchiolar disease characterized histologically by the presence of abundant lymphoid tissue, frequently with prominent germinal centers, situated in the walls of bronchioles and, to some extent, bronchi (Fig. 16.13) (37). In many cases, it probably represents hyperplasia of the airway-associated lymphoid tissue. Most cases are associated with underlying disorders, most often connective-tissue diseases (particularly rheumatoid disease and Sjögren's syndrome), immunodeficiency disorders, and hypersensitivity reactions (37,38).

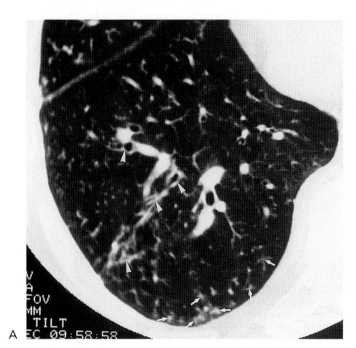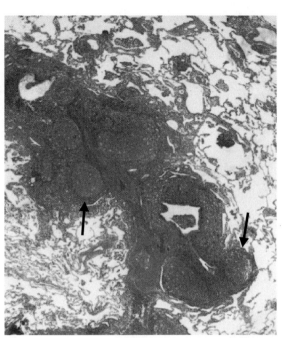

FIGURE 16.13. Follicular bronchiolitis. **A:** HRCT image demonstrates centrilobular nodules (*arrows*) and bronchial wall thickening (arrowheads). **B:** Photomicrograph of a biopsy specimen shows a dense infiltrate of lymphocytes in the wall of a membranous bronchiole. Several germinal centers are evident (*arrows*). (Courtesy by Dr. Kingo Chida, Hamamatsu Medical University, Hamamatsu, Japan.)

The chest radiograph characteristically shows a diffuse reticulonodular pattern (37,38). HRCT demonstrates nodular opacities mainly in a peribronchovascular or subpleural distribution, related to the presence of lymphoid aggregates; these opacities are usually small (1 to 3 mm in diameter) but occasionally are as large as 1 to 2 cm in diameter (38,39) (Fig. 16.13). Other findings include centrilobular branching structures, bronchial wall thickening, and (occasionally) patchy areas of low attenuation (38). In one investigation of 12 patients, the main abnormalities evident on HRCT consisted of bilateral centrilobular nodules (seen in all 12 patients), patchy ground-glass opacities (in nine [75%]), peribronchial nodules (in five [42%]), and subpleural nodules (in three [25%]) (39).

Diffuse Panbronchiolitis

Diffuse panbronchiolitis is a disease of unknown etiology and pathogenesis associated with chronic inflammation of the paranasal sinuses and respiratory bronchioles. The latter is characterized histologically by luminal obliteration and a striking accumulation of foamy macrophages in the walls of bronchioles (particularly respiratory in type), alveolar ducts, and adjacent parenchyma (Fig. 16.14) (40). The disease has been recognized almost exclusively in Japan and South Korea (41). A few cases have been described in North America and Europe (42).

Radiographic abnormalities consist of diffuse nodules smaller than 5 mm in diameter and mild to moderate hyperinflation (42,43). The findings on HRCT are characteristic and include small centrilobular nodules and branching linear opacities, bronchiolectasis, bronchiectasis, and mosaic areas of decreased parenchymal attenuation (14,15) (Fig. 16.15). The presence of these findings is related to the stage of the disease: the earliest manifestation consists of centrilobular nodular opacities, followed by branching linear opacities that connect to the nodules, followed by thick-walled, centrilobular lucencies (44). These findings have been shown to correspond, respectively, to bronchiolar wall and peribronchiolar inflammation and fibrosis, bronchiolar dilatation with the presence of intraluminal secretions, and dilated air-filled bronchioles (14).

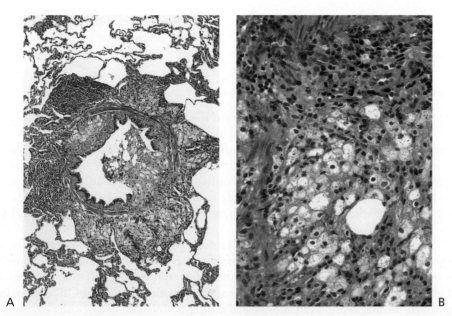

FIGURE 16.14. Diffuse panbronchiolitis. Low- (**A**) and high- (**B**) magnification photomicrographs show marked thickening of the wall of a membranous bronchiole by lymphocytes and numerous macrophages. The latter are distinctly foamy in appearance and, focally, are present in the airway lumen. Similar findings were evident in respiratory bronchioles.

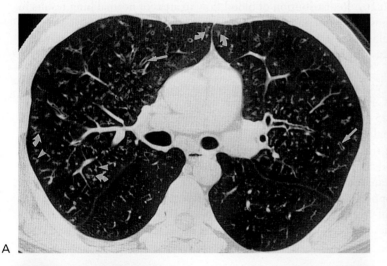

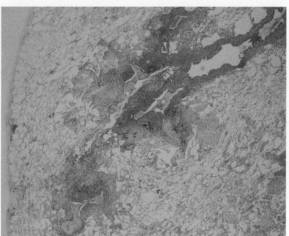

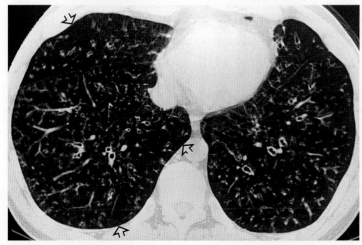

FIGURE 16.15. Diffuse panbronchiolitis. **A:** HRCT image at the level of the main bronchi shows bronchiectasis (*straight arrows*), bronchiolectasis (*curved arrows*) and centrilobular branching linear and nodular opacities (*arrowheads*). **B:** Image at a more caudad level shows more severe abnormalities as well as focal areas of decreased attenuation and vascularity (*arrows*). **C:** Biopsy specimen shows a moderate degree of thickening of the walls of membranous and proximal respiratory bronchioles by a mononuclear inflammatory cell infiltrate accompanied by paler aggregates of macrophages.

Late manifestations of the disease include large, cystic spaces; bullae; and evidence of air trapping with large lung volumes and decreased attenuation of peripheral lung parenchyma (14) (Fig. 16.15).

Obliterative Bronchiolitis

Obliterative bronchiolitis (OB) is characterized histologically by the presence of more or less concentric fibrosis of the mucosa of terminal and respiratory bronchioles, with resulting narrowing or obliteration of the airway lumen (Fig. 16.2). Affected patients usually present with progressive shortness of breath and functional evidence of airway obstruction. The abnormality is the result of a variety of causes and, rarely, is idiopathic (Table 16.3). In clinical practice, it is seen most commonly following childhood viral infection; in patients who have undergone lung, heart–lung, or bone marrow transplantation; and in patients who have rheumatoid disease (45).

The chest radiograph is often normal. In some patients, mild hyperinflation, subtle peripheral attenuation of the vascular markings, and evidence of central airway dilatation may be seen (46,47). HRCT is superior to the radiograph in demonstrating the presence and extent of abnormalities (48,49). In one study of patients who had OB, chest radiographs were normal in one-third and showed mild hyperinflation and vascular attenuation in the remaining two-thirds (48). CT, on the other hand, showed widespread and conspicuous abnormalities in lung attenuation in nearly 90% of the patients.

The main HRCT findings usually consist of areas of decreased lung attenuation associated with vessels of decreased caliber on inspiratory scans and air trapping on expiratory scans (20,23) (Fig. 16.16). Redistribution of blood flow to areas of normal lung results in a pattern known as mosaic attenuation or mosaic perfusion, namely, areas of decreased attenuation and vascularity adjacent to areas of increased attenuation and vascularity (20,23). Bronchiectasis, both central and peripheral, is also commonly present (23,50) (Fig. 16.17).

Air trapping on expiratory HRCT is the most sensitive sign to detect obliterative bronchiolitis on HRCT. In fact, it is often the only abnormal HRCT finding (20,51). In one investigation of 45 patients who had air trapping found on routine expiratory HRCT scans, nine had normal inspiratory HRCT findings; five of the nine had OB (51).

In one study, air trapping (diagnosed on expiratory scans if a total area of more than one segment appeared abnormal) was seen in four of five patients who had biopsy-proven OB and expiratory scans, and in none of three patients who had a negative biopsy (23). In another study, air trapping was found in 10 of 11 patients who had biopsy-diagnosed OB, compared with two of 10 patients who did not have biopsy-diagnosed OB or pulmonary function abnormalities (20). Thus air trapping was found to have a sensitivity of 91%, a

---

TABLE 16.3. DISEASES ASSOCIATED WITH OBLITERATIVE BRONCHIOLITIS

Infection
  Childhood viral infection (e.g., adenovirus, respiratory syncytial virus)
  Infection in adults (e.g., *Mycoplasma pneumoniae, Pneumocystis carinii* in AIDS patients)
Toxic fume inhalation (e.g., nitrogen dioxide [silo-filler's lung], sulfur dioxide)
Connective-tissue diseases, particularly rheumatoid disease
Drug therapy (e.g., penicillamine, gold)
Chronic rejection following lung and heart–lung transplantation
Chronic graft-versus-host disease following bone marrow transplantation
Neuroendocrine cell hyperplasia
Idiopathic

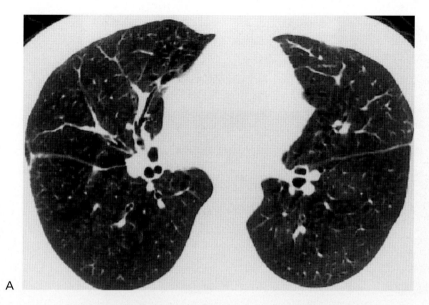

A

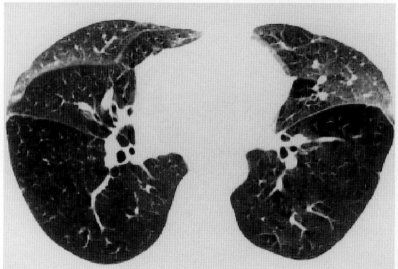

B

FIGURE 16.16. Obliterative bronchiolitis. Inspiratory HRCT image shows subtle areas of decreased attenuation and vascularity mainly in the lower lobes. Increased attenuation and vascularity is evident in the anterior lung regions due to blood flow redistribution. **B:** Expiratory image shows marked air trapping throughout the lower lobes with anterior convexity of the oblique fissures. Patchy areas of air trapping are present in the right middle and right upper lobes and lingula. The patient was a 40-year-old woman who had undergone double lung transplantation.

specificity of 80%, and an accuracy of 86% for diagnosing OB. However, the patients who had OB in this study had established disease; the mean time from lung transplantation to CT in their study was 4.8 years, and the mean duration of a known diagnosis of obliterative bronchiolitis was 1.3 years.

Swyer-James Syndrome

Swyer-James syndrome is an uncommon abnormality characterized radiographically by a hyperlucent lobe or lung and functionally by normal or reduced volume during inspiration and air trapping during expiration (52). The patients may be asymptomatic or present with a history of repeated lower respiratory tract infections (52).

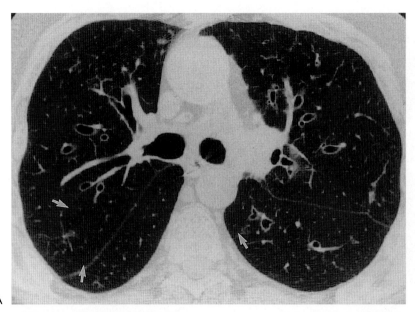

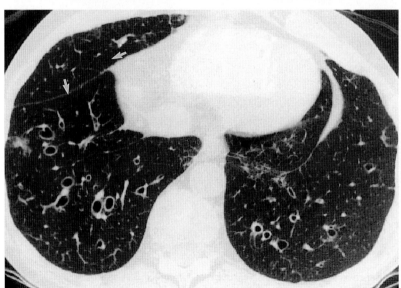

FIGURE 16.17. Obliterative bronchiolitis. HRCT images at the level of main bronchi (**A**) and the lung bases (**B**) show bronchial dilatation and areas of decreased attenuation and vascularity. The patient was a 48-year-old man who had undergone double lung transplantation.

The characteristic radiographic findings consist of a marked difference in the radiolucency of the two lungs (or of the affected and unaffected lobes), caused by decreased vascularity and perfusion. On radiographs exposed at total lung capacity, the volume of the affected lung (or lobe) either is comparable to that of the normal contralateral lung or is reduced. Expiratory chest radiographs show air trapping. This is a reflection of airway obstruction and is helpful in differentiating the syndrome from other conditions that may give rise to unilateral or lobar hyperlucency.

The diagnosis of Swyer-James syndrome can be easily confirmed by CT (53,54) (Fig. 16.18). In one study of nine patients who had the condition, eight of the nine affected lungs had decreased attenuation on CT; the other was small but had normal attenuation (53). Air trapping was present in all cases; on the expiratory CT scan, there was no appreciable change in the volume of the affected lung, whereas the normal lung decreased in vol-

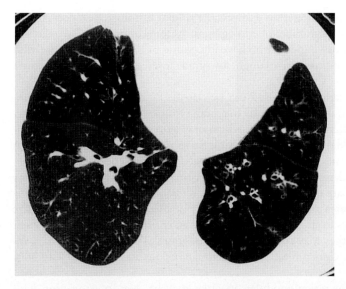

FIGURE 16.18. Swyer-James syndrome. HRCT image shows decreased attenuation and vascularity of left lung and bronchiectasis in left lower lobe and lingula. Note decreased volume of left lung with ipsilateral shift of the mediastinum. Focal bronchiectasis is also seen in right middle lobe. The patient was a 53-year-old man.

ume. All nine patients had evidence of bronchiectasis and decreased size of the pulmonary vessels. In another study of eight patients, five demonstrated bilateral areas of decreased attenuation, and five had areas of normal attenuation within the hyperlucent lung, indicating that the process was much more heterogeneous than suspected (54). Air trapping within the hyperlucent lung was confirmed with the expiratory CT scan in five patients. Bronchiectasis was seen in only three of the eight patients.

Bronchiolitis Obliterans Organizing Pneumonia

BOOP is characterized grossly by patchy, usually poorly delimited foci of consolidation and histologically by the presence of fibroblastic tissue within the lumens of respiratory bronchioles, alveolar ducts and the adjacent alveolar airspaces (Fig. 16.19) (55). Occasionally, a proteinaceous exudate can be identified in the central portion of the fibroblastic tissue, representing a more direct manifestation of prior epithelial/endothelial injury. A variable degree of nonspecific chronic inflammation and interstitial fibrosis is also seen in the parenchyma within and adjacent to the foci of airspace disease.

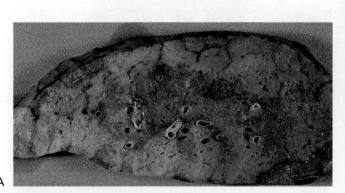

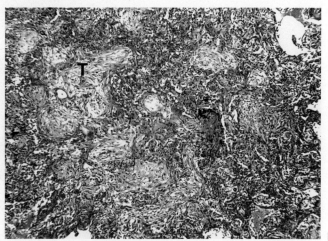

A

B

FIGURE 16.19. Bronchiolitis obliterans organizing pneumonia. **A:** Transverse slice of lung shows patchy, somewhat poorly delimited foci of consolidation in the subpleural parenchyma. **B:** Photomicrograph shows the presence of fibroblastic tissue in the lumens of several transitional airways (*T*) and their associated alveoli. There is a moderate degree of interstitial pneumonitis.

BOOP is most commonly idiopathic. However, a similar histologic reaction pattern can be seen in association with a number of etiologies, including connective-tissue disease, drugs, infection, and aspiration. Patients who have idiopathic BOOP usually present with a 1- to 3-month history of nonproductive cough, low-grade fever, and increasing shortness of breath (56,57).

The radiologic manifestations of BOOP can be classified into four distinctive radiographic and CT patterns: (a) multiple, usually bilateral, symmetric, patchy airspace opacities; (b) diffuse, bilateral interstitial opacities, which may be reticular, nodular, or reticulonodular; (c) focal consolidation; and (d) multiple large nodules or masses (57,58). A mixed pattern of combined airspace and interstitial opacities has also been described.

Patchy airspace consolidation is the most characteristic and the most common of these patterns (57). The opacities are most often peripheral and pleural based (Fig. 16.20). They may decrease in size in one area and appear in previously unaffected regions (59). The size of individual opacities ranges from about 3 cm to almost an entire lobe (Fig. 16.21). Their margins are indistinct, and they may contain air bronchograms. The lung volume may appear preserved or decreased. Concomitant small pleural effusions are seen in 20% to 30% of patients (57,60).

A pattern of reticular or reticulonodular opacities may be seen in association with airspace opacities or, occasionally, as an isolated finding (57,60). A less common radiologic presentation is as a focal area of consolidation. The last and least common manifestation is as multiple large nodules or masses, which may simulate metastatic disease (58).

On HRCT, most patients show areas of airspace consolidation, small nodules, or both (26,27); peripheral reticular areas of increased attenuation and ground-glass opacities are seen less often (26,61). In one study of 43 patients (of whom 32 were immunocompetent and 11 were immunocompromised secondary to a variety of conditions), consolidation was more common in immunocompetent (91%) than in immunocompromised (45%) patients (26). In the former group, such consolidation was most frequently subpleural or peribronchial in distribution. Ground-glass attenuation and nodules were more common in immunocompromised patients (73% and 55%, respectively) than in immunocompetent patients (56% and 23%, respectively).

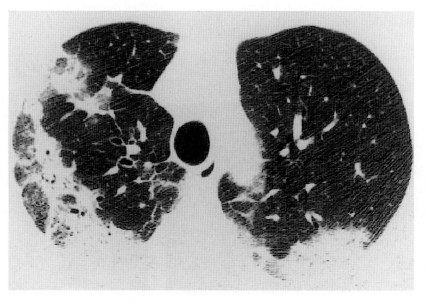

FIGURE 16.20. Bronchiolitis obliterans organizing pneumonia. HRCT image shows bilateral airspace consolidation involving mainly the subpleural lung regions. The patient was a 46-year-old man.

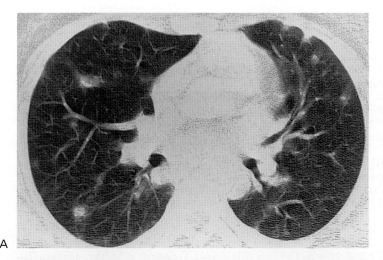

A

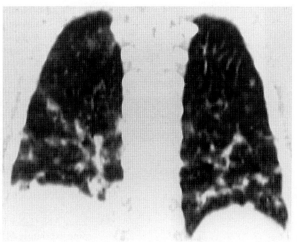

C

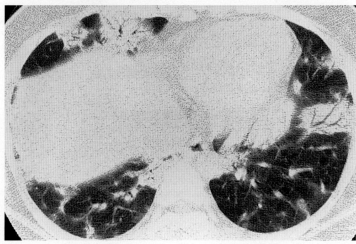

B

FIGURE 16.21. Bronchiolitis obliterans organizing pneumonia. **A:** HRCT image at the level of the lower lobe bronchi shows nodular bilateral areas of airspace consolidation. **B:** Image at the level of the dome of the right hemidiaphragm shows peribronchial areas of consolidation. **C:** Coronal multiplanar reconstruction image shows the patchy nature of the consolidation.

REFERENCES

1. Colby TV. Bronchiolitis: pathologic considerations. *Am J Clin Pathol* 1998;109:101–109.
2. Müller NL, Miller RR: Diseases of the bronchioles: CT and histopathologic findings. *Radiology* 1995;196:3–12.
3. Du Bois RM, Geddes DM. Obliterative bronchiolitis, cryptogenic organizing pneumonia and bronchiolitis obliterans organizing pneumonia: three names for two different conditions. *Eur Respir* 1991;4:774–775.
4. American Thoracic Society/European Respiratory Society International Multidisciplinary Consensus Classification of the Idiopathic Interstitial Pneumonias. *Am J Respir Crit Care Med* 2002;165:277–304.
5. Lynch DA. Imaging of small airways disease. *Clin Chest Med* 1993;14:623–634.
6. Webb WR. High-resolution computed tomography of obstructive lung disease. *Rad Clin N Am* 1994;32:745–757.
7. Collins J, Blankenbaker D, Stern EJ. CT patterns of bronchiolar disease: what is tree-in-bud? *Am J Roentgenol* 1998;171:365–370.
8. Hartman TE, Primack SL, Lee KS, et al. CT of bronchial and bronchiolar diseases. *Radiographics* 1994;14:991–1003.
9. Gruden JF, Webb WR, Warnock M. Centrilobular opacities in the lung on high-resolution CT: diagnostic considerations and pathologic correlation. *Am J Roentgenol* 1994;162:569–574.
10. Desai SR, Hansell DM. Small airways disease: expiratory computed tomography comes of age. *Clin Radiol* 1997;52:332–337.
11. Arakawa H, Webb WR. Expiratory high-resolution CT scan. *Radiol Clin North Am* 1998;36:189–209.

12. Im JG, Itoh H, Shim YS, et al. Pulmonary tuberculosis: CT findings—early active disease and sequential change with antituberculous therapy. *Radiology* 1993;186:653–660.
13. Logan PM, Primack SL, Miller RR, et al. Invasive aspergillosis of the airways: radiographic, CT and pathologic findings. *Radiology* 1994;193:383–388.
14. Nishimura K, Kitaichi M, Izumi T, et al. Diffuse panbronchiolitis: correlation of high-resolution CT and pathologic findings. *Radiology* 1992;184:779–785.
15. Akira M, Higashihara T, Sakatani M, et al. Diffuse panbronchiolitis: follow-up CT examination. *Radiology* 1993;189:559–562.
16. Heyneman LE, Ward S, Lynch DA, et al. Respiratory bronchiolitis, respiratory bronchiolitis-associated interstitial pneumonia: different entities or part of the spectrum of the same disease process? *Am J Roentgenol* 1999;173:1617–1622.
17. Padley SPG, Adler BD, Hansell DM, et al. Bronchiolitis obliterans: high resolution CT findings and correlation with pulmonary function tests. *Clin Radiol* 1993;47:236–240.
18. Worthy SA, Müller NL. Small airways diseases. *Rad Clin North Am* 1998;36:163–173.
19. Stern EJ, Frank MS. Small airway diseases of the lungs: findings at expiratory CT. *Am J Roentgenol* 1994;163:37–41.
20. Leung AN, Fisher K, Valentine V, et al. Bronchiolitis obliterans after lung transplantation: detection using expiratory HRCT. *Chest* 1998;113:365–370.
21. Webb WR, Stern EJ, Nanth N, et al. Dynamic pulmonary CT: findings in healthy adult men. *Radiology* 1993;186:117–124.
22. Park CS, Müller NL, Worthy SA, et al. Airway obstruction in asthmatic and healthy individuals: inspiratory and expiratory tin-section CT findings. *Radiology* 1997;203:361–367.
23. Worthy SA, Park CS, Kim JS, et al. Bronchiolitis obliterans after lung transplantation: high-resolution CT findings in 15 patients. *Am J Roentgenol* 1997;169:673–677.
24. Hansell DM, Wells AU, Padley SP, et al. Hypersensitivity pneumonitis: correlation of individual CT patterns with functional abnormalities. *Radiology* 1996;199:123–128.
25. King GG, Müller NL, Paré PD: Pulmonary perspective: evaluation of airways in obstructive lung disease using high-resolution CT. *Am J Respir Crit Care Med* 1999;159:992–1004.
26. Müller NL, Staples CA, Miller RR. Bronchiolitis obliterans organizing pneumonia: CT features in 14 patients. *Am J Roentgenol* 1990;154:983–987.
27. Lee KS, Kullnig P, Hartman TE, et al. Cryptogenic organizing pneumonia: CT findings in 43 patients. *Am J Roentgenol* 1994;162:543–546.
28. Reittner P, Müller NL, Heyneman L, et al. *Mycoplasma pneumoniae* pneumonia: radiographic and high-resolution CT features in 28 patients. *Am J Roentgenol* 2000;214:73–80.
29. McGuinness G, Gruden JF, Bhalla M, et al. AIDS-related airways disease. *Am J Roentgenol* 1997;168:67–77.
30. Aquino SL, Gamsu G, Webb WR, et al. Tree-in-bud pattern: frequency and significance on thin section CT. *J Comput Assist Tomogr* 1996;20:594–599.
31. Remy-Jardin M, Remy J, Wallaert B, et al. Subacute and chronic bird breeder hypersensitivity pneumonitis: sequential evaluation with CT and correlation with lung function tests and bronchoalveolar lavage. *Radiology* 1993;198:111–118.
32. Cosio MG, Hale KA, Niewoehner DE. Morphologic and morphometric effects of prolonged smoking on the small airways. *Am Rev Respir Dis* 1980;122:265–321.
33. Moon J, du Bois RM, Colby TV, et al. Clinical significance of respiratory bronchiolitis on open lung biopsy and its relationship to smoking-related interstitial lung disease. *Thorax* 1999;54:1009–1014.
34. Yousem SA, Colby TV, Gaensler EA. Respiratory bronchiolitis-associated interstitial lung disease and its relationship to desquamative interstitial pneumonia. *Mayo Clin Proc* 1989;64:1373–1380.
35. Remy-Jardin M, Remy J, Boulenguez C, et al. Morphologic effects of cigarette smoking on airways and pulmonary parenchyma in healthy adult volunteers: CT evaluation and correlation with pulmonary function tests. *Radiology* 1993;186:107–115.
36. Park J, Brown K, Tuder R, et al. Respiratory bronchiolitis associated interstitial lung disease: radiologic features with clinical and pathologic correlation. *J Comput Assist Tomogr* 2002;26:13–20.
37. Yousem SA, Colby TV, Carrington CB. Follicular bronchitis/bronchiolitis. *Hum Pathol* 1985;16:700–706.
38. Hayakawa H, Sato A, Imokawa S, et al. Bronchiolar disease in rheumatoid arthritis. *Am J Respir Crit Care Med* 1996;154:1531–1536.
39. Howling SJ, Hansell DM, Wells AU, et al. Follicular bronchiolitis: thin-section CT and histologic findings. *Radiology* 1999;212:637–642.
40. Iwata M, Colby TV, Kitaichi M. Diffuse panbronchiolitis: diagnosis and distinction from various pulmonary diseases with centrilobular interstitial foam cell accumulations. *Hum Pathol* 1994;25:357–363.
41. Sugiyama Y: Diffuse panbronchiolitis. *Clin Chest Med* 1993;14:765–772.
42. Homma H, Yamanaka A, Tanimoto S, et al. Diffuse panbronchiolitis: a disease of the transitional zone of the lung. *Chest* 1983;83:63–69.

43. Fisher MS Jr, Rush WL, Rosado-de-Christenson ML, et al. Diffuse panbronchiolitis: histologic diagnosis in unsuspected cases involving North American residents of Asian descent. *Arch Pathol Lab Med* 1998;122:156–160.
44. Akira M, Kitatani F, Yong-Sik L, et al. Diffuse panbronchiolitis: evaluation with high-resolution CT1. *Radiology* 1988;168:433–438.
45. King TE. Overview of bronchiolitis. *Clin Chest Med* 1993;14:607–610.
46. Breatnach E, Kerr I. The radiology of cryptogenic obliterative bronchiolitis. *Clin Radiol* 1982;33: 657–661.
47. Skeens JL, Fuhrman CR, Yousem SA. Bronchiolitis obliterans in heart-lung transplantation patients: radiologic findings in 11 patients. *Am J Roentgenol* 1989;153:253–256.
48. Sweatman MC, Millar AB, Strickland B, et al. Computed tomography in adult obliterative bronchiolitis. *Clin Radiol* 1990;41:116–119.
49. Morrish WF, Herman SJ, Weisbrod GL, et al. Bronchiolitis obliterans after lung transplantation: findings at chest radiography and high-resolution CT. *Radiology* 1991;179:487–490.
50. Lentz D, Bergin CJ, Berry GJ, et al. Diagnosis of bronchiolitis obliterans in heart-lung transplantation patients: importance of bronchial dilatation on CT. *Am J Roentgenol* 1992;159:463–467.
51. Arakawa H, Webb WR. Air-trapping on expiratory high-resolution CT scans in the absence of inspiratory scan abnormalities: correlation with pulmonary function tests and differential diagnosis. *Am J Roentgenol* 1998;170:1349–1353.
52. Swyer PR, James GCW. A case of unilateral pulmonary emphysema. *Thorax* 1953;8:133–136.
53. Marti-Bonmati L, Perales FR, Catala F, et al. CT findings in Swyer-James syndrome. *Radiology* 1989;172:477–480.
54. Moore ADA, Godwin JD, Dietrich PA, et al. Swyer-James syndrome: CT findings in eight patients. *Am J Roentgenol* 1992;158:1211–1215.
55. Epler GR, Colby TV, McLoud TC, et al. Bronchiolitis obliterans organizing pneumonia. *N Engl J Med* 1985;312:152–158.
56. Epler GR. Bronchiolitis obliterans organizing pneumonia: definition and clinical features. *Chest* 1992;102:2–6.
57. Müller N, Guerry-Force ML, Staples C, et al. Differential diagnosis of bronchiolitis obliterans with organizing pneumonia and usual interstitial pneumonia: clinical, functional, and radiologic findings. *Radiology* 1987;162:151–156.
58. Akira M, Yamamoto S, Sakatani M. Bronchiolitis obliterans organizing pneumonia manifesting as multiple large nodules or masses. *Am J Roentgenol* 1998;170:291–295.
59. Spiteri M, Klenerman P, Sheppard M, et al. Seasonal cryptogenic organizing pneumonia with biochemical cholestasis: a new clinical entity. *Lancet* 192; 340:281–284.
60. Chandler P, Shin M, Friedman S, et al. Radiographic manifestations of bronchiolitis obliterans with organizing pneumonia vs usual interstitial pneumonia. *Am J Roentgenol* 1986;147:899–906.
61. Bouchardy LM, Kuhlman JE, Ball WC, et al. CT findings in bronchiolitis obliterans organizing pneumonia (BOOP) with radiographic, clinical and histologic correlation. *J Comput Assist Tomogr* 1993;17:352–357.

17

PULMONARY EMBOLISM

ACUTE PULMONARY THROMBOEMBOLISM
Pathologic Characteristics
Radiologic Manifestations

CHRONIC PULMONARY THROMBOEMBOLISM

SEPTIC EMBOLISM

FAT EMBOLISM

EMBOLISM OF TALC (TALCOSIS)

Pulmonary thromboembolism (PE) by definition implies the formation of thrombus elsewhere than the lungs, most commonly in the deep veins of the leg, and its transport in the blood to one or more pulmonary arteries. Such thrombus has two immediate consequences—a decrease or cessation of flow distally and, if the thrombus is large enough, an increase in pressure proximally. The former can result in pulmonary hemorrhage alone or hemorrhage accompanied by necrosis of lung parenchyma (infarction). In both cases, the hemorrhage is related to ischemic damage to endothelial and alveolar epithelial cells, permitting the passage of red blood cells and fluid into the airspaces. The blood can be derived from the bronchial arteries via bronchopulmonary anastomoses (1), from the pulmonary artery itself (following partial or complete lysis of the thrombus), or from the pulmonary veins via retrograde flow.

The radiologic and clinical manifestations of PE are often considered in two categories: those in which the embolic episode is acute and those in which the emboli are chronic and/or repeated.

ACUTE PULMONARY THROMBOEMBOLISM

Most episodes of acute PE are unassociated with symptoms and produce no detectable changes on the chest radiograph. Even if the diagnosis is suspected clinically and confirmed angiographically, no abnormalities are evident radiographically in approximately 10% to 15% of patients (2,3). Even at autopsy, tissue necrosis is documented in only about 10% to 15% of cases (4). In fact, various observations suggest that some abnormality in addition to the vascular obstruction needs to be present to result in significant tissue damage in most cases. The most common underlying condition predisposing to infarction is congestive heart failure, an association possibly explained by increased pulmonary venous pressure and decreased bronchial artery blood flow.

Pathologic Findings

In most instances, the lung parenchyma distal to a PE is either normal or shows only mild atelectasis and minimal intraalveolar hemorrhage or edema. The atelectasis may be secondary to reflex bronchoconstriction or a local deficiency of surfactant. When changes are more marked, they consist of either hemorrhage alone or a combination of hemorrhage and necrosis. In its early stage, isolated parenchymal hemorrhage is grossly similar to infarction and consists of a more or less wedge-shaped area of red, consolidated lung typically abutting the pleura (Fig. 17.1). The blood usually disappears fairly rapidly and the only evidence of the thromboembolic event may be the presence of hemosiderin-laden macrophages.

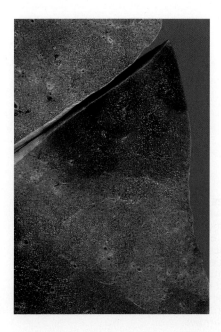

FIGURE 17.1. Acute pulmonary thromboembolism—parenchymal hemorrhage. A magnified view of the superior segment of a lower lobe shows a fairly well-demarcated focus of hemorrhagic consolidation. A thromboembolus was evident in the segmental artery proximally. Histologic examination showed airspace hemorrhage without evidence of tissue necrosis.

Within 1 or 2 days of the embolic event, an infarct becomes more firm than pure hemorrhage. Although it is usually fairly well demarcated and more or less wedge-shaped (Fig. 17.2), patchy areas of parenchymal hemorrhage may be present adjacent to it (Fig. 17.3) (a feature that accounts for the poor definition of some infarcts radiographically and a ground-glass appearance adjacent to a focus of consolidation on high-resolution computed tomography HRCT (see Fig. 17.10). Overlying fibrinous pleuritis is often present. With time, the necrotic parenchyma becomes more sharply demarcated from the adjacent lung by granulation tissue that may be red (reflecting a pronounced vascularity) or white (Fig. 17.4) (as a result of the influx of a large number of polymorphonuclear leukocytes). Release of enzymes from neutrophils may be followed by liquefaction of the necrotic tissue and cavity formation. Eventually, the infarcted parenchyma is completely replaced by

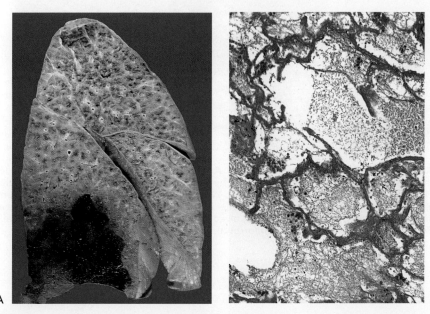

FIGURE 17.2. Pulmonary infarct—recent. **A:** Parasagittal slice of the right lung shows a well-demarcated focus of hemorrhagic consolidation in the posterior basal region of the lower lobe. **B:** Histologic examination shows airspace hemorrhage and necrotic alveolar septa (indicated by the absence of nuclei).

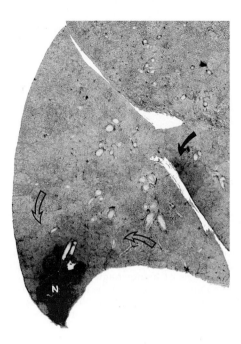

FIGURE 17.3. Pulmonary infarct—recent. Magnified view of a paper-mounted slice of the right lung shows a focus of infarction (N) in the posterior basal region. The necrotic tissue is surrounded by a poorly demarcated region of lung that is consolidated by blood (*open arrows*). Examination of the latter region showed congested but otherwise normal alveolar septa. A smaller focus of embolism-related parenchymal hemorrhage is also evident in the middle lobe (*solid arrow*).

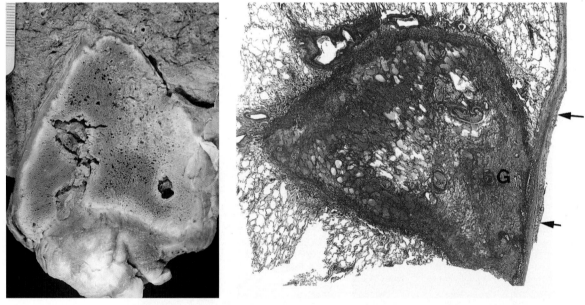

A   B

FIGURE 17.4. Pulmonary infarcts—organizing. **A:** Magnified view of the basal region of a lower lobe shows a well-demarcated region of parenchymal necrosis. A distinct rim of white granulation tissue is evident at the periphery of the infarct. Two foci of early cavitation are also apparent. **B:** Low-magnification photomicrograph of a smaller infarct in the superior segment also shows a rim of granulation tissue (*G*). Residual (necrotic) alveolar septa are still identifiable in the central portion. Fibrinous pleuritis can also be seen (*arrows*).

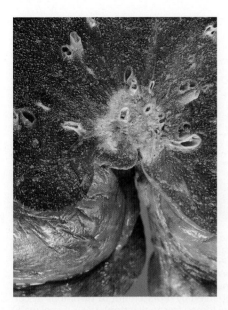

FIGURE 17.5. Pulmonary infarct—remote. A magnified view of a lower lobe shows a nodule of fibrous tissue associated with pleural puckering. The patient had experienced an episode of pulmonary thromboembolism several months before death; organized emboli were identified in the segmental arteries supplying the region of lung that contained the nodule.

fibrous tissue, resulting in a nodular or somewhat elongated scar frequently associated with pleural puckering (Fig. 17.5).

Grossly, recent thromboemboli typically have a distinct laminated appearance as a result of alternating aggregates of red blood cells and fibrin-platelet thrombus (Fig. 17.6). Remote emboli may appear as foci of white fibrous tissue that completely occlude the vessel lumen or that form plaquelike elevations on the wall, fibrous bands that traverse the lumen, or webs that project into it. Histologic examination of thromboemboli shows various degrees of organization, depending on duration the embolus has been in the artery and on the degree of organization that occurred at the initial site of venous thrombosis. With time the thrombus may disappear completely by a process of fibrinolysis or may organize. In the latter situation, it may be incorporated into the vessel wall (resulting in the plaques described earlier) (Fig. 17.7A) or may become recanalized as a result of infiltration by macrophages and endothelial cells (Fig. 17.7B).

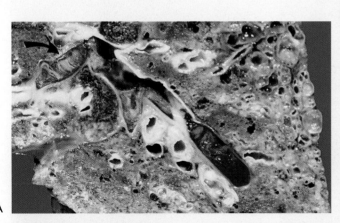

A

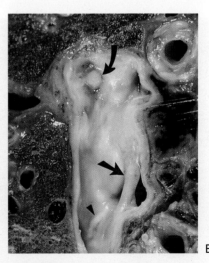

B

FIGURE 17.6. Pulmonary thromboemboli—recent and organized. **A:** Magnified view of a slice of the right lung shows complete occlusion of the middle lobe artery (*arrow*) and two segmental arteries in the lower lobe by thrombus. The latter has a distinct laminated appearance. The lung itself shows fibrosis and cyst formation consistent with idiopathic pulmonary fibrosis; no infarcts were identified. **B:** Magnified view of an interlobar pulmonary artery from another patient shows complete occlusion of the lumen of one small branch by fibrous tissue (*curved arrow*). A fibrous band (*straight arrow*) can be seen traversing the lumen and small foci of intimal fibrosis are evident (*arrowhead*) elsewhere. All three abnormalities are manifestations of organized thrombus.

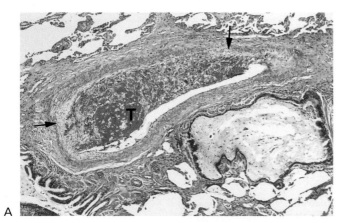
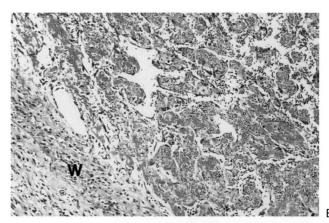

FIGURE 17.7. Pulmonary thromboemboli—organizing. **A:** Photomicrograph shows partial occlusion of a pulmonary artery by thrombus (*T*). Lightly staining fibroblastic tissue (*arrows*) is present in the intima adjacent to the thrombus and within it. Progression of the fibrosis results in the formation of an eccentric plaquelike thickening of the vessel wall. **B:** Magnified view of a thrombus from another patient shows it to be subdivided into numerous irregularly shaped channels lined by endothelial cells. Progression of this process accompanied by replacement of thrombus by collagen results in bands of fibrous tissue within the vessel lumen (recanalization). (*W* = vessel wall.)

Radiologic Manifestations

Radiographic manifestations related to thromboembolism without hemorrhage or infarction include oligemia distal to the obstructed vessels (Westermark's sign), enlargement of a central pulmonary artery (Fleischner's sign), abrupt tapering of the occluded vessel distally (knuckle sign), foci of linear atelectasis, and loss of lung volume (3). The last-named may be manifested by elevation of the hemidiaphragm, downward displacement of the major fissure, or both (2,3).

The radiographic manifestations of acute PE with infarction or hemorrhage consist of segmental areas of consolidation associated with volume loss. In the early stage of infarc-

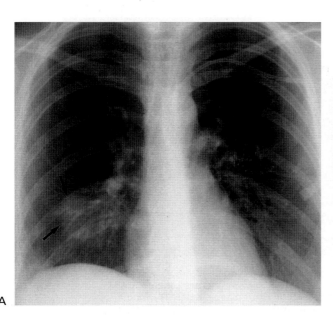
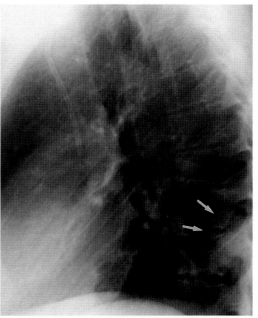

FIGURE 17.8. Acute pulmonary thromboembolism. **A:** Chest radiograph shows a poorly defined area of consolidation (*arrows*). **B:** Lateral radiograph shows a pleural-based opacity (*arrows*) with an appearance resembling a truncated cone (Hampton's hump). Incidental note is made of a central venous line with the tip in the superior vena cava. The patient was a 25-year-old woman.

tion, parenchymal opacities are ill defined. They are most common in the base of the lower lobe, often nestled in the costophrenic sulcus. Their configuration usually resembles a truncated cone (Hampton's hump) (3), consisting of a focus of homogeneous, wedge-shaped consolidation in the lung periphery, with its base contiguous to a visceral pleural surface and its rounded, convex apex toward the hilum (Fig. 17.8). It has been postulated that the latter appearance may be related to sparing of the apex of the cone from infarction as a result of collateral circulation from bronchial arteries (5). The size of the consolidated area is usually from 3 to 5 cm in diameter but may be as large as 10 cm.

Contrast-enhanced CT, MR, and angiography allow direct demonstration of thromboemboli as partial or complete intraluminal filling defects (6–8). On CT, the former is defined as an intravascular central or marginal area of low attenuation surrounded by a variable amount of contrast material. The latter is defined as an intraluminal area of low attenuation that occupies the entire arterial section, that is, by the abrupt absence of contrast material in a visible vessel. The most reliable sign of acute embolism is a filling defect that forms an acute angle with the vessel wall and is outlined by contrast material (Fig. 17.9). Although filling defects associated with a smooth, obtuse angle with the vessel wall

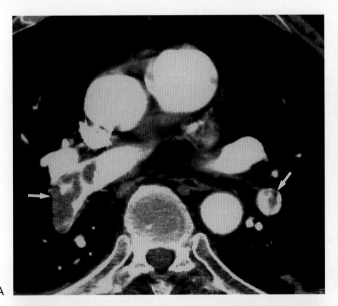

A

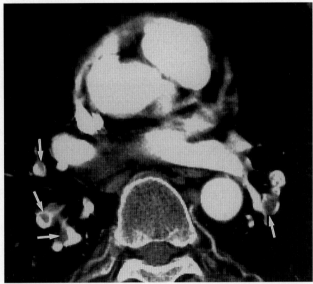

B

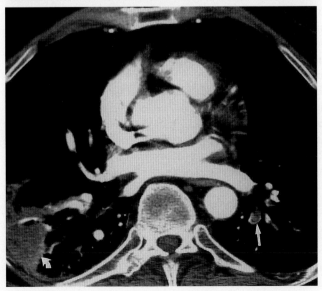

C

FIGURE 17.9. Acute pulmonary thromboembolism. **A:** Contrast-enhanced spiral CT image shows filling defects (*arrows*) within the right interlobar and left lower lobe pulmonary arteries. **B:** Image at a more caudad level shows filling defects (*arrows*) within the segmental arteries of both lower lobes. **C:** Third image at the level of the left atrium shows a filling defect (*straight arrow*) in the posterior basal segmental artery of the left lower lobe and a nonenhancing triangular pleural-based area of consolidation (*curved arrow*) in the right lower lobe. The appearance is characteristic of multiple acute pulmonary emboli associated with an infarct in the lateral basal segment of right lower lobe. The patient was a 63-year-old man.

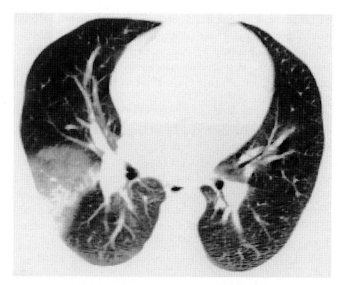

FIGURE 17.10. Acute pulmonary thromboembolism. CT image shows a wedge-shaped pleura-based area of ground-glass attenuation and focal consolidation in the right middle lobe. The patient was a 37-year-old man.

or complete cutoffs of contrast opacification of a vessel may be caused by acute emboli, they can also be seen with chronic emboli.

Parenchymal manifestations of acute PE on CT are similar to those on chest radiography and include oligemia, loss of lung volume, and wedge-shaped pleura-based opacities (9) (Fig. 17.10). Localized areas of decreased attenuation secondary to oligemia are uncommon, except in patients who have massive thromboemboli.

CHRONIC PULMONARY THROMBOEMBOLISM

Although most patients treated for an acute PE improve, some show only partial improvement; others develop chronic or recurrent embolism. The term *chronic pulmonary embolism* is used to refer to these two situations. In one study of 62 patients, spiral CT scans were performed 1 to 53 months (median, 8 months) after initial diagnosis (10). All patients had been admitted to a cardiology intensive care unit and treated with anticoagulants for massive PE; 31 had received fibrinolytic therapy initially. On the follow-up spiral CT scan, emboli were considered acute if they partially or completely occluded the arterial lumen and the arterial diameter was not reduced. They were considered chronic if at least two of the following features were present: (a) an eccentric location contiguous to the vessel wall, (b) evidence of recanalization within the intraluminal filling defect (i.e., circumferential filling defect with central or eccentric patent lumen), (c) arterial stenosis or webs, (d) reduction of more than 50% of the arterial diameter, and (e) complete occlusion at the level of the stenosed arteries (10) (Fig. 17.11). In 30 of 62 patients (48%), there was complete resolution of the initial embolus on the follow-up CT, and in 24 (39%) there was partial resolution; eight (13%) developed CT features of chronic PE. The clinical presentations, risk factors at diagnosis, and treatment did not differ between the patients who had complete resolution and the other patients. However, the group of patients who showed residual abnormalities or developed chronic emboli had more extensive embolization at initial diagnosis.

The angiographic findings of chronic PE were assessed in a study of 250 patients and correlated with findings at thromboendarterectomy (11). The abnormalities consisted of abrupt vascular narrowing, complete vascular obstruction, webs or bands, intimal irregularities, and "pouching" defects. The last was defined as the presence of obstructing or par-

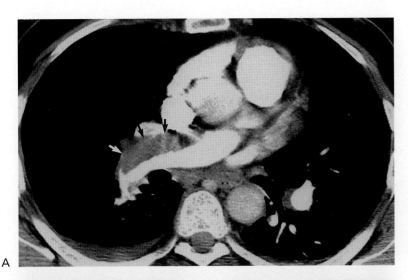

A

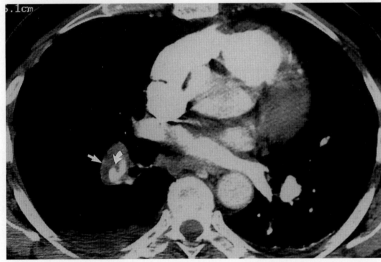

B

FIGURE 17.11. Chronic pulmonary thromboembolism. **A:** Contrast-enhanced spiral CT image shows an eccentric filling defect (*arrows*) in the right interlobar pulmonary artery. **B:** Image at the level of the left atrium shows an eccentric filling defect in the right lower lobe pulmonary artery (*straight arrow*) and an intraluminal web (*curved arrow*). The patient was a 69-year-old man with chronic pulmonary thromboembolism.

tially occlusive thromboemboli that organized in a concave configuration toward the lumen of the artery. Such pouches opacify early in the angiographic sequence and may be associated with partial or complete vascular obstruction. Tapering of vessels usually connotes circumferential organization and recanalization and, therefore, an old embolic episode. Abrupt narrowing of a major pulmonary vessel is also a characteristic finding of chronic PE, the normal gentle tapering of the vessel being replaced by an abrupt decrease in the diameter of the opacified lumen (11). Pulmonary artery webs or bands are lines of low opacity that traverse the width of the contrast material within the pulmonary vessel and are often associated with narrowing of the vessels and poststenotic dilation. Another common finding of chronic PE is the presence of intimal irregularity, which results in a scalloped appearance to the arterial wall. At surgery this abnormality has been shown to be the result of irregularly organized thrombus adherent to the vessel wall (11).

Parenchymal abnormalities are commonly seen on CT in patients who have chronic PE and are often sufficiently characteristic to suggest the diagnosis (12,13). The most common finding consists of localized areas of decreased attenuation and vascularity that are sharply marginated from adjacent areas that have increased or normal attenuation and vessel size, a pattern known as *mosaic perfusion* (Fig. 17.12). The areas with decreased attenuation and vascularity correspond to lung distal to partially or completely occluded vessels, whereas the areas of increased attenuation and vascularity are the result of blood flow redistribution to normal lung.

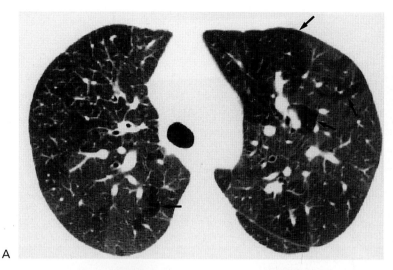

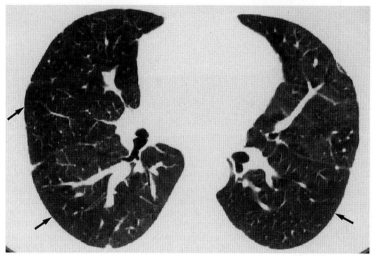

FIGURE 17.12. Chronic pulmonary thromboembolism. **A:** HRCT image at the level of the aortic arch shows focal areas of decreased attenuation and vascularity (*arrows*) in the left upper lobe and (to a lesser extent) in the right upper lobe. **B:** Image at the level of the superior segmental bronchi shows focal areas of decreased attenuation and vascularity (*arrows*) in both lower lobes, right middle lobe and lingula. The patient was a 43-year-old woman with pulmonary arterial hypertension.

In a review of the CT findings in 75 patients who had angiographically proven chronic PE, a mosaic perfusion pattern was found in 58 (77%) (12). The mean attenuation of the areas with decreased attenuation was −868 HU and that of the areas with increased attenuation was −727 HU. After intravenous administration of contrast, the areas with decreased attenuation showed less enhancement (mean 30 HU increase after intravenous contrast) than the areas with increased attenuation (mean 45 HU). In the same study, 54 of 75 patients (72%) had nodular or wedge-shaped, pleura-based areas of increased attenuation on unenhanced scans that remained unchanged after the administration of contrast. These presumably represented residual pulmonary infarcts. In another investigation of 33 patients who had chronic PE, 18 (55%) had areas of mosaic perfusion and 22 (67%) had linear areas of increased attenuation (14).

Chronic PE may also be associated with airway abnormalities (14). In one study of 33 patients who had chronic PE and a control group of 19 patients who had acute PE (14), cylindrical bronchiectasis was seen on HRCT in 21 patients (64%) who had chronic embolism but in only two of those (11%) who had acute disease. The abnormal bronchi were located next to the obstructed pulmonary arteries. It has been postulated that the pathogenesis of the airway dilatation is similar to that of traction bronchiectasis in interstitial pulmonary fibrosis, the ectasia being secondary to retraction of fibrous tissue within the vascular lumen (14).

SEPTIC EMBOLISM

Septic embolism occurs when fragments of thrombus contain organisms, usually bacteria and occasionally fungi or parasites. A predisposing factor is nearly always present, most often drug addiction, generalized infection in patients with immunologic deficiencies (particularly lymphoma), congenital heart disease, and skin infection (15). Most emboli originate from the heart (in association with endocarditis of the tricuspid valve or a ventricular septal defect) (16,17) or the peripheral veins (septic thrombophlebitis).

The pathologic changes in the parenchyma and arteries are similar to those associated with bland thromboemboli (Fig. 17.13). However, the presence of microorganisms tends to result in a greater neutrophil infiltrate and more frequent and extensive liquefaction of necrotic tissue than in noninfected emboli. Drainage of the liquefied necrotic material often results in the formation of cavities. Because the infection tends to extend outward in all directions from its initial site, a nodular appearance to the affected area is frequently seen.

The radiologic manifestations usually consist of multiple, rather ill-defined, round or wedge-shaped opacities in the periphery of the lungs (18,19) (Fig. 17.14). They may be uniform or may vary widely in size, reflecting recurrent showers of emboli. The opacities may be migratory in nature, appearing first in one area and then in another as older lesions resolve and new ones appear (18). Cavitation is frequent and may occur rapidly; the cavities are usually thin-walled, and may contain air–fluid levels. The abnormalities are usually bilateral, although they may be asymmetric and occasionally unilateral (19).

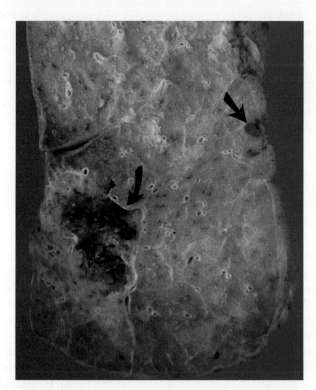

FIGURE 17.13. Septic embolism. Sagittal slice of the right lung shows multiple irregularly shaped foci of yellowish consolidation. Several hemorrhagic lesions are also apparent. One has a wedge shape suggestive of an infarct (*straight arrow*); the other (*curved arrow*) is a cavity lined by granulation tissue. The patient had had staphylococcal septicemia of unknown source about 4 weeks before he died and had radiologic evidence of septic embolism, for which he had been treated.

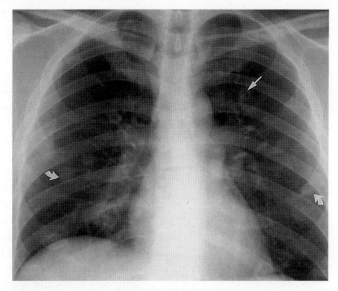

FIGURE 17.14. Septic embolism. Chest radiograph shows poorly defined bilateral cavitated (*straight arrow*) and noncavitated (*curved arrows*) nodules. The patient was a 32-year-old drug addict. Blood cultures grew *Staphylococcus aureus.*

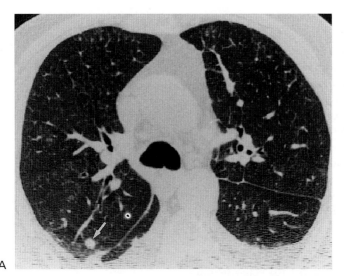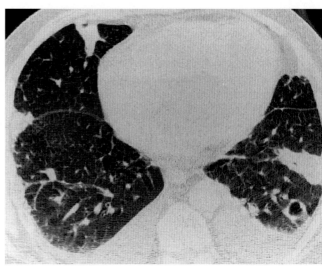

A   B

FIGURE 17.15. Septic embolism. **A:** HRCT image at the level of the tracheal carina shows a small nodule (*arrow*) in the right upper lobe as well as small bilateral pleural effusions. **B:** Image through the lung bases shows a cavitated nodule in the left lower lobe, bilateral wedge-shaped pleural-based areas of consolidation, and bilateral pleural effusions. The patient was a 64-year-old man. Blood cultures grew *Staphylococcus aureus.*

On CT, discrete nodules in various stages of cavitation are identified in approximately 70% of cases (19) (Fig. 17.15). They are often located at the end of a pulmonary vessel (feeding vessel sign) (19,20). Another common manifestation is the presence of bilateral areas of consolidation. In approximately 70% of cases, these are subpleural and wedge-shaped (19). Central regions of heterogeneous lucency or frank cavitation are seen in approximately 90% (19). After administration of intravenous contrast material, a rimlike pattern of peripheral enhancement is frequently seen along the borders, reflecting the presence of highly vascular granulation tissue. Other common findings include pleural effusion and hilar or mediastinal lymph node enlargement (19).

FAT EMBOLISM

The term *fat embolism* refers to the presence of globules of free fat, usually derived from the bone marrow, within the pulmonary vasculature (21,22). The globules may pass from this site into the systemic circulation and embolize to many organs, notably the brain and skin, where they are associated with a variety of neurologic manifestations and cutaneous petechiae. The combination of respiratory, neurologic, and cutaneous disease constitutes the fat embolism syndrome. The commonest underlying condition associated with fat embolism is trauma, which causes disruption of marrow fat cells and laceration of medullary veins. Typically, the full clinical syndrome develops 1 or 2 days after the traumatic event.

The pathogenetic mechanisms involved in the production of the pulmonary component of the fat embolism syndrome are probably twofold. The first is mechanical obstruction of pulmonary vessels, predominantly by fat globules themselves. The second is probably biochemically mediated. Fat appears to be transported to the lungs as neutral triglycerides, and it has been hypothesized that these are converted by endothelial lipases into free fatty acids that then exert a direct toxic effect on cells in the alveolar septa. The resulting damage could in turn lead to the activation of complement or the release of toxins from leukocytes, further exaggerating the injury (23).

Pathologically, the lungs show patchy areas of hemorrhage and edema. Diffuse alveolar damage (proteinaceous airspace exudate and hyaline membranes) is seen histologically in severe cases. Fat can be identified predominantly within arterioles and capillaries as

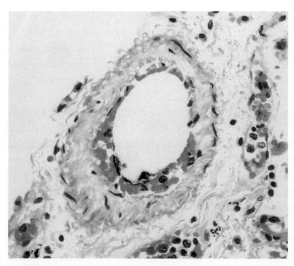
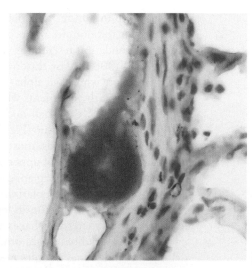

A

B

FIGURE 17.16. Fat embolism. **A:** Photomicrograph shows a round space within a small pulmonary artery, apparently compressing red blood cells to one side. **B:** Oil red O fat stain confirms the presence of intravascular lipid in another vessel. The patient had died 24 hours after severe trauma in a motor vehicle accident.

round-to-oval spaces, 20 to 40 μm in diameter, compressing red blood cells to one side (Fig. 17.16). It can also be seen within macrophages in alveolar airspaces.

Pulmonary fat embolism is unrecognized in many cases if it is not severe, partly because symptoms are mild or absent but also because the chest radiograph is often normal. When present, the radiographic findings are those of acute respiratory distress syndrome (ARDS) of any cause, consisting of widespread airspace consolidation. The distribution tends to be predominantly in the lower lobes and to involve mainly the peripheral rather than the central lung (24). The initial radiologic presentation may consist of poorly defined small nodular opacities (25). HRCT in one patient showed these opacities to have a predominantly centrilobular and subpleural distribution (26). They can progress over the following 24 hours into confluent airspace consolidation (26). In patients with more advanced disease, HRCT shows patchy or confluent ground-glass opacities, areas of consolidation and poorly defined nodules measuring less than 10 mm in diameter (25), findings that presumably reflect the presence of airspace edema and hemorrhage.

EMBOLISM OF TALC (TALCOSIS)

Talc emboli are seen almost invariably in individuals who have engaged in intravenous drug abuse over a long period. In most instances, the complication occurs with medications intended solely for oral use; pills are crushed in a receptacle, water is added, and the mixture is drawn into a syringe and injected. Common oral medications misused in this way include amphetamines, methylphenidate hydrochloride (Ritalin), methadone hydrochloride, pentazocine (Talwin), and meperidine (27,28). All these medications have in common the addition of an insoluble particulate filler to bind the medicinal component and to act as a lubricant during manufacture (27,28). The most widely used filler is talc; cornstarch or microcrystalline cellulose is used in some medications (29).

When injected intravenously, the fillers become trapped within pulmonary arterioles and capillaries, sometimes associated with thrombus. In time, the particles migrate through the vessel wall into the adjacent perivascular interstitial tissue. In early disease, slices of lung can be seen to contain numerous, more or less discrete parenchymal nodules measuring up to 1 mm in diameter (Fig. 17.17) (30). In long-standing disease, there is a tendency for the nodules to become confluent, especially in the upper lobes, producing foci of consolidation resembling the progressive massive fibrosis seen in pneumoconiosis (Fig. 17.18) (30,31). For reasons that are unclear, panacinar emphysema similar to that seen in patients who have alpha-1-antitrypsin deficiency also is commonly present (Fig. 17.19), particularly in patients who have abused Ritalin (28,32,33).

Histologically, the small nodules consist of aggregates of multinucleated giant cells surrounded by fibrous tissue (Fig. 17.17). Although some of these aggregates can be seen in the walls of small vessels, most are present in the perivascular or parenchymal interstitial tissue. The large foci of upper lobe consolidation seen in long-standing disease consist of sheets of multinucleated giant cells separated by a variable amount of fibrous tissue. Talc is readily identifiable by polarization microscopy within the giant cells as birefringent, platelike crystals 5 to 15 μm in length. Cellulose and starch crystals also usually can be identified by characteristic shapes and histochemical reactions (34).

The earliest radiologic abnormality consists of widespread micronodulation, with the diameter of individual nodules ranging from barely visible to about 1 mm (30,35). The opacities have sharply defined margins. The distribution tends to be diffuse and uniform

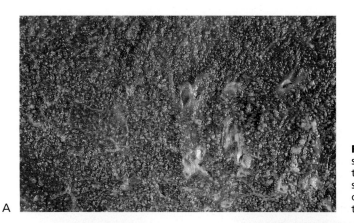

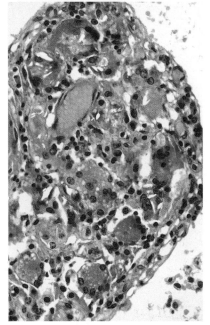

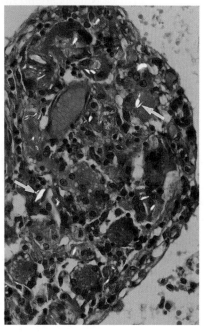

FIGURE 17.17. Talcosis. **A:** Magnified view of a slice of a lower lobe shows innumerable nodules approximately 0.1 to 0.3 mm in diameter. **B, C:** Photomicrographs of a portion of one of the nodules shows it to consist of an aggregate of multinucleated giant cells that contain birefringent platelike crystals (*arrows* in **C**) consistent with talc.

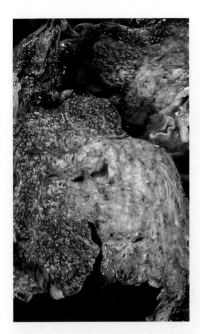

FIGURE 17.18. Talcosis—progressive massive fibrosis-like appearance. Magnified view of a slice of the right lung shows numerous small nodules throughout the parenchyma as well as two fairly well-demarcated areas of dense fibrous tissue.

throughout the lungs. As indicated, the opacities may coalesce in the upper lobes to form an almost homogeneous opacity that closely resembles the progressive massive fibrosis of silicosis except for the frequent presence of an air bronchogram (35,36). HRCT findings consist of diffuse ground-glass attenuation; small, well-defined nodules; and perihilar upper lobe conglomerate areas of fibrosis (28,37) (Figs. 17.20 and 17.21). Localized areas of high attenuation consistent with talc deposition can be seen within the conglomerate masses (Fig. 17.21).

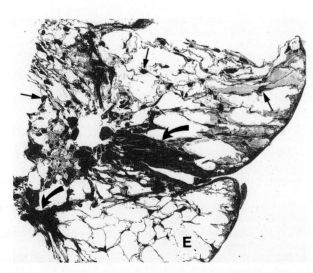

FIGURE 17.19. Talcosis. Low-magnification photomicrograph shows multiple small nodules in the parenchyma (*straight arrows*), corresponding to the multinucleated giant cell aggregates illustrated in Fig. 17.17. Conglomeration of these aggregates has resulted in two larger foci of disease (*curved arrows*), representing an early stage of progressive massive fibrosis. Almost no alveolar septa are evident in one lobule, corresponding to the presence of panacinar emphysema (*E*).

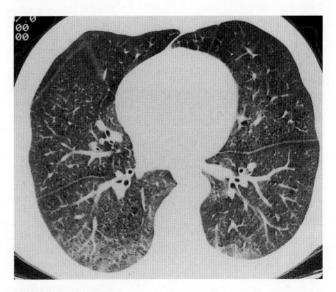

FIGURE 17.20. Talcosis. HRCT image shows extensive bilateral ground-glass opacities with a slightly granular appearance. The patient was a 49-year-old intravenous drug user.

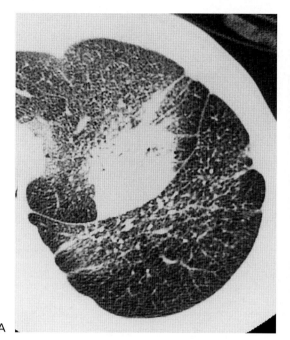
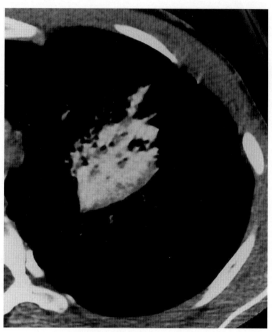

FIGURE 17.21. Talcosis. **A:** HRCT image of the left lung shows numerous small nodules, a conglomerate mass in the left upper lobe associated with volume loss, and evidence of emphysema. **B:** Soft-tissue windows show high attenuation consistent with talc accumulation within the conglomerate mass. The patient was a 27-year-old intravenous drug user.

REFERENCES

1. Dalen JE, Haffajee CI, Alpert JS, et al. Pulmonary embolism, pulmonary hemorrhage and pulmonary infarction. *N Engl J Med* 1977;296:1431–1435.
2. Stein PD, Athanasoulis C, Greenspan RH, et al. Relation of plain chest radiographic findings to pulmonary arterial pressure and arterial blood oxygen levels in patients with acute pulmonary embolism. *Am J Cardiol* 1992;69:394–396.
3. Worsley DF, Alavi A, Aronchick JM, et al. Chest radiographic findings in patients with acute pulmonary embolism: observations from the PIOPED study. *Radiology* 1993;189:133–136.
4. Lindblad B, Sternby NH, Bergqvist D. Incidence of venous thromboembolism verified by necropsy over 30 years. *BMJ* 1991;302:709–714.
5. Sinner WN. Computed tomographic patterns of pulmonary thromboembolism and infarction. *J Comput Assist Tomogr* 1978;2:395–399.
6. Remy-Jardin M, Remy J, Deschildre F, et al. Diagnosis of pulmonary embolism with spiral CT: comparison with pulmonary angiography and scintigraphy. *Radiology* 1996;200:699–706.
7. Mayo JR, Remy-Jardin M, Müller NL, et al. Prospective comparison of spiral CT and ventilation-perfusion scintigraphy in the diagnosis of pulmonary embolism. *Radiology* 1997;205:447–452.
8. Meaney JFM, Weg JG, Chenevert TL, et al. Diagnosis of pulmonary embolism with magnetic resonance angiography. *N Engl J Med* 1997;336:1422–1427.
9. Coche E, Müller NL, Kim KI, et al. Acute pulmonary embolism: ancillary findings on spiral CT. *Radiology* 1998;207:753–758.
10. Remy-Jardin M, Louvegny S, Remy J, et al. Acute central thromboembolic disease: posttherapeutic follow-up with spiral CT angiography. *Radiology* 1997;203:173–180.
11. Auger WR, Fedullo PF, Moser KM, et al. Chronic major-vessel thromboembolic pulmonary artery obstruction: appearance at angiography. *Radiology* 1992;182:393–398.
12. Schwickert HC, Schweden F, Schild HH, et al. Pulmonary arteries and lung parenchyma in chronic pulmonary embolism: preoperative and postoperative CT findings. *Radiology* 1994;191:351–357.
13. Bergin CJ, Rios G, King MA, et al. Accuracy of high-resolution CT in identifying chronic pulmonary thromboembolic disease. *Am J Roentgenol* 1996;166:1371–1377.
14. Remy-Jardin M, Remy J, Louvegny S, et al. Airway changes in chronic pulmonary embolism: CT findings in 33 patients. *Radiology* 1997;203:355–360.
15. Roberts WC, Buchbinder NA. Right-sided valvular infective endocarditis: a clinicopathologic study of twelve necropsy patients. *Am J Med* 1972;53:7–19.
16. Iwama T, Shigemaatsu S, Asami K, et al. Tricuspid valve endocarditis with large vegetations in a non–drug addict without underlying cardiac disease. *Intern Med* 1996;35:203–206.

17. Clifford CP, Eykyn SJ, Oakley CM. Staphylococcal tricuspid valve endocarditis in patients with structurally normal hearts and no evidence of narcotic abuse. *Q J Med* 1994;87:755–757.

18. Jaffe RB, Koschmann EB. Septic pulmonary emboli. *Radiology* 1970;96:527–532.

19. Huang RM, Naidich DP, Lubat E, et al. Septic pulmonary emboli: CT-radiographic correlation. *Am J Roentgenol* 1989;153:41–45.

20. Kuhlman JE, Fishman EK, Teigen C: Pulmonary septic emboli: diagnosis with CT. *Radiology* 1990;174:211–213.

21. Müller C, Rahn BA, Pfister U, et al. The incidence, pathogenesis, diagnosis, and treatment of fat embolism. *Orthop Rev* 1994;23:107–117.

22. Richards RR. Fat embolism syndrome. *Can J Surg* 1997;40:334–339.

23. Kapur MM, Jain P, Gidh M. The effect of trauma on serum C3 activation and its correlation with injury severity score in man. *J Trauma* 1986;26:464–466.

24. Berrigan TJ Jr, Carsky EW, Heitzman ER. Fat embolism: roentgenographic pathologic correlation in 3 cases. *Am J Roentgenol* 1966;96:967–971.

25. Arakawa H, Kurihara Y, Nakajima Y. Pulmonary fat embolism syndrome: CT findings in six patients. *J Comput Assist Tomogr* 2000;24:24–29.

26. Heyneman LE, Müller NL. Pulmonary nodules in early fat embolism syndrome: a case report. *J Thorac Imaging* 2000;15:71–74.

27. Schwartz IS, Bosken C. Pulmonary vascular talc granulomatosis. *JAMA* 1986;256:2584.

28. Ward S, Heyneman LE, Reittner P, et al. Talcosis associated with IV abuse of oral medications: CT findings. *Am J Roentgenol* 2000;174:789–793.

29. Houck RJ, Bailey GL, Daroca PJ Jr, et al. Pentazocine abuse: Report of a case with pulmonary arterial cellulose granulomas and pulmonary hypertension. *Chest* 1980;77:227–230.

30. Paré JP, Cote G, Fraser RS. Long-term follow-up of drug abusers with intravenous talcosis. *Am Rev Respir Dis* 1989;139:233–241.

31. Crouch E, Churg A. Progressive massive fibrosis of the lung secondary to intravenous injection of talc: a pathologic and mineralogic analysis. *Am J Clin Pathol* 1983;80:520–526.

32. Schmidt RA, Glenny RW, Godwin JD, et al. Panlobular emphysema in young intravenous Ritalin abusers. *Am Rev Respir Dis* 1991;143:649–656.

33. Stern EJ, Frank MS, Schmutz JF, et al. Panlobular pulmonary emphysema caused by IV injection of methylphenidate (Ritalin): findings on chest radiographs and CT scans. *Am J Roentgenol* 1994;162:555–560.

34. Tomashefski JF Jr, Hirsch CS. The pulmonary vascular lesions of intravenous drug abuse. *Hum Pathol* 1980;11:133–145.

35. Paré JA, Fraser RG, Hogg JC, et al. Pulmonary "mainline" granulomatosis: talcosis of intravenous methadone abuse. *Medicine* 1979;58:229–239.

36. Sieniewicz DJ, Nidecker AC. Conglomerate pulmonary disease: a form of talcosis in intravenous methadone abusers. *Am J Roentgenol* 1980;135:697–702.

37. Padley SPG, Adler BD, Staples CA, et al. Pulmonary talcosis: CT findings in three cases. *Radiology* 1993;186:125–127.

18

PULMONARY HYPERTENSION

PATHOLOGIC CHARACTERISTICS	Pulmonary Hypertension Associated with Congenital Cardiovascular Disease
RADIOLOGIC MANIFESTATIONS	
	PULMONARY HYPERTENSION ASSOCIATED WITH RESPIRATORY DISEASE
PRIMARY VASCULAR DISEASE	
Primary Pulmonary Hypertension	
Pulmonary Hypertension Associated with Connective Tissue Disease	**PULMONARY VENOUS HYPERTENSION**
	Primary Venoocclusive Disease

Normal pulmonary arteries are composed of an intima of endothelial cells, a media of smooth muscle cells, and an adventitia of collagen. Arteries that have a diameter greater than 0.5 mm also have lamellae of elastic tissue in the media, and are termed *elastic pulmonary arteries.* The latter course in connective tissue adjacent to bronchi down to the subsegmental branches (1). Beyond the subsegmental bronchi, the amount of elastic tissue decreases until there are only single internal and external lamellae separating a media composed entirely of muscle. Many of these muscular arteries accompany the airways down to the level of the terminal bronchioles; additional (supernumerary) branches extend directly into the lung parenchyma. The smooth muscle layer in these vessels progressively thins and eventually disappears, resulting in the formation of arterioles. These measure 15 to 150 μm in diameter and run in connective tissue adjacent to the respiratory bronchioles and in the parenchyma itself, eventually leading to the capillary network in the alveolar walls (1). The latter drains into venules that unite to form veins, which course in the interlobular septa and drain into the left atrium.

The pulmonary vascular circuit is a low-pressure system, the mean arterial pressure normally being only about one-sixth of the systemic arterial pressure. Pulmonary arterial hypertension is considered to be present when the mean pulmonary artery pressure is greater than 25 mm Hg at rest or 30 mm Hg during exercise (1). Pulmonary venous hypertension can be diagnosed when the pressure in the pulmonary veins measured indirectly by a catheter wedged in a pulmonary artery exceeds 12 mm Hg.

An increase in pulmonary arterial pressure can occur because of an increase in resistance to flow through arteries, capillaries, or veins; an increase in blood flow; or an increase in left atrial pressure. Several classifications of pulmonary hypertension have been proposed (2–4). The one recommended at the 1998 World Health Organization meeting considers five main categories (3): (a) pulmonary arterial hypertension that is manifested pathologically as plexogenic arteriopathy (see later), (b) pulmonary venous hypertension, (c) pulmonary hypertension associated with disorders of the respiratory system and/or hypoxemia, (d) pulmonary hypertension due to chronic thrombotic and/or embolic disease, and (e) pulmonary hypertension due to disorders that directly affect the pulmonary vasculature (Table 18.1). In this chapter, we review the most common entities associated with these categories (with the exception of chronic pulmonary embolism, which is discussed in Chapter 17).

TABLE 18.1. WORLD HEALTH ORGANIZATION CLASSIFICATION OF PULMONARY HYPERTENSION (3)

1. Pulmonary arterial hypertension
    1.1. Primary pulmonary hypertension
        a. Sporadic
        b. Familial
    1.2. Related to
        a. Collagen vascular disease
        b. Congenital systemic-to-pulmonary shunts
        c. Portal hypertension
        d. HIV infection
        e. Drugs/toxins
            (1) Appetite-suppressing drugs
            (2) Other
        f. Persistent pulmonary hypertension of the newborn
        g. Other
2. Pulmonary venous hypertension
    2.1. Left-sided atrial or ventricular heart disease
    2.2. Left-sided valvular heart disease
    2.3. Extrinsic compression of central pulmonary veins
        a. Fibrosing mediastinitis
        b. Lymphadenopathy/tumors
    2.4. Pulmonary venoocclusive disease
    2.5. Other
3. Pulmonary hypertension associated with disorders of the respiratory system and/or hypoxemia
    3.1. Chronic obstructive pulmonary disease
    3.2. Interstitial lung disease
    3.3. Sleep-disordered breathing
    3.4. Alveolar hypoventilation disorders
    3.5. Chronic exposure to high altitude
    3.6. Neonatal lung disease
    3.7. Alveolar-capillary dysplasia
    3.8. Other
4. Pulmonary hypertension due to chronic thrombotic and/or embolic disease
    4.1. Thromboembolic obstruction of proximal pulmonary arteries
    4.2. Obstruction of distal pulmonary arteries
        a. Pulmonary embolism (thrombus, tumor, ova and/or parasites, foreign material)
        b. *In situ* thrombosis
        c. Sickle cell disease
5. Pulmonary hypertension due to disorders directly affecting the pulmonary vasculature
    5.1. Inflammatory
        a. Schistosomiasis
        b. Sarcoidosis
        c. Other

PATHOLOGIC CHARACTERISTICS

When sufficiently severe, pulmonary arterial hypertension often can be appreciated on gross specimens by thickening of the walls of elastic and large muscular arteries (Fig. 18.1). Atherosclerotic plaques, sometimes complicated by calcification, also may be evident. Dilatation of the elastic arteries, especially the main pulmonary branch, is also common and may result in a diameter larger than that of the aorta. The thickening seen grossly is predominantly the result of intimal fibrosis in the larger vessels and a combination intimal fibrosis and medial muscle hypertrophy and hyperplasia in the smaller muscular branches (Fig. 18.2).

In primary pulmonary hypertension and in hypertension secondary to conditions such as congenital cardiac shunts and cirrhosis, additional abnormalities are seen in the muscular pulmonary arteries that are collectively known as plexogenic pulmonary arteriopathy. The most characteristic of these is the plexiform lesion (Fig. 18.3). Typically, this is seen a short distance beyond the origin of a small supernumerary branch (usually 100 to

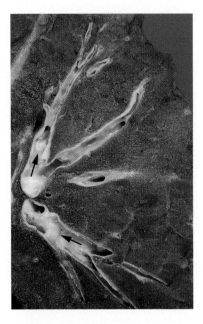

FIGURE 18.1. Pulmonary arterial hypertension—gross appearance. A magnified view of a slice of an upper lobe shows a moderate degree of thickening of the walls of several subsegmental pulmonary arteries. Foci of atherosclerosis (*arrows*) are evident.

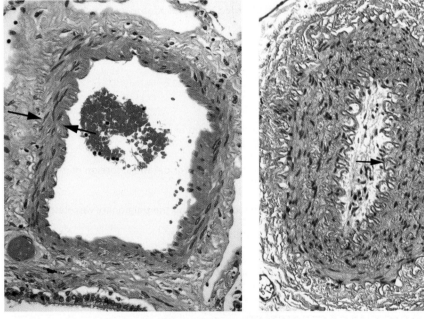

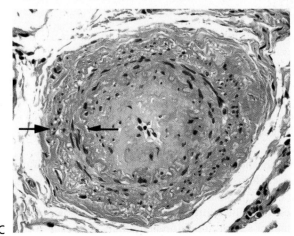

FIGURE 18.2. Pulmonary arterial hypertension—microscopic appearance. **A:** Photomicrograph shows a normal pulmonary artery whose wall is composed of a thin muscular media (*arrows*) and an inconspicuous intima. Pulmonary arteries from a patient with primary pulmonary hypertension show marked medial hypertrophy and intimal thickening by fibroblastic tissue (**B**) and mature fibrous tissue (**C**). (*Arrows* indicate media.)

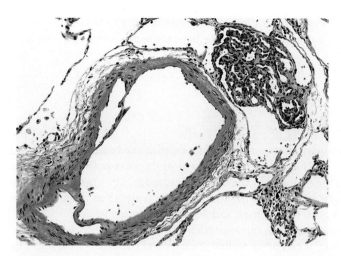

FIGURE 18.3. Pulmonary arterial hypertension—plexiform lesion. The photomicrograph shows a pulmonary artery with mild medial hypertrophy. A complex of irregularly shaped capillary-like vessels (plexiform lesion) is present in the adjacent tissue.

200 μm in diameter) (5) and consists of a localized focus of vascular dilation associated with an intraluminal plexus of slitlike vascular channels separated by a variable number of fibroblast-like cells. The plexus itself often continues distally into a thin-walled, somewhat tortuous and dilated vascular channel. Additional histologic findings that may be seen in plexogenic arteriopathy are vasculitis and the presence of loose connective tissue accompanied by concentric layers of fibroblast-like cells in the intima.

In most cases of pulmonary hypertension, arterial intimal fibrous tissue has a solid appearance and is distributed in a more or less concentric fashion in the vessel lumen. Occasionally, it is eccentric in location or traverses the lumen (Fig. 18.4), in which case the

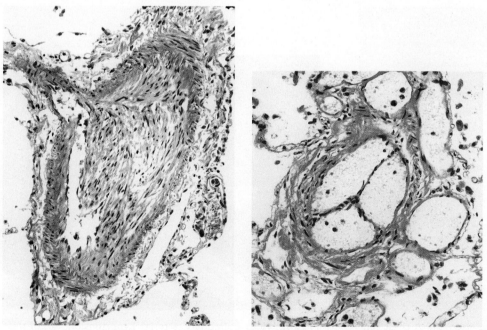

A   B

FIGURE 18.4. Pulmonary arterial hypertension—organized thrombi. Photomicrographs show two small pulmonary arteries, one (**A**) with a focus of intimal fibrosis located on one side of the vessel lumen and the other (**B**) with thin fibrous strands traversing the lumen in a "spoke-wheel" pattern. Both appearances suggest organized thrombus. The patient was a 32-year old woman with primary pulmonary hypertension.

pathogenesis of the fibrosis is likely organization of thrombus formed *in situ* or embolized. Both such processes have been hypothesized to be the basis for some cases of primary pulmonary hypertension.

RADIOLOGIC MANIFESTATIONS

The characteristic radiologic features of pulmonary arterial hypertension consist of enlargement of the central pulmonary arteries and rapid tapering of the vessels as they extend to the periphery of the lungs (1) (Fig. 18.5). Enlargement of the hilar pulmonary arteries can be assessed by measuring the diameter of the interlobar arteries. The upper limit of the transverse diameter of the right interlobar artery from its lateral aspect to the air column of the intermediate bronchus is 16 mm in men and 15 mm in women (6).

Because the main pulmonary artery is intrapericardial, it cannot be measured on conventional radiography; however, it can be identified readily on CT and MR imaging. The possibility of pulmonary hypertension should be suspected on CT or MR when the diameter of the main pulmonary artery is greater than 2.8 cm (7–9) or when the diameter of the pulmonary artery is greater than that of the aorta (10) (Fig. 18.6). The diameter of the main pulmonary artery is measured in the scan plane of the pulmonary artery bifurcation, at a right angle to its long axis and just lateral to the ascending aorta. Another common finding on CT in patients who have pulmonary hypertension is enlargement of the segmental pulmonary arteries. This feature is visually assessed by comparing the diameter of the segmental pulmonary arteries to that of the adjacent bronchus. The presence of segmental artery-to-bronchus diameter ratios greater than 1:1 in three or four lobes is highly suggestive of hypertension (1,9).

Patients who have pulmonary hypertension due to primary vascular disease often have patchy areas of increased attenuation and vascularity adjacent to areas of decreased atten-

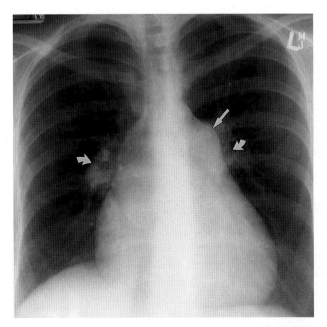

FIGURE 18.5. Pulmonary arterial hypertension. A chest radiograph shows enlargement of the main (*straight arrow*) and interlobar (*curved arrows*) pulmonary arteries. Note rapid tapering of the pulmonary arteries distal from the hila. The patient was a 27-year-old woman.

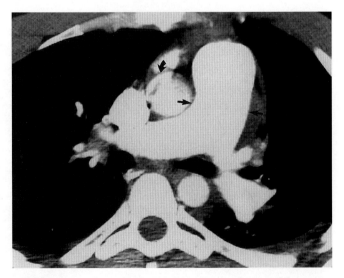

FIGURE 18.6. Pulmonary arterial hypertension. A contrast-enhanced spiral CT image shows enlarged main (straight arrows), right and left pulmonary arteries. The diameter of the main pulmonary artery measured 3.2 cm while that of the ascending aorta (*curved arrow*) was 2.5 cm. The patient was a 25-year-old man.

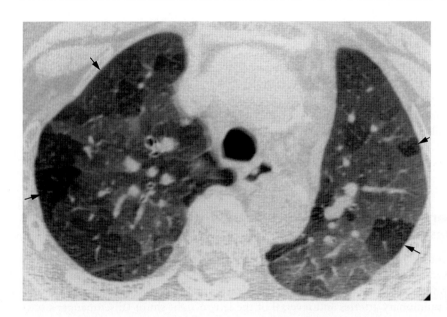

FIGURE 18.7. Mosaic perfusion in pulmonary arterial hypertension. HRCT image shows areas of decreased attenuation and perfusion (*straight arrows*) and areas with increased attenuation and vascularity. The patient was a 73-year-old woman with pulmonary arterial hypertension secondary to chronic thromboembolism.

uation and vascularity. This pattern is known as mosaic perfusion and is seen most commonly in patients with hypertension secondary to chronic pulmonary embolism (11,12) (Fig. 18.7). It is presumably related to variability in the severity of vasculature obstruction, with blood flow being greater in some lobules than in others.

The MR imaging findings in pulmonary hypertension include right ventricular hypertrophy, reversal of the interventricular septal curvature, enlargement of the central pulmonary arteries and increased intravascular signal on spin-echo images due to slow pulmonary arterial flow (1,13).

PRIMARY VASCULAR DISEASE

Primary Pulmonary Hypertension

Primary pulmonary hypertension (i.e., hypertension for which no cause can be identified) is uncommon, having an incidence of only about 1 per 1 million population (14). It is seen most commonly in patients 25 to 45 years of age; the female-to-male predominance is 1.7:1 (14). The main symptom is dyspnea on exertion, which is often insidious in onset. Plexiform arteriopathy is found histologically in virtually all patients. Organizing thrombi or foci of eccentric or recanalized fibrous tissue consistent with organized thrombi are identified in more than 50% (1,15); their role in the pathogenesis of the condition is controversial.

The radiographic findings consist of enlargement of the central pulmonary arteries, rapid tapering, and peripheral oligemia (14). In one study, the chest radiographs of 187 patients were graded subjectively. Prominence of the main pulmonary artery was found in 90%; enlarged hilar vessels, in 80%; right ventricular hypertrophy, in 74%; and decreased peripheral vascularity, in 51%. The radiographic appearance was felt to be normal in 6% (14). CT demonstrates enlargement of the main, hilar, and segmental pulmonary arteries (1). A mosaic pattern of lung attenuation is seen on CT in approximately 50% of patients, compared with 80% of patients who have pulmonary hypertension secondary to chronic pulmonary embolism (16). Radionuclide ventilation–perfusion scans are typically interpreted as normal or low probability for pulmonary embolism (1).

Pulmonary Hypertension Associated with Connective Tissue Disease

Pulmonary arterial hypertension, unaccompanied by parenchymal lung disease and manifested pathologically by plexogenic arteriopathy, occurs occasionally in immunologically mediated connective tissue disorders, particularly progressive systemic sclerosis (PSS), mixed connective tissue disease, and systemic lupus erythematosus (SLE). Pulmonary hypertension also occurs in some individuals with immunologically mediated interstitial lung disease such as rheumatoid disease and PSS; in these cases, radiographic and pathologic features are identical to those associated with chronic interstitial lung disease of other etiologies.

Pulmonary Hypertension Associated with Congenital Cardiovascular Disease

The most common congenital diseases associated with a left-to-right shunt are atrial septal defect, ventricular septal defect, and patent ductus arteriosus. The shunting can lead to the development of severe, irreversible pulmonary arterial hypertension with dilation of the central pulmonary arteries and reversal of the left-to-right shunt (Eisenmenger's syndrome) (17). The pathologic features are those of plexogenic arteriopathy.

The main radiographic sign of a left-to-right shunt is an increase in caliber of all the pulmonary arteries throughout the lungs (Fig. 18.8). The degree of enlargement of the main and hilar pulmonary arteries usually is proportional to the degree of distention of the intrapulmonary vessels. Tapering of the peripheral pulmonary vessels as a result of luminal narrowing by intimal fibrosis and medial hyperplasia is common (1). Linear calcification of the central pulmonary arteries (as a result of dystrophic calcification of intimal fibrous tissue) and thrombus formation may be seen on CT (1). Both echocardiography and MR imaging can readily demonstrate the presence of the shunt and the anatomic features of the underlying cardiovascular anomalies (18,19)

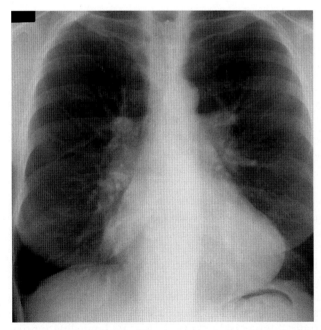

FIGURE 18.8. Pulmonary arterial hypertension secondary to atrial septal defect. Chest radiograph shows enlargement of the central and peripheral pulmonary arteries. The patient was a 47-year-old woman with an atrial septal defect.

PULMONARY HYPERTENSION ASSOCIATED WITH RESPIRATORY DISEASE

A wide variety of primary diseases of the lungs, pleura, chest wall, and respiratory control center may cause a rise in pulmonary arterial pressure without significant change in pulmonary venous pressure. However, pulmonary arterial pressures seldom reach the levels attained in cases of primary vascular disease, and the arterial and arteriolar narrowing due to intimal thickening and medial hypertrophy is less. Histologic features of plexogenic arteriopathy are absent. In fact, the hypertension may be transient, reflecting episodes of pulmonary infection and its associated hypoxia.

It is probable that the main cause of pulmonary arterial hypertension in this group of conditions is hypoxemia, with or without respiratory acidosis. The reduction in arterial oxygen saturation may be secondary to ventilation–perfusion inequality, shunt, or generalized alveolar hypoventilation.

The radiologic manifestations of pulmonary hypertension in these patients are identical to those of primary vascular disease, except for the presence of the findings related to the underlying pulmonary or pleural abnormality.

PULMONARY VENOUS HYPERTENSION

Pulmonary venous hypertension results most commonly from diseases of the left side of the heart, usually those that cause left ventricular failure, such as systemic hypertension and coronary artery disease. Less common causes include mitral stenosis, fibrosing mediastinitis, atrial myxoma, and primary venoocclusive disease.

Morphologic abnormalities in chronic venous hypertension can be seen in the arteries, veins, and lung parenchyma. Muscular arteries show medial hypertrophy and intimal fibrosis, although usually less severe than in plexogenic arteriopathy. Extension of muscle into the media of pulmonary arterioles (muscularization of arterioles) is common (20). Plexiform lesions do not occur. Medial hypertrophy and intimal fibrosis also are common in the pulmonary veins (Fig. 18.9) (20). In addition, the elastic laminae, which are normally irregular in distribution, may become concentrated into internal and external laminae, similar to the appearance of pulmonary arteries ("arterialization" of pulmonary veins). In severe disease, the alveolar interstitium often shows patchy fibrosis, possibly as a reaction to chronic transudation of fluid across the capillaries. Evidence of recent or remote airspace hemorrhage is common, the latter manifested grossly as foci of brown discoloration and histologically as the accumulation of hemosiderin-laden macrophages in alveolar airspaces. Foci of bone are also frequent (Fig. 18.9) and may be sufficient in size to be seen radiologically. They may be caused by metaplasia of fibrous tissue resulting from organization of airspace blood.

A characteristic radiographic manifestation of pulmonary venous hypertension is an increase in size of the upper lobe vessels (Fig. 18.10). Because this increase in size is caused by increased resistance to blood flow through the lower zones, it affects the arteries and veins. Other common findings include septal (Kerley B) lines, small pleural effusions, enlargement of the central pulmonary arteries, and cardiomegaly (1).

Pulmonary Venoocclusive Disease

Pulmonary venoocclusive disease is a rare abnormality characterized pathologically by evidence of repeated pulmonary venous thrombosis and clinically by slowly progressive dyspnea interspersed by episodes of acute deterioration related to acute pulmonary edema. It is most common in children and young adults. The etiology is usually unknown; however, the disease has been observed in patients using oral contraceptives, receiving treatment with some chemotherapeutic agents, following bone marrow transplantation, or having autoimmune disease (21,22).

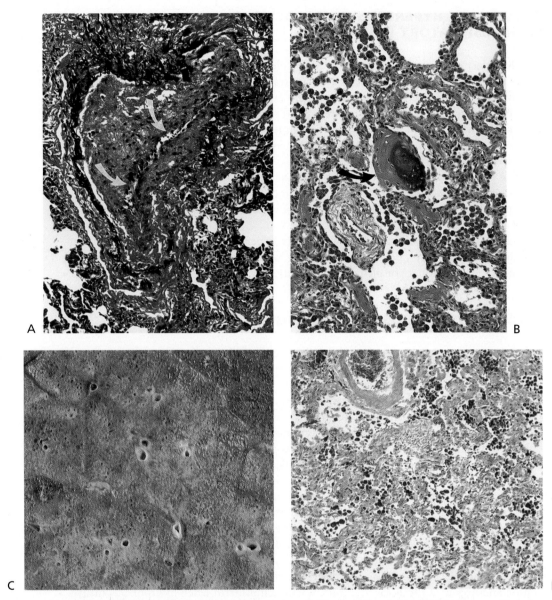

FIGURE 18.9. Pulmonary venous hypertension. **A:** Elastic stain of a small pulmonary vein shows marked intimal fibrosis, only a small, slitlike lumen remaining (*arrows*). **B:** Magnified view of lung parenchyma shows mild alveolar interstitial fibrosis and numerous macrophages in the airspaces. A small fragment of bone is present in one airspace (*arrow*). **C:** Magnified view of a slice of lung shows numerous foci of brown discoloration. **D:** Photomicrograph of one of the brown foci shows numerous hemosiderin-containing macrophages (stained blue) in alveolar airspaces. The patient was a 65-year-old man with mitral stenosis.

The most prominent histologic feature is stenosis or complete obliteration of the lumens of small to intermediate-sized pulmonary veins and venules by intimal fibrous tissue (Fig. 18.11) (23,24). The fibrous tissue may have a loose (active) or mature appearance; not uncommonly, it appears as trabeculae that subdivide the lumen into several channels, suggesting recanalized thrombus. Evidence of pulmonary arterial hypertension is usually present in the form of medial hypertrophy of small pulmonary arteries, with or without intimal proliferation, fibrosis, and thrombi (21). The lung parenchyma may show evidence of remote hemorrhage (interstitial and airspace hemosiderin-laden macrophages); some degree of interstitial fibrosis and chronic inflammation are also often evident (25).

The characteristic radiologic manifestations consist of enlargement of the central pulmonary arteries (reflecting the presence of pulmonary arterial hypertension) and interlob-

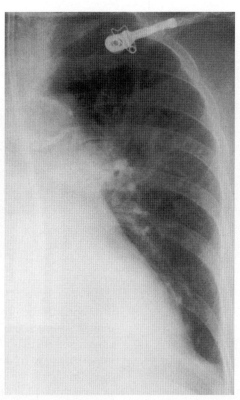

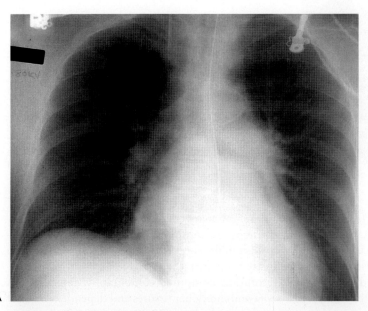

A B

FIGURE 18.10. Pulmonary venous hypertension. **A:** Chest radiograph shows prominence of the upper lobe vessels and cardiomegaly. **B:** View of the left lung the following day shows further increase in size of the upper lobe vessels and hazy perihilar ground glass opacities secondary to pulmonary edema. The patient was a 64-year-old woman with left heart failure and fluid overload.

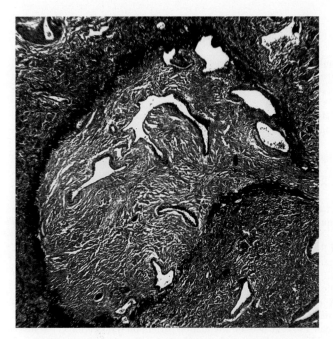

FIGURE 18.11. Pulmonary venoocclusive disease. An elastic stain of an intermediate size pulmonary vein shows almost complete obliteration of the lumen by mature fibrous tissue. Several irregularly shaped vascular channels are present in the fibrous tissue, suggesting that it developed by organization of thrombus.

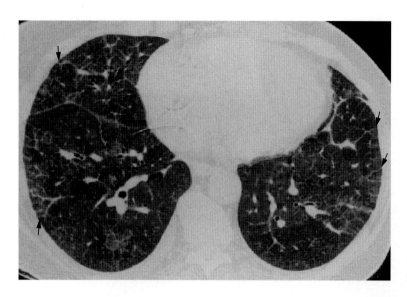

FIGURE 18.12. Pulmonary venoocclusive disease. An HRCT image shows smooth thickening of interlobular septa (*arrows*) and bilateral ground-glass opacities due to pulmonary edema. The patient was a 50-year-old woman.

ular septal thickening (reflecting interstitial pulmonary edema and/or thickening of pulmonary veins) (26,27). Small pleural effusions are common. The left atrium is not enlarged, and there is no evidence of redistribution of blood flow to upper lung zones, both important signs in distinguishing the disease from mitral stenosis (1,26).

Similar to the radiograph, high-resolution computed tomography demonstrates smooth thickening of the interlobular septa and interlobar fissures and dependent areas of ground-glass attenuation consistent with interstitial edema (22,28) (Fig. 18.12). A mosaic pattern of lung attenuation is seen in approximately 50% of cases (22). Other characteristic findings seen include enlargement of the central pulmonary arteries, small or normal-sized central pulmonary veins, and normal-sized left atrium (1,22).

REFERENCES

1. Frazier AA, Galvin JR, Franks TJ, et al. Pulmonary vasculature: hypertension and infarction. *Radiographics* 2000;20:491–524.
2. Wagenvoort CA. Classifying pulmonary vascular disease. *Chest* 1973;64:503–504.
3. Peacock AJ. Primary pulmonary hypertension. *Thorax* 1999;54:1107–1118.
4. Voelkel NF, Tuder RM. Severe pulmonary hypertensive diseases: a perspective. *Eur Respir J* 1999;14:1246–1250.
5. Yaginuma G, Mohri H, Takahashi T. Distribution of arterial lesions and collateral pathways in the pulmonary hypertension of congenital heart disease: a computer aided reconstruction study. *Thorax* 1990;45:586–590.
6. Chang CH: The normal roentgenographic measurement of the right descending pulmonary artery in 1,085 cases. *Am J Roentgenol* 1962;87:929–935.
7. Kuriyama K, Gamsu G, Stern RG, et al. CT-determined pulmonary artery diameters in predicting pulmonary artery hypertension. *Invest Radiol* 1984;19:16–22.
8. Murray TI, Boxt LM, Katz J, et al. Estimation of pulmonary artery pressure in patients with primary pulmonary hypertension by quantitative analysis of magnetic resonance images. *J Thorac Imag* 1994;9:198–204.
9. Tan RT, Kuzo R, Goodman LR, et al. Utility of CT scan evaluation for predicting pulmonary hypertension in patients with parenchymal lung disease. *Chest* 1998;113:1250–1256.
10. Ng CS, Wells AU, Padley SPG. A CT sign of chronic pulmonary arterial hypertension: the ratio of main pulmonary artery to aortic diameter. *J Thorac Imag* 1999;14:270–278.
11. Bergin CJ, Rios G, King MA, et al. Accuracy of high-resolution CT in identifying chronic pulmonary thromboembolic disease. *Am J Roentgenol* 1996;166:1371–1377.
12. Worthy SA, Muller NL, Hartman TE, et al. Mosaic attenuation pattern on thin-section CT scans of the lung: differentiation among infiltrative lung, airway, and vascular diseases as a cause. *Radiology* 1997;205:465–470.
13. White RD, Higgins CB. Magnetic resonance imaging of thoracic vascular disease. *J Thorac Imaging* 1989;4:34–50.

14. Rich S, Dantzker DR, Ayres SM, et al. Primary pulmonary hypertension: a national prospective study. *Ann Intern Med* 1987;107:216–223.
15. Burke A, Virmani R. Mini-symposium: pulmonary pathology: evaluation of pulmonary hypertension in biopsies of the lung. *Curr Diagn Pathol* 1996;3:14–26.
16. Sherrick AD, Swensen SJ, Hartman TE. Mosaic pattern of lung attenuation on CT scans: frequency among patients with pulmonary artery hypertension of different causes. *Am J Roentgenol* 1997;169: 79–82.
17. Hopkins WE. Severe pulmonary hypertension in congenital heart disease: a review of Eisenmenger syndrome. *Curr Opin Cardiol* 1995;10:517–523.
18. Wexler L, Higgins CB, Herfkens RJ. Magnetic resonance imaging in adult congenital heart disease. *J Thorac Imag* 1994;9:219–229.
19. Rebergen SA, Niezen RA, Helbing WA, et al. Cine gradient-echo MR imaging and MR velocity mapping in the evaluation of congenital heart disease. *Radiographics* 1996;16:467–481.
20. Wagenvoort CA. Pathology of congestive pulmonary hypertension. *Prog Resp Res* 1975;9:195–202.
21. Chazova I, Robbins I, Loyd J, et al. Venous and arterial changes in pulmonary veno-occlusive disease, mitral stenosis and fibrosing mediastinitis. *Eur Respir J* 2000;15:116–122.
22. Swensen SJ, Tashjian JH, Myers JL, et al. Pulmonary venoocclusive disease: CT findings in eight patients. *Am J Roentgenol* 1996;167:937–940.
23. Hasleton PS, Ironside JW, Whittaker JS, et al. Pulmonary veno-occlusive disease: a report of four cases. *Histopathology* 1986;10:933–944.
24. Wagenvoort CA, Wagenvoort N, Takahashi T. Pulmonary veno-occlusive disease: involvement of pulmonary arteries and review of the literature. *Hum Pathol* 1985;16:1033–1041.
25. Wagenvoort CA, Wagenvoort N. The pathology of pulmonary veno-occlusive disease. *Virchows Arch* 1974;364:69–79.
26. Shackleford GD, Sacks EJ, Mullins JD, et al. Pulmonary veno-occlusive disease: case report and review of the literature. *Am J Roentgenol* 1977;128:643–648.
27. Holcomb BW Jr, Loyd JE, Ely EW, et al. Pulmonary veno-occlusive disease: a case series and new observations. *Chest* 2000;118:1671–1679.
28. Cassart M, Gevenois PA, Kramer M, et al. Pulmonary venoocclusive disease: CT findings before and after single-lung transplantation. *Am J Roentgenol* 1993;160:759–760.

PULMONARY VASCULITIS AND HEMORRHAGE

This chapter includes a variety of conditions the sole or predominant histologic feature of which is inflammation of pulmonary vessels and in which the inflammatory reaction is directed primarily against the vessel wall and is of proven or presumed immunologic origin. Vasculitis associated with connective tissue diseases (such as systemic lupus erythematosus) is discussed in Chapter 6.

WEGENER'S GRANULOMATOSIS

Wegener's granulomatosis is a multisystem disease with variable clinical expression. In its full-blown state, it is characterized pathologically by necrotizing granulomatous inflammation of the upper and lower respiratory tracts, glomerulonephritis, and necrotizing vasculitis of the lungs and a variety of systemic organs and tissues. In some patients it is manifested primarily or solely in the respiratory tract and is known as *limited (nonrenal) Wegener's granulomatosis* (1).

The disease is rare; the prevalence in the United States has been estimated to be about three per 100,000 (2). It typically affects adults in their 30s to 50s.

Pathologic Characteristics

Grossly, pulmonary involvement by Wegener's granulomatosis usually takes the form of more or less well-circumscribed, nodular or masslike foci of consolidation ranging in diameter from 1 to 4 cm. Necrosis and cavitation are frequent (Fig. 19.1). Less commonly, the disease appears as focal or diffuse hemorrhagic consolidation (3).

Microscopically, the earliest finding is parenchymal infiltration by an inflammatory cell infiltrate composed predominantly of lymphocytes, plasma cells, and histiocytes, with lesser numbers of eosinophils, multinucleated giant cells, and polymorphonuclear leukocytes (Fig. 19.2) (4,5). The neutrophils tend to be aggregated in small, microabscess-like clusters that, as disease progresses, become necrotic and bordered by a rim of macrophages or epithelioid histiocytes. With further progression, these foci enlarge and coalesce, re-

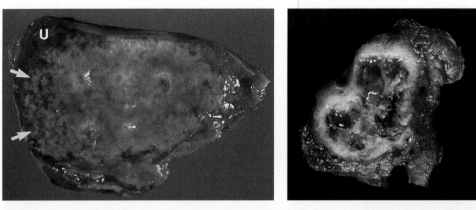

FIGURE 19.1. Wegener's granulomatosis—gross appearance. **A:** Open-lung biopsy specimen shows extensive consolidation and necrosis. (Only a small amount of unaffected lung [u] is apparent.) The tan necrotic foci at the edge of the biopsy (*arrows*) have a distinctive serpiginous outline. The appearance suggests active disease. **B:** Biopsy specimen from another patient shows a more well-circumscribed focus of disease that has a white periphery (suggesting the presence of fibroblastic tissue) and a central cavity. The appearance suggests a more advanced stage of disease than that in **A.**

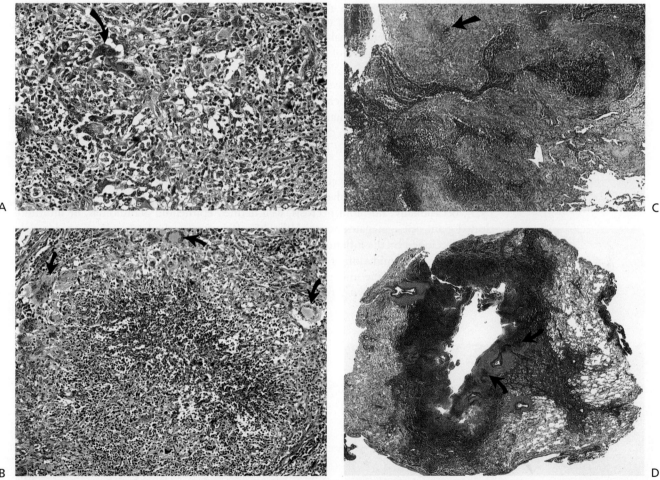

FIGURE 19.2. Wegener's granulomatosis—microscopic appearance. **A:** Photomicrograph shows consolidation of lung parenchyma by a polymorphous inflammatory cell infiltrate composed of lymphocytes, plasma cells, neutrophils and histiocytes; occasional multinucleated giant cells (*arrow*) can be seen. **B:** Photomicrograph from the same biopsy specimen shows a focus of necrotic tissue containing numerous neutrophils and surrounded by a granulomatous inflammatory cell infiltrate (*arrows* indicate giant cells). **C:** Low-magnification view shows the small focus of necrotic tissue seen in **B** (*arrow*), as well as other much larger foci. Enlargement and coalescence of the small foci of disease result in a distinctive serpiginous outline to the larger necrotic regions. **D:** Erosion of the inflammatory infiltrate into an airway has been followed by drainage of necrotic tissue and cavity formation. Small foci of serpiginous necrotic tissue can be identified in the cavity wall (*arrows*).

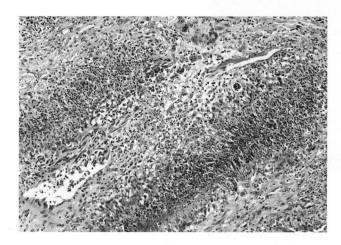

FIGURE 19.3. Wegener's granulomatosis. Photomicrograph shows two linear foci of necrotic tissue located in the media of a small pulmonary artery. The appearance is similar to that of the parenchymal necrosis illustrated in Fig. 19.2B.

sulting in a characteristic serpiginous outline to the necrotic areas. Erosion of one of these areas into an airway leads to drainage of the necrotic tissue and cavity formation (Fig. 19.2). Additional parenchymal findings include airspace filling by blood or fibroblastic tissue (sometimes in a pattern of BOOP) and obstructive pneumonitis (6,7); usually, these are limited in extent.

Involvement of the airways is also common, either by direct extension from a focus of parenchymal disease or independently (8). This involvement usually takes the form of mucosal or submucosal inflammation identical to that in the parenchyma. The epithelium may be intact or ulcerated; in the latter case, an endobronchial polyp of granulation tissue may cause airway obstruction. The subglottic trachea is a relatively common site of the latter complication.

Pulmonary arteries and veins of small to medium size show focal or extensive inflammation. Most often this involves the media and is similar to that in the parenchyma (Fig. 19.3); occasionally, fibrinoid necrosis, well-defined epithelioid granulomas, or multinucleated giant cell aggregates occur. Although often patent, the lumen of affected vessels may be occluded by the inflammatory cell infiltrate or by thrombus.

Histologic examination of cases characterized grossly by focal or diffuse hemorrhagic consolidation shows the underlying lung architecture to be maintained and the alveolar airspaces to be filled with red blood cells (Fig. 19.4) (9,10). Hemosiderin-laden

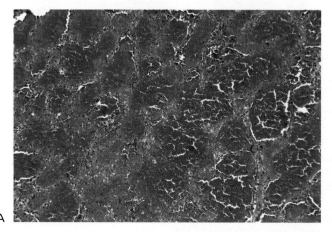

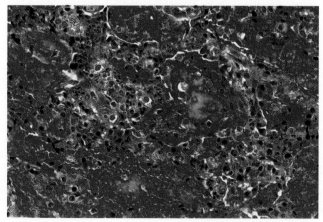

FIGURE 19.4. Wegener's granulomatosis—capillaritis. **A:** Photomicrograph of a biopsy specimen of an area of parenchymal consolidation shows extensive alveolar airspace hemorrhage and mild interstitial thickening. **B:** Higher magnification shows the thickening to be the result of an infiltrate of neutrophils centered on alveolar septa.

macrophages indicative of prior hemorrhage and foci of organizing fibrinous exudate reflecting healing alveolar wall damage also may be seen. Alveolar septa are thickened by an infiltrate of polymorphonuclear leukocytes, and fibrin thrombi may be evident in the capillary lumen (capillaritis). Arterioles and venules often show similar changes (microangiitis). These abnormalities may be the only histologic manifestation of Wegener's granulomatosis or may be seen in association with the necrotizing parenchymal and vascular changes described previously.

Radiologic Manifestations

The typical radiographic pattern consists of nodules measuring 1 to 4 cm in diameter (11–13). In most cases, they are fewer than 10 (11,12). They are bilateral in approximately 75% of cases and are usually widely distributed, with no predilection for any lung zone (11). With progression of disease, the nodules tend to increase in size and number. Cavitation of one or more nodules occurs eventually in approximately 50% of cases (11,14). The cavities are usually thick-walled and tend to have an irregular, shaggy inner lining, reflecting the serpiginous appearance described histologically (11,13).

CT may demonstrate nodules that are not apparent on radiography and is superior in demonstrating the presence of cavitation (15,16). In fact, cavitation is evident on CT in the majority of nodules that measure more than 2 cm (Fig. 19.5) (13). As on radiography, the nodules tend to have a random distribution (13); occasionally, they are predominantly or exclusively subpleural in location (17) or have a peribronchovascular distribution (14,18).

Airspace consolidation or ground-glass opacities are the next most common radiographic findings in Wegener's granulomatosis and may occur with or without the presence of nodules (11,14) (Fig. 19.6). The areas of consolidation are quite variable in appearance, some being dense and localized (11), some involving a whole lobe (19), and others being bilateral and patchy or confluent (14). They are often secondary to pulmonary hemorrhage but sometimes are related to necrotizing granulomatous inflammation similar to that associated with nodules. In one review of the radiographic findings in 77 patients with pulmonary Wegener's granulomatosis, nodules were identified on the radiograph in 69% and areas of consolidation in 53%; 49% of nodules and 17% of areas of consolidation had evidence of cavitation (11). Diffuse bilateral areas of ground-glass opacity or consolidation were seen in 8% of cases. On CT, the areas of consolidation may be random in distribution; sometimes they appear as peripheral wedge-shaped lesions abutting the pleura, mimicking pulmonary infarcts (18) (Fig. 19.7), or have a peribronchoarterial distribution (Fig. 19.6) (13, 20).

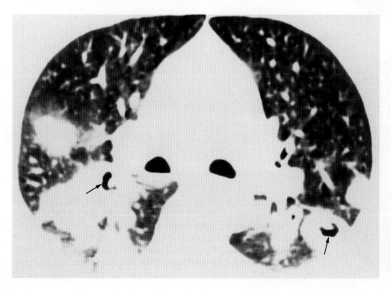

FIGURE 19.5. Wegener's granulomatosis. CT image demonstrates bilateral cavitating (*arrows*) and noncavitating nodules of various sizes and focal areas of consolidation. The patient was a 45-year-old man.

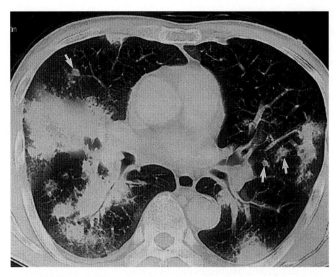

FIGURE 19.6. Wegener's granulomatosis. HRCT image demonstrates peribronchovascular areas of airspace consolidation and ill-defined nodules (*arrows*). The patient was a 58-year-old man. (Courtesy of Dr. Kazuto Ashizawa, Department of Radiology, Nagasaki University School of Medicine, Nagasaki, Japan.)

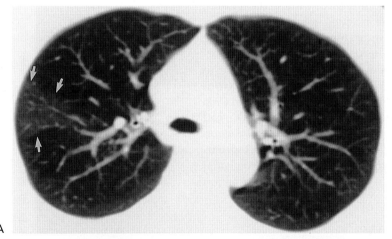

A

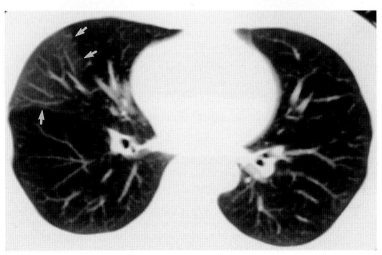

B

FIGURE 19.7. Wegener's granulomatosis. Conventional CT images at level of aortic arch (**A**) and inferior pulmonary veins (**B**) demonstrate segmental areas of ground-glass attenuation (*arrows*) in right upper and middle lobes. The patient was a 49-year-old woman with pulmonary hemorrhage due to Wegener's granulomatosis.

Bronchial wall involvement by Wegener's granulomatosis may result in airway narrowing and lead to segmental, lobar, or total lung atelectasis (11,21). The bronchial abnormalities themselves or those affecting the trachea are seldom visible on the radiograph (12) but can usually be detected on CT (12,14,22). Unilateral or bilateral pleural effusions are present in about 10% of patients (11). Hilar or mediastinal lymph node enlargement, or both, has been reported on radiography or CT in 2% to 15% of cases (11,14).

CHURG-STRAUSS SYNDROME

Churg-Strauss syndrome is characterized clinically by asthma, fever, and blood eosinophilia and pathologically by necrotizing vasculitis and extravascular granulomatous inflammation (23). The condition is rare (24). It develops most often in middle-aged adults, the mean age of onset being 40 to 50 years (25,26).

Pathologic Characteristics

The characteristic microscopic findings consist of a combination of vasculitis and extravascular necrotizing granulomas (7,27). The vasculitis is manifested by a transmural infiltrate of lymphocytes, plasma cells, histiocytes, multinucleated giant cells, and a large number of eosinophils in small-to-medium-sized arteries and veins (Fig. 19.8). Granulomas occasionally occur.

Extravascular parenchymal disease typically consists of foci of necrotic material, frequently containing numerous eosinophils and surrounded by epithelioid histiocytes and multinucleated giant cells (Fig. 19.8). Alveolar interstitial and airspace infiltration by eosinophils and macrophages in a pattern similar to eosinophilic pneumonia is also fre-

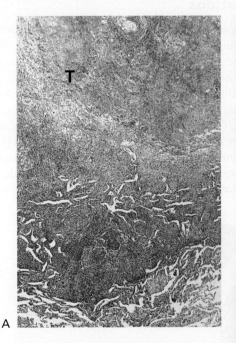
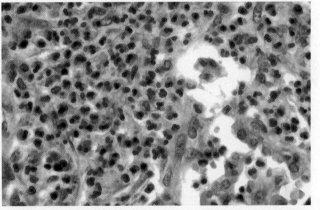
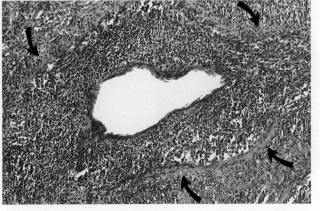

FIGURE 19.8. Churg-Strauss syndrome. **A:** Photomicrograph of a poorly delimited parenchymal nodule shows a focus of necrotic tissue (*T*) surrounded by a dense inflammatory cell infiltrate. **B:** Magnified view shows many of the inflammatory cells to be eosinophils. **C:** Section of a medium-sized vessel adjacent to the necrotic region shows marked inflammation of the media. (*Arrows* indicate the smooth muscle of the vessel wall.)

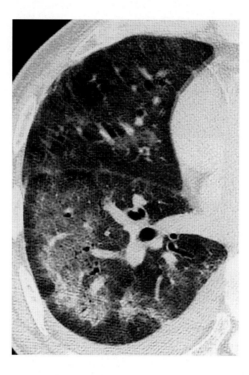

FIGURE 19.9. Churg-Strauss syndrome. HRCT image of the right lung demonstrates areas of ground-glass attenuation and airspace consolidation. The patient was a 71-year-old man.

quent (27). Histologic changes of chronic asthma (goblet cell metaplasia, basement membrane thickening, and muscle hypertrophy) are usually evident in bronchioles and small bronchi (27).

Radiologic Manifestations

The most common radiographic abnormalities consist of transient patchy nonsegmental areas of consolidation without predilection for any lung zone (25,28). These areas tend to be symmetric and may have a nonsegmental distribution similar to that observed in chronic eosinophilic pneumonia (25,28). Occasionally, there are bilateral small and large nodular opacities, or a reticulonodular pattern (25,29). Unilateral or bilateral pleural effusions occur in approximately 30% of patients (25).

The most common HRCT findings consist of areas of ground-glass attenuation or consolidation in either a patchy or a predominantly subpleural distribution (Fig. 19.9) (29,30), findings that correspond to interstitial and airspace infiltration by eosinophils. Less common abnormalities include small centrilobular nodules and larger nodules measuring 0.5 to 3.5 cm in diameter without specific intralobular localization (Fig. 19.10) (29,30). The

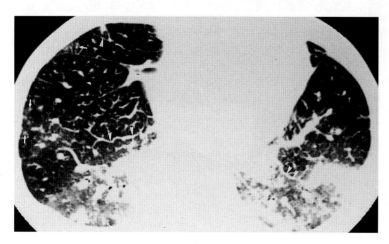

FIGURE 19.10. Churg-Strauss syndrome. HRCT image demonstrates areas of ground-glass attenuation and airspace consolidation involving mainly the dorsal lung regions. Small centrilobular nodules (*arrows*) and smooth thickening of interlobular septa (*arrowheads*) are also evident. The patient was a 32-year-old woman.

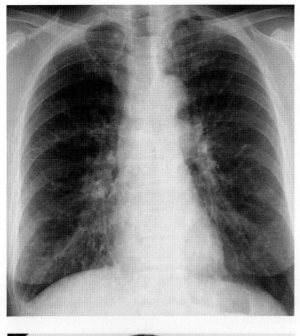

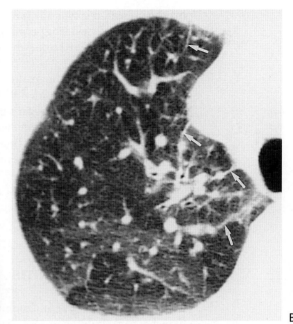

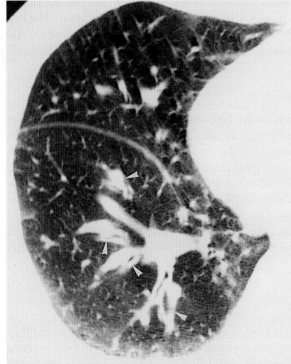

FIGURE 19.11. Churg-Strauss syndrome. **A:** Chest radiograph shows prominence of vascular markings, septal (Kerley B) lines, and a small right pleural effusion. **B:** HRCT image through the right upper lobe demonstrates smooth thickening of interlobular septa (*arrows*) and areas of ground-glass attenuation. **C:** Another image through the right lower lobe shows thickening of bronchovascular bundles (*arrowheads*). The findings are those of hydrostatic pulmonary edema secondary to left-sided heart failure. The patient was a 58-year-old man.

latter may cavitate. Both forms of nodule correspond to foci of necrotizing inflammation, the former in intralobular arteries and their immediate vicinity and the latter more extensively in the parenchyma (30). Interlobular septal thickening may be seen as a result of interstitial pulmonary edema secondary to cardiac involvement (Fig. 19.11) (29,30).

MICROSCOPIC POLYANGIITIS

The term *microscopic polyangiitis* refers to a systemic disease characterized histologically by inflammation of arterioles, venules, and capillaries; although large vessel involvement also may be present, it is typically minimal. The most common and important effects are in the kidneys; clinically evident pulmonary involvement develops in about 15% to 30% of patients. Men are affected somewhat more commonly than women; the average age of onset is about 50 years (31).

Histologically, the lungs show patchy foci of alveolar airspace filling by blood and a variable number of hemosiderin-laden macrophages (32). Alveolar septa show capillaritis similar to that seen in Wegener's granulomatosis (Fig. 19.4), consisting of an infiltrate of neutrophils associated with edema, necrosis, and fibrin thrombi. Similar changes may be seen in arterioles and venules. Bronchial vessels are also commonly affected (32). Fibroblast proliferation indicative of healing also can be seen in the alveolar septal interstitium or adjacent airspace.

Radiographic features consist of patchy, bilateral airspace opacities, corresponding to the airspace hemorrhage (33). Pleural effusion has been reported in approximately 15% of cases and pulmonary edema in 5% (33).

TAKAYASU'S ARTERITIS

Takayasu's arteritis is an uncommon disorder that affects mainly the aorta and its major branches (34). Pulmonary artery involvement is found in an appreciable number of cases; for example, in one review of 76 autopsies, the main pulmonary artery was found to be affected in 34 (45%) and the intrapulmonary arterial branches in 21 (28%) (35). The disease has a marked predilection for women (approximately 90% to 95% of cases) (36) and usually begins between 10 and 40 years of age. It is most common in Southeast Asia.

Pathologic Characteristics

The most prominent changes are seen in the large elastic vessels. The adventitia shows fibrosis and a largely mononuclear inflammatory cell infiltrate; fibrous obliteration of the vasa vasorum associated with a perivascular mononuclear infiltrate is frequent (37). The media contains necrotizing or nonnecrotizing granulomas and scattered multinucleated giant cells; fibrosis, dystrophic calcification, and disruption of the elastic laminae are seen in long-standing disease. These abnormalities are associated with weakening of the vessel wall and may be manifested by more or less diffuse vascular ectasia or by localized aneurysm formation. Intimal fibrosis is also frequent and may be present in the smaller arteries; if severe enough, it may result in localized or diffuse impairment of pulmonary flow.

Radiologic Manifestations

The most common radiographic abnormalities involve the aorta and consist of contour irregularities (reported in about 10% to 75% of patients) and calcification (in 10% to 25%) (Fig. 19.12) (38,39). Less common abnormalities include dilation of the ascending aorta, aneurysms of the descending aorta, oligemia distal to obstructed pulmonary arteries, and changes of pulmonary hypertension (38).

In one study of the contrast-enhanced spiral CT (CT angiography) findings in 12 patients, arterial-phase images demonstrated circumferential thickening of 1 to 4 mm of the aortic wall in all patients and enhancement in five (40). Delayed-phase CT obtained 20 to 40 minutes after intravenous injection demonstrated circumferential enhancement of the aortic wall in eight (Fig. 19.12). (Precontrast images revealed high attenuation of the aortic wall in 10 patients and mural calcification in the aorta in nine. The wall of the aorta in the 10 healthy control subjects was less than 1 mm thick or was imperceptible, demonstrated no calcification, and could not be visualized on the precontrast and

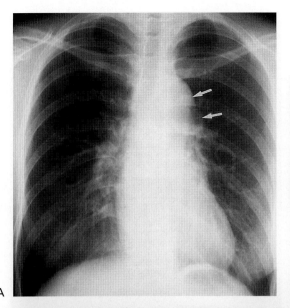

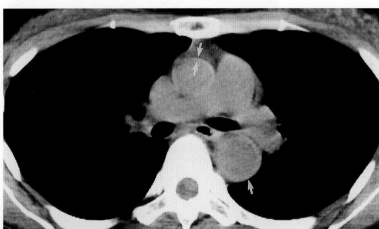

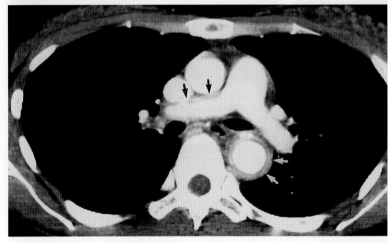

FIGURE 19.12. Takayasu's arteritis. **A:** Chest radiograph demonstrates prominence of the aortic arch (*arrows*). **B:** CT image prior to intravenous injection of contrast shows increased attenuation of the aortic wall (*arrows*). **C:** Contrast-enhanced CT image demonstrates thickening of the wall of the aorta (*white arrows*) and of the main pulmonary artery (*black arrows*). The patient was a 30-year-old-woman.

delayed images.) In two patients, the pulmonary trunk and right and left main pulmonary arteries demonstrated variable wall thickening with both early and delayed enhancement.

The main parenchymal abnormalities seen on CT consist of localized areas of low attenuation and decreased vascularity, which are present in approximately 40% of patients (40–42). These have been shown to correspond to areas of decreased vascularity distal to pulmonary arteritis on pulmonary angiography and to perfusion defects on technetium 99m–macroaggregated albumin perfusion scintigraphy (40). Perfusion defects can also be seen on MR imaging (Fig. 19.13).

BEHÇET'S DISEASE

Behçet's disease is an uncommon systemic disorder characterized by exacerbations and remissions of uveitis and oral and genital ulcers. Pulmonary involvement occurs in 1% to 10% of patients (43,44) and is usually manifested several years after the onset of systemic disease (45). Men are affected more often than women, and the age of onset is

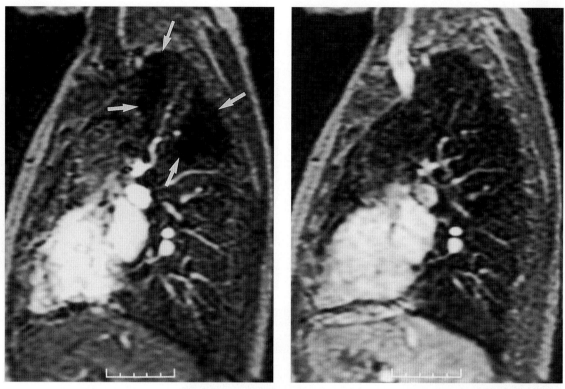

FIGURE 19.13. Takayasu's arteritis. **A:** Sagittal perfusion MRI in the pulmonary arterial phase demonstrates perfusion defects (*arrows*) in the right apical and posterior segments. **B:** Image in the systemic arterial phase shows the intensity of the right posterior apical segment is almost the same as that of other lung zones. The patient was a 32-year-old-woman.

usually between 20 and 30 years. The incidence is highest in the Middle East and Japan (45).

Pulmonary vessels of virtually any size or type may be infiltrated by lymphocytes, plasma cells, and neutrophils. Destruction of the media is associated with weakening of its wall and localized aneurysm formation. Thrombosis secondary to the inflammation also can be seen and may result in parenchymal infarction. Extension of the inflammation outside the vessel wall into the adjacent airway may result in a bronchovascular fistula and repeated or massive hemoptysis.

Pulmonary artery aneurysms are manifested radiographically by round perihilar opacities or the rapid development of unilateral hilar enlargement (45–47). The aneurysms may be single or multiple, and unilateral or bilateral; they usually measure from 1 to 3 cm in diameter (45–47). Their margins are often poorly defined as a result of surrounding hemorrhage (46). The presence, size, and location of the aneurysms can be assessed with CT, MR, or angiography (45,46,48).

Thrombotic occlusion of the pulmonary vasculature most commonly involves the right interlobar artery, followed in decreasing order by lobar and segmental arteries (49). Such occlusion may result in localized areas of consolidation as a result of pulmonary infarction (50), areas of oligemia (50), and areas of atelectasis (46). Pulmonary hemorrhage as a result of vasculitis or pulmonary artery rupture can also result in focal, multifocal, or diffuse airspace consolidation (45,46).

Involvement of the superior vena cava or brachiocephalic veins may be manifested by mediastinal widening on the chest radiograph (47). CT scans in five patients with such widening showed it to be secondary to thrombosis or narrowing of the superior vena cava leading to collateral circulation and mediastinal edema (47). Mediastinal widening also may result from aortic aneurysm formation (46).

GOODPASTURE'S SYNDROME AND IDIOPATHIC PULMONARY HEMORRHAGE

Goodpasture's syndrome and idiopathic pulmonary hemorrhage (IPH) are both characterized by repeated episodes of pulmonary hemorrhage, iron-deficiency anemia, and acute or chronic pulmonary insufficiency. Goodpasture's syndrome includes renal disease in addition to the pulmonary manifestations. It is distinguished from other pulmonary–renal syndromes associated with diffuse alveolar hemorrhage and glomerulonephritis by the presence of an anti–basement membrane antibody in the circulation (51). The etiology and pathogenesis of IPH are unknown.

Goodpasture's syndrome is primarily a disease of young adults (52). It occurs twice as commonly in men as in women (51). IPH, on the other hand, occurs most commonly in children, usually younger than 10 years of age (53). Twenty percent to 40% of patients are young adults (54). In the younger age group, the disease shows no sex predominance; in adults it occurs twice as often in men as in women.

Pathologic Characteristics

The histologic findings in the lung in Goodpasture's syndrome and IPH are similar (7,55,56) The most prominent abnormality is hemorrhage, confined largely to the alveolar airspaces (Fig. 19.14). Other histologic changes include the presence of hemosiderin-

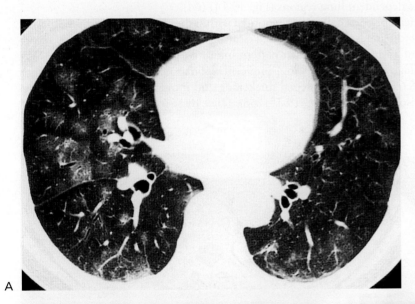

A

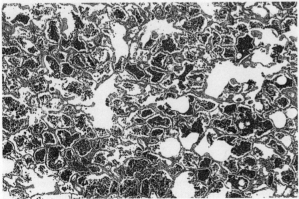

B

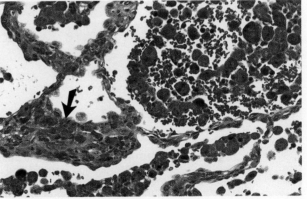

C

FIGURE 19.14. Idiopathic pulmonary hemorrhage. **A:** HRCT image demonstrates bilateral patchy bilateral ground-glass opacities. **B, C:** Photomicrographs show filling of alveolar airspaces by blood and numerous hemosiderin-laden macrophages. The latter are also present in the parenchymal interstitium, which shows mild fibrosis (*arrow* in **C**). The patient was a 35-year-old man.

laden macrophages in both alveolar airspaces and interstitium, mild to moderate interstitial fibrosis, and type II cell hyperplasia. An infiltrate of lymphocytes, typically mild, is seen in the alveolar interstitium in some cases. Focal or (less commonly) diffuse acute interstitial inflammation (capillaritis) can also be seen (10).

Immunofluorescence study of fresh lung tissue from patients who have Goodpasture's syndrome shows a diffuse linear reaction to IgG in the alveolar septum (57,58). The reaction in tissue from patients who have IPH is almost always negative (56,59).

Radiologic Manifestations

The radiologic manifestations of Goodpasture's syndrome and IPH are identical and depend in large measure on the number of hemorrhagic episodes that have occurred. In the early stages of the disease, the radiographic pattern is one of patchy areas of airspace consolidation scattered fairly evenly throughout the lungs. An air bronchogram is usually identifiable in areas of major consolidation. Opacities are usually widespread but may be more prominent in the perihilar areas and in the middle and lower lung zones. The apices and costophrenic angles are almost invariably spared (60). Although parenchymal involvement is usually bilateral, it is commonly asymmetric; occasionally, it is unilateral (60). Less common findings include ground-glass opacities and migratory areas of consolidation (61,62). The chest radiograph also may be normal. In one review of 25 patients with Goodpasture's syndrome, normal findings were documented in seven (18%) of 39 episodes (60).

The CT manifestations of acute pulmonary hemorrhage consist of areas of ground-glass attenuation or consolidation; these may be patchy or diffuse (62,63) but tend to involve mainly the dependent lung regions (Fig. 19.14) (64).

With repeated episodes, collagen is deposited within the alveolar interstitium. In most cases, the chest radiograph shows only partial clearing after each fresh hemorrhage, revealing persistence of a fine reticulonodular pattern indicative of the interstitial disease (65). HRCT at this stage demonstrates 1- to 3-mm centrilobular nodules throughout the lung parenchyma (66,67). Interlobular septal thickening and intralobular reticulation as a result of fibrosis also may be seen (Fig. 19.15) (68). Once these irreversible changes have de-

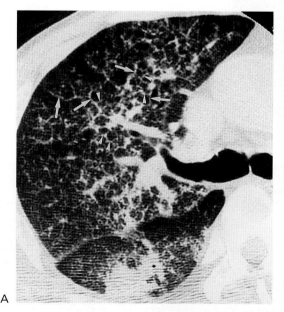
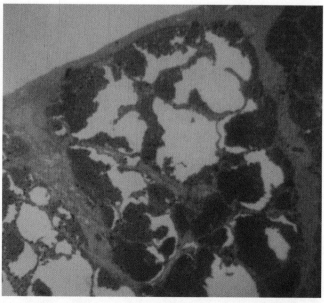

FIGURE 19.15. Idiopathic pulmonary hemorrhage. **A:** HRCT image demonstrates interlobular septal thickening (*arrows*) and intralobular reticular opacities (*arrowheads*) superimposed on areas that have ground-glass attenuation. **B:** Histologic examination shows airspace hemorrhage and interlobular septal thickening by fibrous tissue. The patient was a 42-year-old man.

veloped, fresh episodes of pulmonary hemorrhage usually result in airspace consolidation superimposed on the reticulonodular pattern.

REFERENCES

1. Luqmani RA, Bacon PA, Beaman M, et al. Classical versus nonrenal Wegener's granulomatosis. *Q J Med* 1994;87:161–167.
2. Cotch MF, Hoffman GS, Yerg DE, et al. The epidemiology of Wegener's granulomatosis: estimates of the five-year period prevalence, annual mortality, and geographic disease distribution from population-based data sources. *Arthritis Rheum* 1996;39:87–92.
3. Yoshikawa Y, Watanabe T. Pulmonary lesions in Wegener's granulomatosis: a clinicopathologic study of 22 autopsy cases. *Hum Pathol* 1986;17:401–410.
4. Travis WD, Hoffman GS, Leavitt RY, et al. Surgical pathology of the lung in Wegener's granulomatosis: review of 87 open lung biopsies from 67 patients. *Am J Surg Pathol* 1991;15:315–333.
5. Mark EJ, Matsubara O, Tan-Liu NS, et al. The pulmonary biopsy in the early diagnosis of Wegener's (pathergic) granulomatosis: a study based on 35 open lung biopsies. *Hum Pathol* 1988;19: 1065–1071.
6. Uner AH, Rozum-Slota B, Katzenstein AL. Bronchiolitis obliterans-organizing pneumonia (BOOP)–like variant of Wegener's granulomatosis: a clinicopathologic study of 16 cases. *Am J Surg Pathol* 1996;20:794–801.
7. Colby TV. Pulmonary pathology in patients with systemic autoimmune diseases. *Clin Chest Med* 1998;19:587–612.
8. Yousem SA. Bronchocentric injury in Wegener's granulomatosis: a report of five cases. *Hum Pathol* 1991;22:535–540.
9. Myers JL, Katzenstein AA. Wegener's granulomatosis presenting with massive pulmonary hemorrhage and capillaritis. *Am J Surg Pathol* 1987;11:895–898.
10. Travis WD, Colby TV, Lombard C, et al. A clinicopathologic study of 34 cases of diffuse pulmonary hemorrhage with lung biopsy confirmation. *Am J Surg Pathol* 1990;14:1112–1125.
11. Cordier JF, Valeyre D, Guillevin L, et al. Pulmonary Wegener's granulomatosis: a clinical and imaging study of 77 cases. *Chest* 1990;97:906–912.
12. Aberle DR, Gamsu G, Lynch D. Thoracic manifestations of Wegener granulomatosis: diagnosis and course. *Radiology* 1990;174:703–709.
13. Weir IH, Müller NL, Chiles C, et al. Wegener's granulomatosis: findings from computed tomography of the chest in 10 patients. *Can Assoc Radiol J* 1991;43:31–34.
14. Papiris SA, Manoussakis MN, Drosos AA, et al. Imaging of thoracic Wegener's granulomatosis: the computed tomographic appearance. *Am J Med* 1992;93:529–536.
15. Frazier AA, Rosado-de-Christenson ML, Galvin JR, et al. Pulmonary angiitis and granulomatosis: Radiologic-pathologic correlation. *Radiographics* 1998;18:687–710.
16. Reuter M, Schnabel A, Wesner F, et al. Pulmonary Wegener's granulomatosis: correlation between high-resolution CT findings and clinical scoring of disease activity. *Chest* 1998;114:500–506.
17. Maskell GF, Lockwood CM, Flower CDR. Computed tomography of the lung in Wegener's granulomatosis. *Clin Radiol* 1993;48:377–380.
18. Kuhlman JE, Hruban RH, Fishman ER. Wegener granulomatosis: CT features of parenchymal lung disease. *J Comput Assist Tomogr* 1991;15:948–952.
19. Gohel VK, Dalinka MK, Israel HL, et al. The radiological manifestations of Wegener's granulomatosis. *Br J Radiol* 1973;46:427–432.
20. Foo SS, Weisbrod GL, Herman SJ, et al. Wegener granulomatosis presenting on CT with atypical bronchovasocentric distribution. *J Comput Assist Tomogr* 1990;14:1004–1006.
21. Maguire R, Fauci AS, Doppman JL, et al. Unusual radiographic features of Wegener's granulomatosis. *Am J Roentgenol* 1978;130:233–238.
22. Stein MG, Gamsu G, Webb WR, et al. Computed tomography of diffuse tracheal stenosis in Wegener granulomatosis. *J Comput Assist Tomogr* 1986;10:868–870.
23. Masi AT, Hunder GG, Lie JT, et al. The American College of Rheumatology 1990 criteria for the classification of Churg-Strauss syndrome (allergic granulomatosis and angiitis). *Arthritis Rheum* 1990;33:1094–1100.
24. Watts RA, Carruthers DM, Scott DG: Epidemiology of systemic vasculitis: changing incidence or definition? *Semin Arthritis Rheum* 1995;25:28–34.
25. Lanham JG, Elkon KB, Pusey CD, et al. Systemic vasculitis with asthma and eosinophilia: a clinical approach to the Churg-Strauss syndrome. *Medicine* 1984;63:65–81.
26. Guillevin L, Lhote F, Gayraud M, et al. Prognostic factors in polyarteritis nodosa and Churg-Strauss syndrome: a prospective study in 342 patients. *Medicine* 1996;75:17–28.
27. Koss MN, Antonovych T, Hochholzer L. Allergic granulomatosis (Churg-Strauss syndrome) pulmonary and renal morphologic findings. *Am J Surg Pathol* 1981;5:21–28.

28. Chumbley LC, Harrison EG, DeRemee RA. Allergic granulomatosis and angiitis (Churg-Strauss syndrome): report and analysis of 30 cases. *Mayo Clin Proc* 1977;52:477–484.

29. Worthy SA, Müller NL, Hansell DM, et al. Churg-Strauss syndrome: the spectrum of pulmonary CT findings in 17 patients. *Am J Roentgenol* 1998;170:297–300.

30. Choi YH, Im JG, Han BK, et al. Thoracic manifestation of Churg-Strauss syndrome: radiologic and clinical findings. *Chest* 2000;117:117–124.

31. Lhote F, Guillevin L. Polyarteritis nodosa, microscopic polyangiitis, and Churg-Strauss syndrome: clinical aspects and treatment. *Rheum Dis Clin North Am* 1995;21:911–947.

32. Akikusa B, Sato T, Ogawa M, et al. Necrotizing alveolar capillaritis in autopsy cases of microscopic polyangiitis: Incidence, histopathogenesis, and relationship with systemic vasculitis. *Arch Pathol Lab Med* 1997;121:144–149.

33. Haworth SJ, Savage COS, Carr D, et al. Pulmonary hemorrhage complicating Wegener's granulomatosis and microscopic polyarteritis. *Br Med J* 1985;290:1175–1178.

34. Dabague J, Reyes PA. Takayasu arteritis in Mexico: a 38-year clinical perspective through literature review. *Int J Cardiol* 1996;54:S103–S109.

35. Nasu T. Takayasu's truncoarteritis in Japan: a statistical observation of 76 autopsy cases. *Pathol Microbiol* 1975;43:140–146.

36. Ishikawa K. Diagnostic approach and proposed criteria for the clinical diagnosis of Takayasu's arteriopathy. *J Am Coll Cardiol* 1988;12:964–972.

37. Saito Y, Hirota K, Ito I, et al. Clinical and pathological studies of five autopsied cases of aortitis syndrome: Part I. Findings of the aorta and its branches, peripheral arteries and pulmonary arteries. *Jpn Heart J* 1972;13:20–33.

38. Yamato M, Lecky JW, Hiramatsu K, et al. Takayasu arteritis: radiographic and angiographic findings in 59 patients. *Radiology* 1986;161:329–334.

39. Hachiya J. Current concept of Takayasu's arteritis. *Semin Roentgenol* 1970;5:245–259.

40. Park JH, Chung JW, Im JG, et al. Takayasu arteritis: Evaluation of mural changes in the aorta and pulmonary artery with CT angiography. *Radiology* 1995;196:89–93.

41. Matsunaga N, Hayashi K, Sakamoto I, et al. Takayasu arteritis: Protean radiologic manifestations and diagnosis. *Radiographics* 1997;17:579–594.

42. Takahashi K, Honda M, Furuse M, et al. CT findings of pulmonary parenchyma in Takayasu arteritis. *J Comput Assist Tomogr* 1996;20:742–748.

43. Lakhanpal S, Tani K, Lie JT, et al. Pathologic features of Behçet's syndrome: a review of Japanese autopsy registry data. *Hum Pathol* 1985;16:790–795.

44. Raz I, Okon E, Chajek-Shaul T. Pulmonary manifestations in Behçet's syndrome. *Chest* 1989;95:585–589.

45. Erkan F, Cavdar T. Pulmonary vasculitis in Behçet's disease. *Am Rev Respir Dis* 1992;146:232–239.

46. Tunaci A, Berkmen YM, Gokmen E. Thoracic involvement in Behçet's disease: pathologic, clinical, and imaging features. *Am J Roentgenol* 1995;164:51–56.

47. Ahn JM, Im JG, Ryoo JW, et al. Thoracic manifestations of Behçet syndrome: radiographic and CT findings in nine patients. *Radiology* 1995;194:199–203.

48. Puckette TC, Jolles H, Proto AV. Magnetic resonance imaging confirmation of pulmonary artery aneurysm in Behçet's disease. *J Thorac Imaging* 1994;9:172–175.

49. Numan F, Islak C, Berkmen T, et al. Behçet disease: pulmonary arterial involvement in 15 cases. *Radiology* 1994;192:465–468.

50. Grenier P, Bletry O, Cornud F, et al. Pulmonary involvement in Behçet disease. *Am J Roentgenol* 1981;137:565–569.

51. Kelly PT, Haponik EF. Goodpasture syndrome: molecular and clinical advances. *Medicine* 1994;73:171–185.

52. Proskey AJ, Weatherbee L, Easterling RE, et al. Goodpasture's syndrome: a report of five cases and review of the literature. *Am J Med* 1970;48:162–173.

53. Rezkalla MA, Simmons JL. Idiopathic pulmonary hemosiderosis and alveolar hemorrhage syndrome: case report and review of the literature. *S D J Med* 1995;48:79–85.

54. Specks U. Diffuse alveolar hemorrhage syndromes. *Curr Opin Rheumatol* 2001;13:12–17.

55. Teague CA, Doak PB, Simpson IJ, et al. Goodpasture's syndrome: an analysis of 29 cases. *Kidney Int* 1978;13:492–504.

56. Irwin RS, Cottrell TS, Hsu KC, et al. Idiopathic pulmonary hemosiderosis: an electron microscopic and immunofluorescent study. *Chest* 1974;65:41–45.

57. Abboud RT, Chase WH, Ballon HS, et al. Goodpasture's syndrome: diagnosis by transbronchial lung biopsy. *Ann Intern Med* 1978;89:635–638.

58. Briggs WA, Johnson JP, Teichman S, et al. Antiglomerular basement membrane antibody–mediated glomerulonephritis and Goodpasture's syndrome. *Medicine* 1979;58:348–361.

59. Donald KJ, Edwards RL, McEvoy JDS. Alveolar capillary basement membrane lesions in Goodpasture's syndrome and idiopathic pulmonary hemosiderosis. *Am J Med* 1975;59:642–649.

60. Bowley NB, Steiner RE, Chin WS. The chest x-ray in antiglomerular basement membrane antibody disease (Goodpasture's syndrome). *Clin Radiol* 1979;30:419–429.

61. Albelda SM, Gefter WB, Epstein DM, et al. Diffuse pulmonary hemorrhage: a review and classification. *Radiology* 1985;154:289–297.
62. Müller NL, Miller RR. Diffuse pulmonary hemorrhage. *Radiol Clin North Am* 1991;29:965–971.
63. Cheah FK, Sheppard MN, Hansell DM. Computed tomography of diffuse pulmonary hemorrhage with pathologic correlation. *Clin Radiol* 1993;48:89–93.
64. Niimi A, Amitani R, Kurasawa T, et al. Two cases of idiopathic pulmonary hemosiderosis: analysis of chest CT findings. *Nippon Kyobu Shikkan Gakkai Zasshi* 1992;30:1749–1755.
65. Sybers RG, Sybers JL, Dickie HA, et al. Roentgenographic aspects of hemorrhagic pulmonary-renal disease (Goodpasture's syndrome). *Am J Roentgenol* 1965;94:674–680.
66. Engeler CE. High-resolution CT of airspace nodules in idiopathic pulmonary hemosiderosis. *Eur Radiol* 1995;5:663–665.
67. Seely JM, Effmann EL, Müller NL. High-resolution CT in pediatric lung disease: Imaging findings. *Am J Roentgenol* 1997;168:1269–1275.
68. Lynch DA, Brasch RC, Hardy KA, et al. Pediatric pulmonary disease: assessment with high-resolution ultrafast CT. *Radiology* 1990;176:243–248.

MISCELLANEOUS PULMONARY DISEASES

SARCOIDOSIS

Sarcoidosis is a systemic disorder of unknown cause characterized histologically by the presence of nonnecrotizing granulomatous inflammation (1). Although it may involve virtually any tissue or organ, the most commonly affected structures are the mediastinal and hilar lymph nodes, lungs, skin, and eyes. Pulmonary manifestations are present in 90% of patients; as many as 20% to 25% develop functional impairment (2).

Pathologic Characteristics

The pathologic hallmark of sarcoidosis in the lungs is the presence of granulomatous inflammation (3). The granulomas are usually formed of compact clusters of epithelioid histiocytes and occasional multinucleated giant cells surrounded by a rim of lymphocytes (Fig. 20.1) (1). Necrosis may be evident (4); however, it is usually minimal in amount and present in a minority of granulomas. Although the granulomatous inflammation may resolve completely, some residual fibrosis is not uncommon. The fibrous tissue is deposited initially as concentric lamellae of collagen located between the histologically "active" central portion of the granuloma and the adjacent normal connective tissue (Fig. 20.2). With time, it appears to proceed inward until the entire granuloma is converted into a scar.

Inflammation in the lungs is characteristically most prominent in airway mucosa and perivascular, interlobular septal, and pleural interstitial tissue (Figs. 20.1 and 20.3) (3,5). In the early stages, granulomas in these sites are discrete; as the disease progresses they often become confluent and associated with fibrous tissue. Because the inflammation and fibrosis vary in severity in different areas, the resulting interstitial thickening often has a lobulated or nodular appearance at low-power microscopy (Fig. 20.3).

The lung parenchyma itself is typically unaffected or shows only small foci of granulomatous or lymphocytic inflammation (6). Rarely, parenchymal disease is more extensive, in which case individual granulomas can conglomerate with each other and with granulomas in the peribronchovascular and septal interstitium to form relatively discrete masses several centimeters or more in diameter ("nodular sarcoidosis"). Fibrosis in such areas may be associated with traction bronchiectasis (Fig. 20.4), sometimes severe enough to result

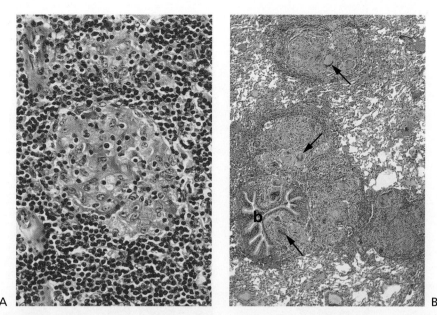

FIGURE 20.1. Sarcoidosis. **A:** Photomicrograph of a portion of a mediastinal lymph node shows a discrete aggregate of epithelioid histiocytes unassociated with necrosis. **B:** Low-magnification view of the corresponding lung biopsy specimen shows confluent granulomas in the mucosa and adjacent interstitial tissue of a membranous bronchiole (*b*). (*Arrows* indicate multinucleated giant cells.)

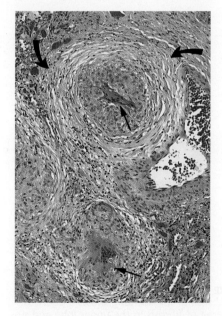

FIGURE 20.2. Sarcoidosis—active fibrosis. Photomicrograph shows two granulomas in the interstitial tissue adjacent to a pulmonary artery. A rim of somewhat concentrically oriented fibroblasts and loose connective tissue is evident around one of the granulomas (*curved arrows*). (*Straight arrows* indicate multinucleated giant cells.)

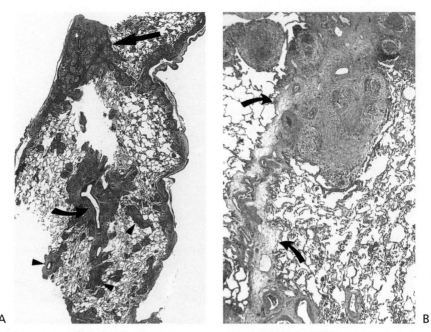

FIGURE 20.3. Sarcoidosis. **A:** Low-magnification view of lung shows confluent granulomatous inflammation in the interstitial tissue of the pleura, an interlobular septum (*straight arrow*) and a centrilobular artery (*curved arrow*) and its branches (*arrowhead*). **B:** Photomicrograph of another biopsy specimen shows a somewhat nodular focus of granulomatous inflammation and fibrosis in one area of an interlobular septum (*arrows*). Note that the pulmonary parenchyma is relatively unaffected in both specimens.

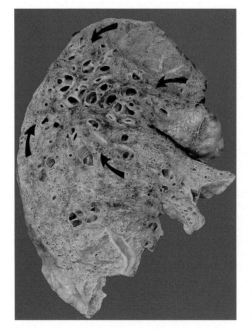

FIGURE 20.4. Sarcoidosis—bronchiectasis. Parasagittal slice of the left lung shows a poorly defined area of fibrosis in the upper lobe and superior segment of the lower lobe (*arrows*). A moderate degree of traction bronchiectasis is evident.

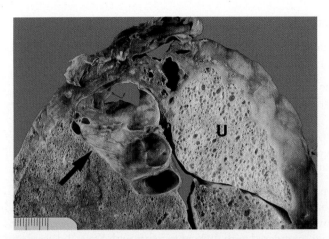

FIGURE 20.5. Sarcoidosis—interstitial fibrosis and saccular bronchiectasis. Magnified view of a parasagittal slice of the right lung shows diffuse interstitial fibrosis in the upper lobe (*U*) and a large (bronchiectatic) "cavity" in the superior segment of the lower lobe (*arrow*).

in the formation of discrete "cavities." The latter are relatively common sites for the formation of fungus balls (7). Solitary or (rarely) multiple cavities and diffuse interstitial fibrosis unassociated with bronchiectasis also can be seen (Fig. 20.5).

Granulomatous inflammation of pulmonary vessels is common (8,9), usually as a result of extension of perivascular interstitial disease into the media. Necrosis of the vessel wall does not occur, and thrombosis is rare. Granulomatous inflammation and associated fibrosis in the airway mucosa is rarely sufficient to cause airway stenosis (10).

Lymph node involvement takes the form of more or less diffuse replacement of the node by granulomas (Fig. 20.6). Initially, they are discrete and appear active; as in pulmonary disease, however, they can become confluent and undergo progressive fibrosis, eventually resulting in complete replacement of the node by fibrous tissue (Fig. 20.6).

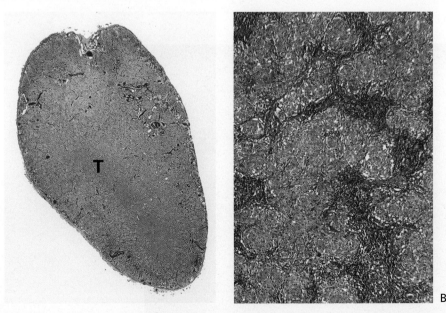

A　　B

FIGURE 20.6. Sarcoidosis—mediastinal lymph node involvement. **A:** Low-magnification view shows almost complete replacement of a mediastinal lymph node by fibrous tissue (*T*); granulomas are few in number. **B:** Magnified view of another node shows an earlier stage of disease, consisting of confluent granulomas and almost no fibrous tissue.

Radiologic Manifestations

The radiographic changes in thoracic sarcoidosis can be classified for descriptive purposes into four groups or stages (11):

Stage 0: No demonstrable abnormality
Stage 1: Hilar and mediastinal lymph node enlargement unassociated with pulmonary abnormality
Stage 2: Hilar and mediastinal lymph node enlargement associated with pulmonary abnormality
Stage 3: Diffuse pulmonary disease unassociated with node enlargement

In one survey of 3,676 patients from nine countries, 8% had normal chest radiographs at presentation, 51% had Stage 1 disease, 29% had Stage 2 disease, and 12% had Stage 3 disease (12). On follow-up, 65% of patients with Stage 1 disease showed resolution of the radiographic findings, compared with 49% of patients with Stage 2 disease and only 20% with Stage 3 disease. (It should be emphasized that this staging system is only a means to describe the radiographic findings and patients do not necessarily progress sequentially from one stage to the next.)

Lymph Node Enlargement without Pulmonary Abnormality

On the chest radiograph, this is seen at presentation in approximately 50% of patients (12,13) (Fig. 20.7). The combination of bilateral hilar and right paratracheal lymph node enlargement is a characteristic manifestation; the former is evident on chest radiographs in more than 95% of patients and the latter, in about 70% who have intrathoracic lymph node enlargement (13,14). Other common sites of lymphadenopathy include the aortopulmonary window (approximately 50% of cases) and subcarinal region (20%) (13,14).

The prevalence and distribution of lymphadenopathy just described refer to the findings on the chest radiograph. As might be expected, hilar and mediastinal lymphadenopathy is seen more commonly on CT (5,15). Furthermore, the mediastinal lymphadenopathy can be seen to involve more nodal stations than are apparent on radiography (15,16).

It is important to appreciate that Stages 0 and 1 refer only to radiographically evident disease and not to disease determined by pathologic examination. As in other interstitial

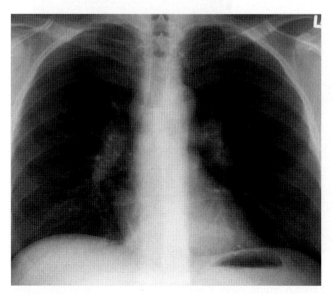

FIGURE 20.7. Sarcoidosis. Chest radiograph shows bilateral hilar and paratracheal lymph node enlargement. The patient was a 42-year-old man.

diseases, the lungs can be involved in the absence of a demonstrable abnormality on the chest radiograph (17). In fact, the chest radiograph is normal (Stage 0) in about 10% of patients who have biopsy-proven intrathoracic sarcoidosis (12,17). As might be expected, parenchymal abnormalities are seen more commonly on high-resolution computed tomography (HRCT) than on the radiograph (5). For example, in one study of 44 patients, mild parenchymal abnormalities were detected on HRCT in all six (14%) patients with radiographic Stage 1 disease (18).

Diffuse Pulmonary Disease with or without Lymph Node Enlargement

Parenchymal disease is seen on the chest radiograph at presentation in approximately 40% of patients and occurs at some time during the course of the disease in 50% to 65% (12,13). At presentation, the pulmonary disease is associated with lymph node enlargement (Stage 2) in approximately 30% of patients; the remaining 10% have no evidence of lymph node enlargement (Stage 3) (12,19).

The parenchymal abnormalities are typically bilateral and symmetric; although they may be diffuse, in 50% to 80% of patients they involve mainly the upper lung zones (5,20). The most frequent patterns are nodular and reticulonodular (Fig. 20.8); less commonly, a reticular pattern, airspace consolidation, or ground-glass opacities predominate (21,22).

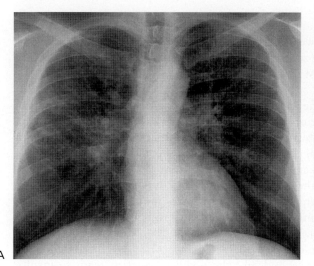

A

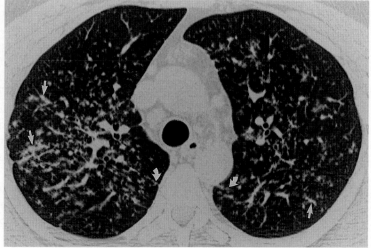

B

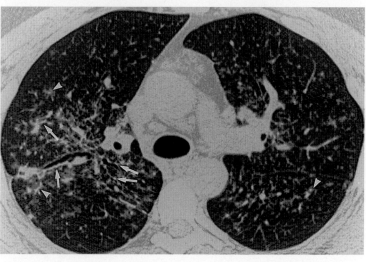

C

FIGURE 20.8. Sarcoidosis. **A:** Chest radiograph shows a reticulonodular pattern involving mainly the middle and upper lung zones, as well as bilateral hilar lymph node enlargement. **B:** HRCT image through the upper lobes shows nodules along the pulmonary vessels (*straight arrows*) and interlobular septa (*curved arrows*). **C:** Another image at a slightly more caudad level shows nodular thickening of bronchi (*arrows*) and along pulmonary vessels (*arrowheads*). The patient was a 35-year-old man.

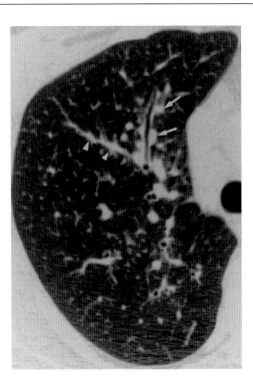

FIGURE 20.9. Sarcoidosis. HRCT image shows nodular thickening of a bronchus (*arrows*) and along a pulmonary vessel (*arrowheads*). The patient was a 31-year-old man.

A *nodular pattern* is present on the chest radiograph in 30% to 60% of patients (23,24). The nodules usually are well circumscribed, have irregular margins, and involve mainly the middle and upper lung zones. They vary in size and frequently range from 1 to 10 mm in diameter, although most measure less than 3 mm.

On HRCT, nodules are seen at presentation in 90% to 100% of patients with pulmonary abnormalities (18,25). They are most numerous along the bronchovascular bundles and adjacent to the costal pleura and interlobar fissures (5,18) (Fig. 20.9). They are also commonly seen along interlobular septa (Fig. 20.10) and in the centrilobular region (5,25). Correlation of HRCT with pathologic findings has shown that they represent interstitial aggregates of granulomas and associated fibrous tissue (5,26).

A *reticular pattern* is seen on the radiograph in 15% to 20% of patients (21,24) (Fig. 20.11). It may result from thickening of interlobular septa, intralobular irregular lines, traction bronchiectasis, or, less commonly, honeycombing. On HRCT, smooth or nodular thickening of interlobular septa has been described in 20% to 90% of patients, and nonseptal irregular lines have been described in 20% to 70% (5,25,27). The interlobular septal thickening is seldom extensive and, like the nodular opacities, tends to involve

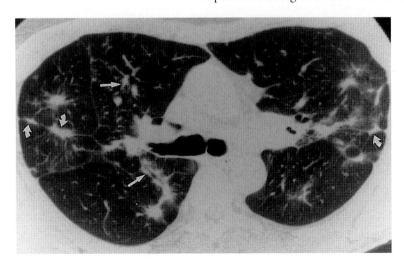

FIGURE 20.10. Sarcoidosis. HRCT image shows irregular nodules along bronchi (*straight arrows*) and interlobular septa (*curved arrows*). The patient was a 59-year-old man.

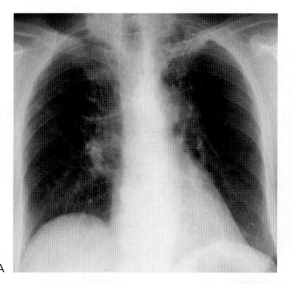

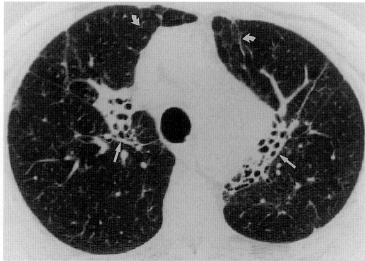

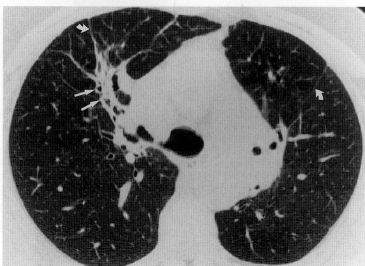

FIGURE 20.11. Sarcoidosis. **A:** Chest radiograph shows a reticular pattern involving mainly the medial aspects of the upper lobes. Note associated volume loss with cephalad retraction of the hila. **B:** HRCT image at the level of the aortic arch shows central conglomeration of ectatic bronchi (traction bronchiectasis; straight arrows), irregular thickening of interlobular septa (*curved arrows*) and distortion of lobular architecture. These findings indicate the presence of fibrosis. **C:** Image at the level of the right upper lobe bronchus shows irregular thickening and distortion of bronchi (straight arrows) and interlobular septa (curved arrows). The patient was a 67-year-old woman.

mainly the central regions of the middle and upper lung zones. Irregular linear opacities seen within a secondary lobule are usually associated with distortion of lobular architecture, indicating the presence of fibrosis of the peribronchovascular interstitium. Occasionally, these opacities are reversible (5,28). The histologic correlate in this situation is unclear but presumably relates to resolution of granulomatous inflammation with minimal or absent fibrosis. Fibrosis also leads to dilatation and distortion of bronchi (traction bronchiectasis), predominantly in the perihilar regions of the upper lung zones, and, occasionally, to honeycombing (29) (Fig. 20.11). The latter usually involves the subpleural lung regions of the middle and upper lung zones (29).

A *reticulonodular pattern* is present in 25% to 50% of patients with radiographically evident pulmonary abnormalities (21,24). As might be expected, this pattern results from a combination of nodules and thickening of the interlobular septa or of nodules and irregular (intralobular) linear opacities.

Parenchymal consolidation is the predominant finding on the chest radiograph in approximately 10% of patients with sarcoidosis (5,24) (Fig. 20.12). The consolidation typically has a bilateral and symmetric distribution, again involving mainly the upper lung zones. On HRCT, the areas of consolidation may be peribronchial or, less commonly, peripheral in distribution (30). The "consolidation" is predominantly the result of expansion of parenchymal and peribronchovascular interstitial tissue by the granulomatous inflam-

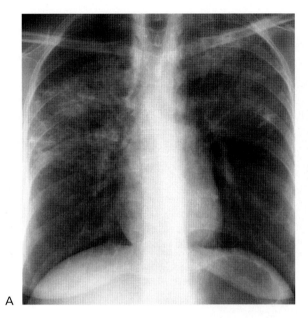

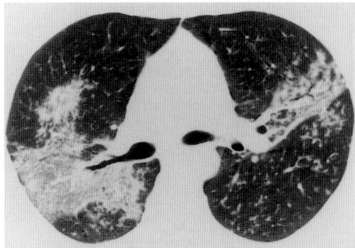

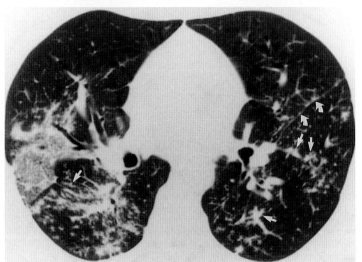

FIGURE 20.12. Sarcoidosis. **A:** Chest radiograph shows patchy areas of consolidation and ground glass opacities involving the middle and upper lung zones. **B:** HRCT image at the level of the right upper lobe bronchus demonstrates bilateral ground-glass opacities in a predominantly peribronchial distribution. Also noted are a few small nodules. **C:** Image at the level of the right lower lobe bronchi shows patchy ground-glass opacities and irregular nodules along vessels (*straight arrows*) and interlobar fissure (*curved arrow*). The patient was a 35-year-old woman with longstanding sarcoidosis.

matory infiltrate and fibrous tissue rather than airspace disease itself. Air bronchograms can be seen in the majority of cases; when the fibrous tissue is predominant, traction bronchiectasis may be seen. In one review of the HRCT findings in 10 patients, additional findings of small nodules, thickening of the bronchoarterial interstitium, and interlobular septa were present in all cases (30).

Hazy areas of increased opacity without obscuration of the vascular markings (*ground-glass opacities*) are seldom seen on the radiograph but are commonly present on HRCT (Fig. 20.13). In one review of the chest radiographs in 1,652 patients, only 10 (0.6%) showed diffuse ground-glass abnormalities; all had associated hilar or mediastinal lymphadenopathy (31). By contrast, areas of ground-glass attenuation have been reported on HRCT in 20% to 60% of patients (23,25,32). In most of these cases, the ground-glass attenuation is seen in association with small nodules; rarely, it is the predominant abnormality (26). Correlation of HRCT and pathologic findings has shown the pattern to be related to granulomatous inflammation in the interstitial tissue surrounding small vessels and bronchioles and, to a lesser extent, alveolar septa (6,26).

Bronchial abnormalities have been reported in as many as 65% of patients on HRCT. The most common findings are regular or nodular bronchial wall thickening and bronchial luminal narrowing (33). The thickening likely reflects the presence of granulomas and fibrous tissue in the peribronchial interstitium. The luminal narrowing correlates with the presence of mucosal thickening at bronchoscopy (33) and presumably reflects prominent inflammation in this location. Obstruction of lobar or segmental bronchi by

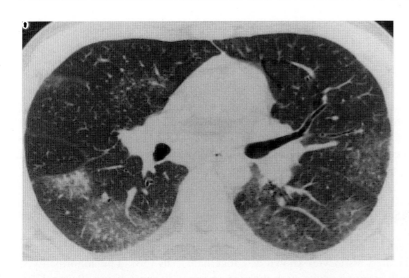

FIGURE 20.13. Sarcoidosis. HRCT image shows bilateral areas of ground-glass attenuation, poorly defined small nodules, and bilateral hilar and subcarinal lymph node enlargement. The patient was a 32-year-old man.

either airway wall fibrosis and inflammation or peribronchial lymph node compression may result in atelectasis. Air trapping on expiratory HRCT is also a common finding as a result of small airway obstruction, again by granulomas and fibrosis (34,35).

Approximately 20% of patients with sarcoidosis and radiographic evidence of pulmonary involvement develop findings consistent with *pulmonary fibrosis* (11) (Fig. 20.14). The fibrosis typically involves mainly the upper lung lobes (11). It is usually associated

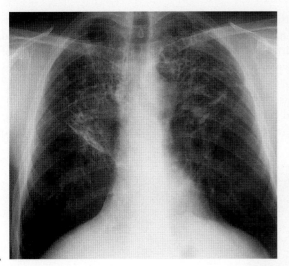

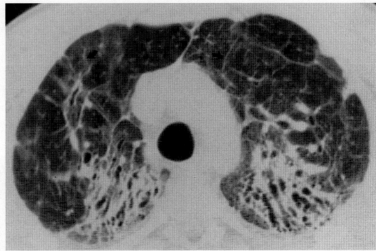

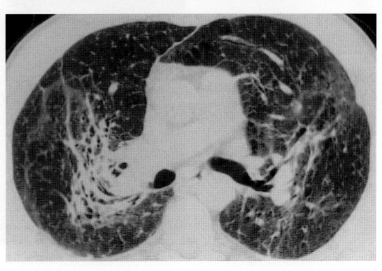

FIGURE 20.14. Sarcoidosis. **A:** Chest radiograph shows a reticulonodular pattern throughout the middle and upper lung zones. Volume loss with cephalad retraction of the hila is evident in the upper lobes and overexpansion is evident in the lower lobes. **B:** HRCT image at the level of the aortic arch shows posterior displacement of distorted and ectatic bronchi (traction bronchiectasis), peribronchial fibrosis, irregular thickening of interlobular septa (*arrows*), distortion of lobular architecture, and extensive ground-glass opacification. **C:** Image at the level of the left upper lobe bronchus shows irregular thickening and distortion of bronchi, interlobular septal thickening and patchy ground-glass opacities. The patient was a 35-year-old man.

with upward retraction of the hila and with well-defined structural changes, including traction bronchiectasis, bulla formation, and compensatory overinflation of the lower lobes.

On HRCT, the fibrosis has a characteristic peribronchovascular distribution radiating from the hila to the upper lobes (28,29) (Fig. 20.14). Additional findings include irregular lines of attenuation with associated architectural distortion, central conglomeration of ectatic bronchi, conglomerate masses, and (in approximately 40% of cases) subpleural honeycombing (29). The last named is usually limited to patients who have severe fibrosis and central conglomeration of bronchi (32); it involves mainly the middle and upper lung zones, with relative sparing of the lung bases (29).

LANGERHANS CELL HISTIOCYTOSIS

Pulmonary Langerhans cell histiocytosis (PLCH) is characterized pathologically by a proliferation of specialized histiocytes known as Langerhans cells (36). The abnormality is seen predominantly in young adults, with the median age at diagnosis being 39 years (37). It is an uncommon condition; in one investigation it accounted for only 3.4% of diagnosis in 502 patients who had open-lung biopsy for chronic, diffuse lung disease (38). The vast majority of affected patients are cigarette smokers (39,40); for example, in one review of 87 patients, only three were nonsmokers (37).

Pathologic Characteristics

Gross examination of the lungs in the early stage of PLCH shows multiple nodules measuring 1 to 10 mm in diameter. With time, these relatively discrete nodular lesions tend to become confluent, resulting in irregularly shaped areas of fibrosis containing cysts of variable size. These abnormalities typically involve mainly the upper and mid-lung zones (Fig. 20.15) (41).

The earliest histologic finding is a cellular infiltrate located predominantly in the interstitial tissue of membranous and proximal respiratory bronchiolar walls (Fig. 20.16) (40). The infiltrate consists of several types of cell, the proportion varying from area to

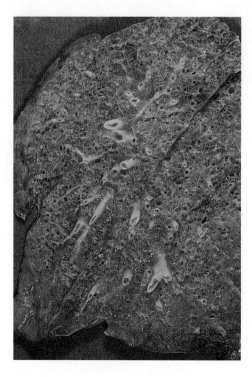

FIGURE 20.15. Langerhans cell histiocytosis. Parasagittal slice of the left lung shows patchy but extensive fibrosis associated with small cystic spaces. The basal portion of the lower lobe is less severely affected than its superior segment and the upper lobe.

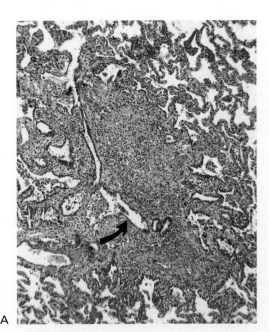
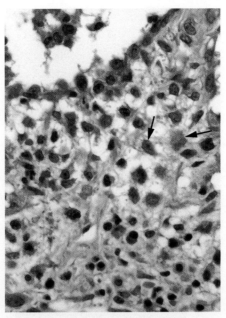

FIGURE 20.16. Langerhans cell histiocytosis. **A:** Photomicrograph shows marked narrowing of the lumen of a membranous bronchiole (*arrow*) by a cellular infiltrate associated with a small amount of fibrous tissue. The infiltrate extends into the adjacent alveolar interstitial tissue, resulting in a stellate appearance. **B:** Magnified view of the infiltrate shows it to consist of histiocyte-like cells with pale staining, notched nuclei (*arrows*) (Langerhans cells) and lesser numbers of lymphocytes and plasma cells (eosinophils are not evident in this view).

area. As might be expected, Langerhans cells—characterized by vesicular, often grooved nuclei and a moderate amount of pale, eosinophilic cytoplasm—are frequently abundant. Admixed among these cells are numerous eosinophils and lesser numbers of neutrophils, plasma cells, lymphocytes, and multinucleated giant cells. Necrosis is very uncommon.

In more advanced disease, the infiltrate typically extends into the alveolar interstitium adjacent to affected airways and the central portion of the lesion undergoes fibrosis, resulting in a characteristic stellate shape (Fig. 20.16). With further progression, individual foci of disease coalesce, fibrous tissue becomes more prominent, and an increasing amount of lung is destroyed. In advanced disease, the lung may consist almost entirely of fibrous tissue and cystic spaces, with only scattered Langerhans cells and few or no eosinophils.

Cystic spaces several millimeters to several centimeters in diameter are commonly seen (Fig. 20.17). Their pathogenesis is uncertain and may be related to more than one mechanism. Because of the intimate association of the cellular infiltrate with small airways, it is possible that some arise by peripheral airspace dilatation secondary to bronchiolar obstruction. It is also conceivable that they develop by progressive apoptosis or necrosis of the central portion of the cellular nodules, followed by drainage of the necrotic material via the associated airway.

Radiologic Manifestations

On the chest radiograph, pulmonary involvement is characteristically bilaterally symmetric and diffuse throughout the upper and mid-lung zones with sparing of the costophrenic angles (42) (Fig. 20.18). Early on, the appearance consists of a nodular pattern, with individual lesions ranging from 1 to 10 mm in diameter. Cavitated nodules are only occasionally seen on the radiograph during this stage but can be identified on high-resolution computed tomography (HRCT) in about 10% of cases (43,44). In more advanced disease, the pattern becomes reticulonodular. The end stage is characterized by a coarse reticular pattern that, in the upper-lung zones particularly, often assumes a cystic appearance. Usually, the cysts are about 1 cm in diameter, but they may measure up to 3 cm, especially in the lung periphery.

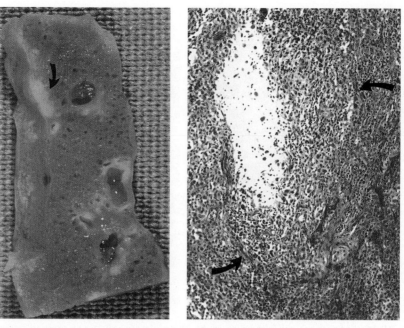

FIGURE 20.17. Langerhans cell histiocytosis. **A:** Magnified view of a biopsy specimen shows three small cystic spaces surrounded by a small amount of solid tissue. A small nodule of similar tissue unassociated with a cyst is also evident adjacent to the pleura (*arrow*). **B:** Photomicrograph shows a membranous bronchiole whose wall and mucosa are markedly infiltrated by a cellular infiltrate. (*Arrows* indicate residual muscularis mucosa.) The cells appear to be discohesive in the region of the airway lumen. It is possible that continued sloughing of such cells leads to the cystic spaces seen in **A.**

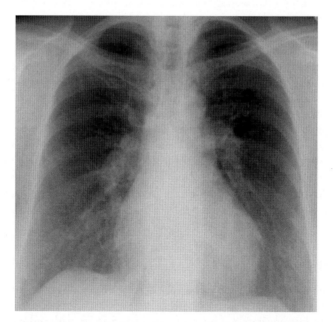

FIGURE 20.18. Langerhans cell histiocytosis. Chest radiograph shows a fine reticulonodular pattern throughout the middle and upper lung zones and sparing of the costophrenic angles. There is enlargement of the central pulmonary arteries secondary to pulmonary arterial hypertension. The patient was a 50-year-old woman.

The most common abnormalities on HRCT are cysts (present in approximately 80% of patients) and nodules (present in 60% to 80%; Fig. 20.19) (44,45). Less common findings, seen in approximately 10% of cases each, include cavitated nodules, reticulation, and areas of ground-glass attenuation. As might be expected, the incidence of these findings depends on the stage of disease. In patients who have recent symptoms, the predominant abnormality consists of small nodules, which may vary from a few in number to a myriad (43,44) (Fig. 20.20). Most measure 1 to 5 mm in diameter, although larger nodules are seen in approximately 30% of cases. The nodules tend to have a centrilobular distribution corresponding to the peribronchiolar distribution of the cellular infiltrate seen histologically (44). Their margins may be smooth or irregular. Some nodules, particularly those larger than 1 cm in diameter, may show lucent centers. Some of these lesions correspond to a dilated bronchiole surrounded by thickened peribronchiolar interstitium (44). Progression of such nodules to clear-cut cysts can be seen in some patients (46), presumably corresponding to a process of necrosis and cavitation, as discussed previously (47).

With progression of disease, cysts become the predominant feature (Fig. 20.21). They range from a few millimeters to several centimeters in diameter and may be round or irregular in shape (43,45). Unusual shapes, such as bilobed, cloverleaf, or branched, may result from fusion of several cysts or correspond to the presence of ectatic and thick-walled bronchi (43). The reticular and reticulonodular opacities that are frequently identified on the chest radiograph are relatively uncommon on CT (44,45), with many of the opacities probably representing the walls of the cysts (43). In fact, the pulmonary parenchyma between the cysts appears remarkably normal on CT in many cases (43).

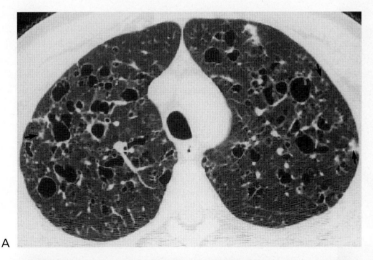

A

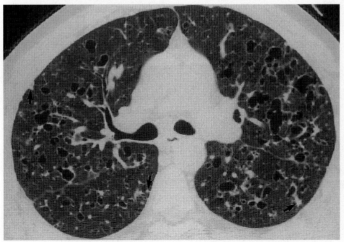

B

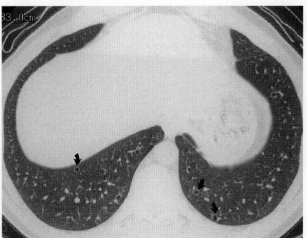

C

FIGURE 20.19. Langerhans cell histiocytosis. **A:** HRCT image at the level of the aortic arch shows thin-walled cystic spaces and a few irregular small nodules (*arrows*). **B:** Image at the level of the right upper lobe bronchus shows similar findings. **C:** Image through lung bases shows only a few small cysts (*arrows*). The patient was a 30-year-old man.

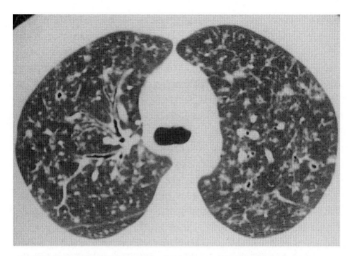

FIGURE 20.20. Langerhans cell histiocytosis. HRCT image shows numerous small nodules and a few small cysts. The patient was a 39-year-old woman. (Case courtesy of Dr. Jim Barrie, University of Alberta Medical Centre, Edmonton, Alberta, Canada.)

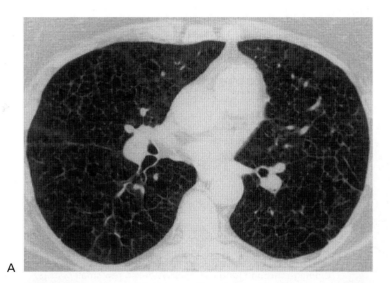

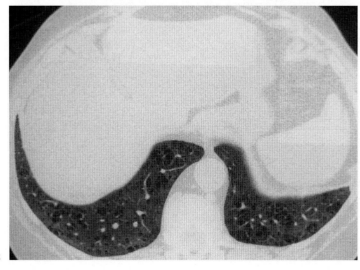

FIGURE 20.21. Langerhans cell histiocytosis. **A:** HRCT image at the level of the right middle lobe bronchus shows thin-walled cystic spaces throughout both lungs. **B:** Image through lung bases shows relative sparing. The patient was a 56-year-old woman.

With further progression of disease, there is evidence of fibrosis and, eventually, extensive honeycombing. Regardless of the stage, the abnormalities are most severe in the upper- and mid-lung zones; the lung bases are relatively spared (41,43). Spontaneous pneumothorax is a relatively common complication, being seen in approximately 10% of patients (43).

LYMPHANGIOLEIOMYOMATOSIS

Lymphangioleiomyomatosis is a rare condition of uncertain etiology characterized histologically by a proliferation of smooth muscle predominantly around small airways and vessels. The disease is confined to women; the average age at presentation is 30 to 35 years (46).

Pathologic Characteristics

The earliest histologic abnormality in lymphangioleiomyomatosis is a cellular proliferation in the interstitial tissue of small bronchioles, blood and lymphatic vessels, and pleura (Fig. 20.22). Although the abnormal cells may have a spindle shape reminiscent of typical smooth muscle cells, many are round or polygonal in shape and have large, somewhat pleomorphic nuclei (48). The smooth muscle phenotype of the latter cells is demonstrated by their immunohistochemical reactivity for muscle-specific actin (49).

Examination of slices of the lungs in advanced disease (i.e., at autopsy or pneumonectomy for transplantation) shows innumerable cystic spaces 0.2 to 2.0 cm in diameter separated by solid interstitial tissue or apparently normal lung parenchyma (Fig. 20.23) (48). The former is the result of muscle proliferation. The pathogenesis of the development of the cysts is not clear. Some investigators have suggested that degradation of elastic fibers in the airway wall by alpha-1-antiprotease may be involved (50); it is also possible that obstruction of small airways by the proliferating smooth muscle cells results in

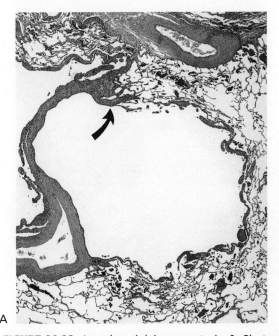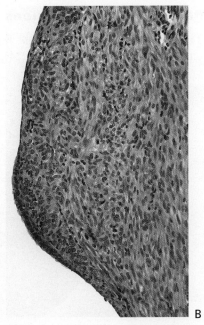

A   B

FIGURE 20.22. Lymphangioleiomyomatosis. **A:** Photomicrograph shows marked dilatation of a membranous bronchiole associated with mild thickening of its wall. The adjacent lung parenchyma is normal except for focal accumulation of airspace macrophages. **B:** Magnified view of the region indicated by the *arrow* in **A** shows the thickening to be the result of a proliferation of spindle-shaped cells resembling smooth muscle cells.

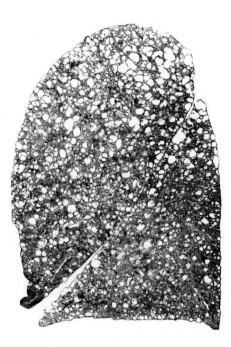

FIGURE 20.23. Lymphangioleiomyomatosis. A parasagittal slice of the left lung shows innumerable cystic spaces throughout both lobes.

distal airway dilatation (51). Histologic examination of the cyst walls may show only a thin rim of abnormal muscle or a thick, eccentric or concentric proliferation.

Evidence of pulmonary hemorrhage (hemosiderin-laden macrophages) is common, most likely as a result of vascular obstruction (48). Dilation of lymphatic vessels is also frequently present. Small (1- to 3-mm) foci of alveolar interstitial fibrosis associated with type II cell hyperplasia are present in some patients.

Smooth muscle proliferation also may be seen in the thoracic duct, which may be totally obliterated, and in mediastinal lymph nodes. Such involvement frequently results in disturbance in pleuropulmonary lymph flow and chylothorax.

Radiologic Manifestations

The most common radiographic finding in lymphangioleiomyomatosis is a bilateral reticular pattern (52,53) (Fig. 20.24). In approximately 80% of cases, it involves all lung

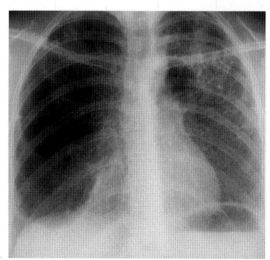

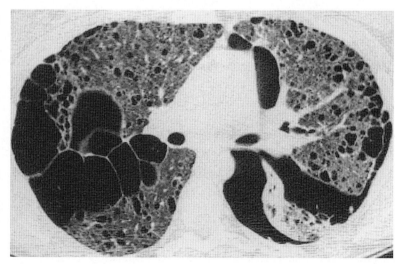

FIGURE 20.24. Lymphangioleiomyomatosis. **A:** Chest radiograph shows thin-walled cystic spaces throughout both lungs and a small left apical pneumothorax. **B:** HRCT image shows numerous thin-walled cysts, large right subpleural cysts and bullae, and a small, partially loculated left pneumothorax. The patient was a 29-year-old woman.

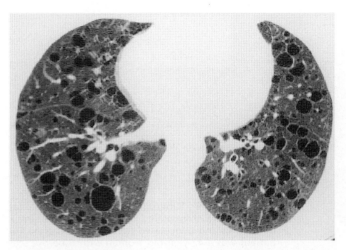

FIGURE 20.25. Lymphangioleiomyomatosis. HRCT image shows thin-walled cysts randomly distributed in both lungs. The parenchyma between the cysts is normal. The patient was a 50-year-old woman.

zones to a similar degree; in the remainder, it is more marked in the lower lung zones (52). Evidence of hyperinflation with increase in the retrosternal airspace or flattening of the diaphragm is seen at presentation in many patients (52,53). Pneumothorax (presumably related to rupture of one of the cystic spaces) has been reported in 30% to 40% (52,54), and unilateral or bilateral pleural effusions (chylothorax) have been found in 10% to 20% (52,54). In 10% to 20% of cases, the chest radiograph is normal (52,53).

The characteristic HRCT finding consists of numerous air-filled cysts surrounded by normal lung parenchyma (52,53) (Fig. 20.25). Cysts can be seen in patients who have normal radiographs or who have radiographs showing only reticular opacities (52,53). They usually measure between 0.2 and 2.0 cm in diameter, although they may be as large as 6 cm (52,53). Their size varies with severity of disease, the majority of patients with relatively mild involvement having cysts less than 1 cm in diameter (52). Most cysts are round and have smooth walls that may be faintly perceptible or measure up to 4 mm in thickness (52,53). They are distributed diffusely throughout the lungs, without central, peripheral, or lower lung zone predominance (52). In most cases, the parenchyma between the cysts appears normal. Occasionally, there is a slight increase in interstitial markings (55), interlobular septal thickening (53), or patchy areas of ground-glass attenuation (presumably the result of pulmonary hemorrhage) (52). Sometimes, a few small nodular opacities can be seen (54), reflecting the presence of focal type II cell proliferation.

TUBEROUS SCLEROSIS

Tuberous sclerosis is an autosomal dominant disorder characterized clinically by mental retardation, epilepsy, and adenoma sebaceum. It affects males and females equally. Pulmonary involvement occurs in about 1% to 2% of patients, almost all of whom are women (56). The manifestations are identical to those of lymphangioleiomyomatosis histologically (57) and radiologically (56,58) (Fig. 20.26). As in that condition, pneumothorax is common, having been reported in up to 50% of patients (56). By contrast, chylous pleural effusion is distinctly unusual (58).

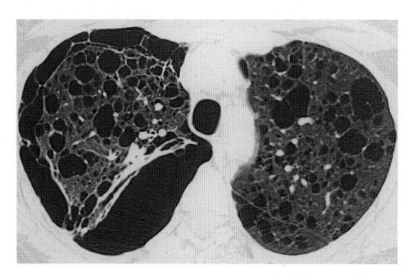

FIGURE 20.26. Tuberous sclerosis. HRCT image demonstrates thin-walled cystic spaces throughout both lungs and a loculated right pneumothorax. The patient was a 42-year-old woman with tuberous sclerosis and recurrent right pneumothorax.

ASPIRATION OF GASTRIC OR OROPHARYNGEAL SECRETIONS

The pulmonary manifestations of aspiration are influenced by the amount and nature of the aspirated material. Aspiration of bacteria-laden oropharyngeal secretions frequently leads to the development of pneumonia (see Chapter 2). However, aspiration of oropharyngeal or gastric secretions, with or without admixed food particles, can also cause significant pulmonary disease in the absence of infection. Pulmonary damage occurs predominantly when the pH of the aspirate is less than 2.5 and the volume of fluid is greater than 25 mL (59). However, it also may occur when the pH of aspirated fluid is greater than 2.5 (59). Disease is seen particularly in the elderly and in patients who have esophageal abnormalities (e.g., achalasia, Zenker diverticulum, or carcinoma) or conditions predisposing to loss of consciousness (e.g., alcoholism or epilepsy).

The initial reaction to aspirated gastric or oropharyngeal contents is an acute inflammatory exudate (Fig. 20.27). The cause of the exudate often can be identified histologi-

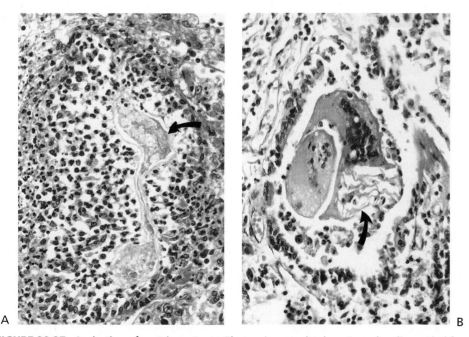

A   B

FIGURE 20.27. Aspiration of gastric contents. Photomicrographs show two alveoli sampled from different areas of an upper lobe. One (**A**) is filled with neutrophils and the other (**B**) contains two multinucleated giant cells. Partially digested food particles (*arrows*) can be seen in each airspace. The patient was a 76-year-old man who had carcinoma of the esophagus and a history of repeated aspiration.

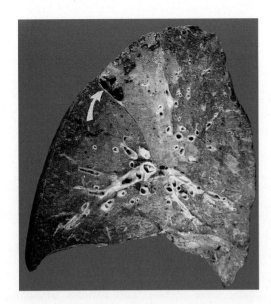

FIGURE 20.28. Aspiration of gastric contents. Parasagittal slice of the left lung shows a well-demarcated area of consolidation in the posterior segment of the upper lobe. Focal cavitation is evident (*arrow*). The patient had metastatic carcinoma of the colon and had been observed to aspirate approximately 3 weeks prior to death.

cally by the presence of foreign particles consistent with partially digested food. In time, these particles incite a granulomatous inflammatory reaction, characteristically associated with prominent multinucleated giant cells. A pattern of bronchiolitis obliterans organizing pneumonia also may be seen. Localization of the pneumonia to the posterior segment of an upper lobe is frequent (Fig. 20.28). Cavitation may be seen in the consolidated regions if there is concomitant infection (often by anaerobic bacteria).

The predominant radiographic abnormality is airspace consolidation, which may be unilateral or bilateral, and patchy or diffuse. The consolidation tends to involve mainly the dependent lung regions (Fig. 20.29). When the patient is supine, the most frequently involved sites are the posterior segments of the upper lobes and the superior segments of the lower lobes (60). Aspiration of large amounts of gastric secretions (Mendelson syndrome) results in diffuse alveolar damage and increased permeability pulmonary edema. This is reflected radiologically by the presence of widespread bilateral airspace consolidation.

The reaction to aspirated food is usually more or less diffusely distributed throughout the affected pulmonary lobules. Occasionally, however, inflammation tends to be localized around small membranous or respiratory bronchioles (Fig. 20.30), a situation that has been termed *aspiration bronchiolitis* (60,61) or *lentil aspiration pneumonia* (62). The radiologic manifestations consist of 1- to 5-mm-diameter nodular opacities involving the dependent lung regions (62). HRCT demonstrates centrilobular nodular and branching linear opacities (62) (Fig. 20.31).

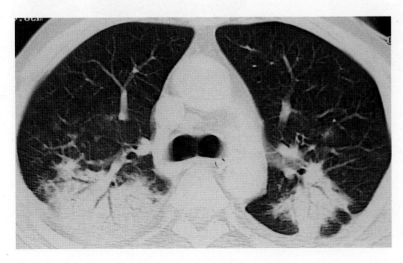

FIGURE 20.29. Aspiration of gastric contents. HRCT image shows bilateral airspace consolidation involving the dorsal regions of both upper lobes. The patient was a 43-year-old man.

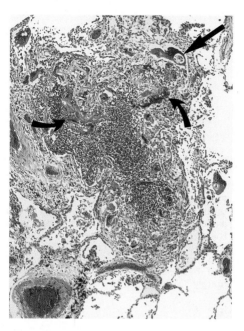

FIGURE 20.30. Aspiration of gastric contents—bronchiolitis. Photomicrograph shows filling of the lumen of a membranous bronchiole with neutrophils. Numerous irregularly shaped multinucleated giant cells (*curved arrows*) surround the exudate; some contain food particles (*straight arrow*). The surrounding lung parenchyma is relatively unaffected.

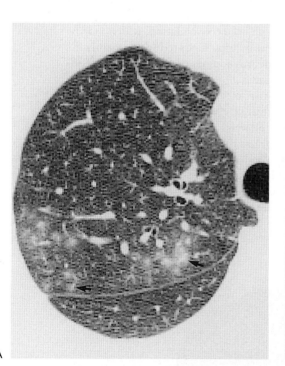

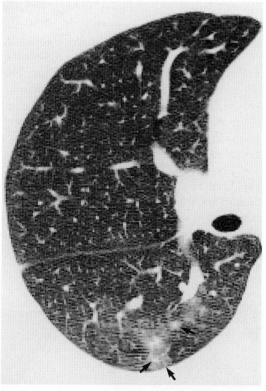

A   B

FIGURE 20.31. Aspiration of gastric contents—bronchiolitis. **A:** HRCT image at the level of the aortic arch demonstrates centrilobular nodular (*arrows*) and patchy ground-glass opacities in the dependent regions of the right upper lobe. **B:** Image at the level of the bronchus intermedius shows centrilobular nodular opacities (*arrows*) in the superior segment of right lower lobe.

LIPOID PNEUMONIA

Aspiration of mineral oil or of the various vegetable or animal oils present in food or medications can result in focal or diffuse *lipid (lipoid) pneumonia.* The most common cause is the use of mineral oil for treatment of constipation. Pulmonary abnormalities usually result from repeated subclinical episodes of aspiration.

Pathologic findings depend on the time after aspiration at which the lung is examined. Mineral oil is relatively inert and causes little, if any, acute inflammatory reaction. Instead, it is ingested by macrophages which, in early disease, are located entirely within the airspaces and appear finely vacuolated (Fig. 20.32). In time, the lipid-laden macrophages and some of the free lipid itself migrate into the alveolar and perivascular interstitial tissue. At this stage, the intracytoplasmic lipid droplets tend to coalesce, resulting in a single large lipid vacuole engulfed by a multinucleated giant cell. Possibly as a result of profibrotic and inflammatory mediators released by functionally altered macrophages/giant cells, lymphocytes are recruited and collagen is deposited, resulting in a grossly poorly defined area of parenchymal fibrosis/consolidation (Fig. 20.33).

The radiologic manifestations depend on the amount of aspirated lipid and whether the process is acute or chronic. Acute aspiration results in patchy or confluent airspace consolidation that tends to have a segmental distribution (59). HRCT may demonstrate extensive ground-glass opacities or areas of consolidation with attenuation values between those of fat (-90 HU) and water (0 HU) (63,64). The higher-than-fat attenuation is presumably due to the associated inflammatory reaction and pulmonary edema (64).

Chronic lipoid pneumonia most commonly results in a focal, masslike area of consolidation (63) (Fig. 20.34). The consolidation most commonly is seen within the dependent portions of the lung, although it may also occur in the middle lobe or lingula (63). Linear shadows radiating from the periphery of such a mass result from the interlobular septal thickening caused by infiltration of lipid-laden macrophages and secondary fibrosis

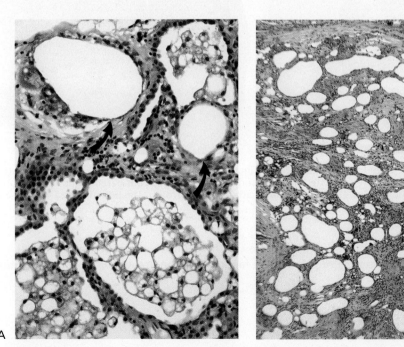

A   B

FIGURE 20.32. Lipoid pneumonia. **A:** Photomicrograph shows several alveolar airspaces almost completely filled by macrophages whose cytoplasm contains clear vacuoles of variable size. The adjacent alveolar interstitium contains two large lipid vacuoles (*arrows*), each surrounded by a multinucleated giant cell. **B:** Low-magnification view of another region of lung shows numerous irregularly shaped, large lipid vacuoles separated by abundant fibrous tissue and scattered lymphocytes. The patient was a chronic schizophrenic who repeatedly aspirated mineral oil.

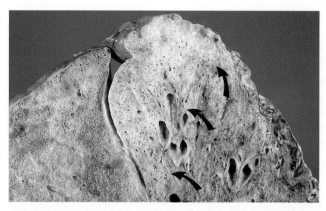

FIGURE 20.33. Lipoid pneumonia. Magnified view of the right lung shows a poorly delimited focus of consolidation/fibrosis in the posterior segment of the upper lobe (*arrows*). Histologic examination showed a pattern identical to that in Figure 20.32B.

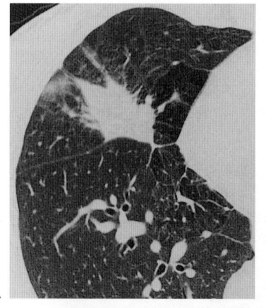

A

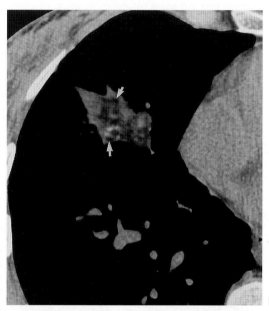

B

FIGURE 20.34. Lipoid pneumonia. **A:** HRCT image shows a masslike area of consolidation in the right middle lobe. Note spiculated margins and distortion of adjacent parenchyma due to fibrosis. **B:** Soft-tissue windows show areas of fat attenuation (*arrows*). The patient was a 48-year-old woman.

and chronic inflammation. The diagnosis of lipid pneumonia can often be made on HRCT by demonstrating the presence of focal areas of fat attenuation (-90 HU) within the lesion (63).

REFERENCES

1. Colby T, Carrington C. Interstitial lung disease. In: Thurlbeck WM, Churg AM, eds. *Pathology of the lung.* New York: Thieme Medical Publishers, 1994:589–737.
2. Crystal RG, Bitterman PB. Rennard SI, et al. Interstitial lung diseases of unknown cause: disorders characterized by chronic inflammation of the lower respiratory tract. *N Engl J Med* 1984;310:154–166.

3. Colby TV, Swensen SJ. Anatomic distribution and histopathologic patterns in diffuse lung disease: correlation with HRCT. *J Thorac Imag* 1996;11:1–26.
4. Rosen Y, Vuletin JC, Pertschuk LP, et al. Sarcoidosis: from the pathologist's vantage point. *Pathol Ann* 1979;14:405–439.
5. Müller NL, Kullnig P, Miller RR. The CT findings of pulmonary sarcoidosis: analysis of 25 patients. *Am J Roentgenol* 1989;152:1179–1187.
6. Müller NL, Miller RR. Ground-glass attenuation, nodules, alveolitis, and sarcoid granulomas (editorial). *Radiology* 1993;189:31–32.
7. Wollschlager C, Khan F: Aspergillomas complicating sarcoidosis: a prospective study in 100 patients. *Chest* 1984;86:585–588.
8. Rosen Y, Moon S, Huang C-T, et al. Granulomatous pulmonary angiitis in sarcoidosis. *Arch Pathol Lab Med* 1977;101:170–174.
9. Takemura T, Matsui Y, Saiki S, et al. Pulmonary vascular involvement in sarcoidosis: a report of 40 autopsy cases. *Hum Pathol* 1992;23:1216–1223.
10. Hadfield JW, Page RL, Flower CDR, et al. Localized airways narrowing in sarcoidosis. *Thorax* 1982;37:443–447.
11. DeRemee RA. The roentgenographic staging of sarcoidosis: historic and contemporary perspectives. *Chest* 1983;83:128–133.
12. James DG, Neville E, Siltzbach LE, et al. A worldwide review of sarcoidosis. *Ann NY Acad Sci* 1976;278:321–334.
13. Chiles C. Putman CE. Pulmonary sarcoidosis. *Semin Resp Med* 1992;13:345–356.
14. Bein ME, Putman CE, McLoud TC. et al. A reevaluation of intrathoracic lymphadenopathy in sarcoidosis. *Am J Roentgenol* 1978;131:409–415.
15. Sider L, Horton ES Jr. Hilar and mediastinal adenopathy in sarcoidosis as detected by computed tomography. *J Thorac Imag* 1990;5:77–80.
16. Kuhlman JE, Fishman EK, Hamper UM, et al. The computed tomographic spectrum of thoracic sarcoidosis. *Radiographics* 1989;9:449–466.
17. Epler GR, McLoud TC, Gaensler EA. et al. Normal chest roentgenograms in chronic diffuse infiltrative lung disease. *N Engl J Med* 1978;298:934–939.
18. Brauner MW, Grenier P, Mompoint D, et al. Pulmonary sarcoidosis: evaluation with high-resolution CT. *Radiology* 1989;172:467–471.
19. Hillerdal G, Nou E, Osterman K, et al. Sarcoidosis: epidemiology and prognosis. *Am Rev Resp Dis* 1984;130:29–32.
20. Mathieson JR, Mayo JR, Staples CA, et al. Chronic diffuse infiltrative lung disease: comparison of diagnostic accuracy of CT and chest radiography. *Radiology* 1989;171:111–116.
21. Müller NL, Mawson JB, Mathieson JR, et al. Sarcoidosis: correlation of extent of disease at CT with clinical, functional, and radiographic findings. *Radiology* 1989;171:613–618.
22. Traill ZC, Maskell GF, Gleeson FV. High-resolution CT findings of pulmonary sarcoidosis. *Am J Roentgenol* 1997;168:1557–1560.
23. Grenier P, Valeyre D, Cluzel P, et al. Chronic diffuse interstitial lung disease: diagnostic value of chest radiography and high-resolution CT. *Radiology* 1991;179:123–132.
24. McLoud TC, Epler GR, Gaensler E, et al. A radiographic classification for sarcoidosis: physiologic correlation. *Invest Radiol* 1982;17:129–138.
25. Remy-Jardin M, Giraud F, Remy J, et al. Pulmonary sarcoidosis: role of CT in the evaluation of disease activity and functional impairment and in prognosis assessment. *Radiology* 1994;191:675–680.
26. Nishimura K, Itoh H, Kitaichi M, et al. Pulmonary sarcoidosis: correlation of CT and histopathologic findings. *Radiology* 1993;189:105–109.
27. Grenier P, Chevret S, Beigelman C, et al. Chronic diffuse infiltrative lung disease: determination of the diagnostic value of clinical data, chest radiography, and CT with Bayesian analysis. *Radiology* 1994;191:383–390.
28. Murdoch J, Müller NL. Pulmonary sarcoidosis: changes on follow-up CT examination. *Am J Roentgenol* 1992;159:473–477.
29. Primack SL, Hartman TE, Hansell DM, et al. End-stage lung disease: CT findings in 61 patients. *Radiology* 1993;189:681–686.
30. Johkoh T, Ikezoe J, Takeuchi N, et al. CT findings in "pseudoalveolar" sarcoidosis. *J Comput Assist Tomogr* 1992;16:904–907.
31. Tazi A, Desfemmes-Baleyte T, Soler P, et al. Pulmonary sarcoidosis with a diffuse ground glass pattern on the chest radiograph. *Thorax* 1994;49:793–797.
32. Lynch DA, Webb WR, Gamsu G, et al. Computed tomography in pulmonary sarcoidosis. *J Comput Assist Tomogr* 1989;13:405–410.
33. Lenique F, Brauner MW, Grenier P, et al. CT assessment of bronchi in sarcoidosis: endoscopic and pathologic correlations. *Radiology* 1995;194:419–423.
34. Gleeson FV, Traill ZC, Hansell DM. Evidence of expiratory CT scans of small-airway obstruction in sarcoidosis. *Am J Roentgenol* 1996;166:1052–1054.
35. Hansell DM, Milne DG, Wilsher ML, et al. Pulmonary sarcoidosis: morphologic associations of airflow obstruction at thin-section CT. *Radiology* 1998;209:697–704.

36. Chu T, Jaffe R. The normal Langerhans cell and the LCH cell. *Br J Cancer Suppl* 1994;23:S4–S10.
37. Howarth DM, Gilchrist GS, Mullan BP, et al. Langerhans cell histiocytosis: diagnosis, natural history, management, and outcome. *Cancer* 1999;85:2278–2290.
38. Gaensler EA, Carrington CB. Open biopsy for chronic diffuse infiltrative lung disease: clinical, roentgenographic, and physiologic correlations in 502 patients. *Ann Thorac Surg* 1980;30:411–426.
39. Hance AJ, Basset F, Saumon G, et al. Smoking and interstitial lung disease: the effect of cigarette smoking on the incidence of pulmonary histiocytosis X and sarcoidosis. *Ann NY Acad Sci* 1986;465:643–656.
40. Travis WD. Borok Z, Roum JH, et al. Pulmonary Langerhans cell granulomatosis (histiocytosis X): a clinicopathologic study of 48 cases. *Am J Surg Pathol* 1993;17:971–986.
41. Müller NL, Miller RR. Computed tomography of chronic diffuse infiltrative lung disease. Part 2. *Am Rev Respir Dis* 1990;142:1440–1448.
42. Lacronique J, Roth C, Battesti J-P, et al. Chest radiological features of pulmonary histiocytosis X: a report based on 50 adult cases. *Thorax* 1982;37:104–109.
43. Moore ADA, Godwin JD, Müller NL, et al. Pulmonary histiocytosis X: comparison of radiographic and CT findings. *Radiology* 1989;172:249–254.
44. Brauner MW, Grenier P, Mouelhi MM, et al. Pulmonary histiocytosis X: evaluation with high-resolution CT. *Radiology* 1989;172:255–258.
45. Kulwiec EL, Lynch DA, Aguayo SM, et al. Imaging of pulmonary histiocytosis X. *Radiographics* 1992;12:515–526.
46. Taylor JR, Ryu J, Colby TV, et al. Lymphangioleiomyomatosis: clinical course in 32 patients. *N Engl J Med* 1990;323:1254–1260.
47. Taylor DB, Joske D, Anderson J, et al. Cavitating pulmonary nodules in histiocytosis-X high resolution CT demonstration. *Australas Radiol* 1990;34:253–255.
48. Corrin B, Liebow AA, Friedman PJ. Pulmonary lymphangiomyomatosis. *Am J Pathol* 1975;79:348–382.
49. Guinee DG Jr, Feuerstein I, Koss MN, et al. Pulmonary lymphangioleiomyomatosis: diagnosis based on results of transbronchial biopsy and immunohistochemical studies and correlation with high-resolution computed tomography findings. *Arch Pathol Lab Med* 1994;118:846–849.
50. Fukuda Y, Kawamoto M, Yamamoto A, et al. Role of elastic fiber degradation in emphysema-like lesions of pulmonary lymphangiomyomatosis. *Hum Pathol* 1990;21:1252–1261.
51. Sobonya RE, Quan SF, Fleishman JS. Pulmonary lymphangioleiomyomatosis: quantitative analysis of lesions producing airflow limitation. *Hum Pathol* 1985;16:1122–1128.
52. Müller NL, Chiles C, Kullnig P. Pulmonary lymphangiomyomatosis: correlation of CT with radiographic and functional findings. *Radiology* 1990;175:335–339.
53. Lenoir S, Grenier P, Brauner MW, et al. Pulmonary lymphangiomyomatosis and tuberous sclerosis: comparison of radiographic and thin-section CT findings. *Radiology* 1990;175:329–334.
54. Kitaichi M, Nishimura K, Itoh H, et al. Pulmonary lymphangioleiomyomatosis: a report of 46 patients including a clinicopathologic study of prognostic factors. *Am J Resp Crit Care Med* 1995;151:527–533.
55. Templeton PA. McLoud TC, Müller NL, et al. Pulmonary lymphangioleiomyomatosis: CT and pathologic findings. *J Comput Assist Tomogr* 1989;13:54–57.
56. Castro M, Shepherd CW, Gomez MR, et al. Pulmonary tuberous sclerosis. *Chest* 1995;107:189–195.
57. Capron F, Ameille J, Leclerc P, et al. Pulmonary lymphangioleiomyomatosis and Bourneville's tuberous sclerosis with pulmonary involvement: the same disease? *Cancer* 1983;52:851–855.
58. Kullnig P, Melzer G, Smolle-Jüttner FM. High-resolution computed tomography of the thorax in lymphangioleiomyomatosis and tuberous sclerosis. *Rofo Fortschr Geb Rontgenstr Neuen Bildgeb Verfahr* 1989;151:32–35.
59. Fraser RF, Müller NL, Colman N, et al. *Diagnosis of diseases of the chest.* Philadelphia: WB Saunders, 1999:2485–2516.
60. Franquet T, Gimenez A, Roson N, et al. Aspiration diseases: findings, pitfalls, and differential diagnosis. *Radiographics* 2000;20:673–685.
61. Matsuse T, Oka T, Kida K, et al. Importance of diffuse aspiration caused by chronic occult aspiration in the elderly. *Chest* 1996;110:1289–1293.
62. Marom EM, Page McAdams H, et al. Lentil aspiration pneumonia: radiographic and CT findings. *J Comput Assist Tomogr* 1998;22:598–600.
63. Lee KS, Müller NL, Hale V, et al. Lipoid pneumonia: CT findings. *J Comput Assist Tomogr* 1995;19:48–51.
64. Lee JY, Lee KS, Kim TS, et al. Squalene-induced extrinsic lipoid pneumonia: serial radiologic findings in nine patients. *J Comput Assist Tomogr* 1999;23:730–735.

SUBJECT INDEX

Page numbers followed by *f* refer to figures, page numbers followed by *t* refer to tables.